Penguin Handbooks
The Massage Book

D0610505

George Downing *illustrated by* Anne Kent Rush

Penguin Books

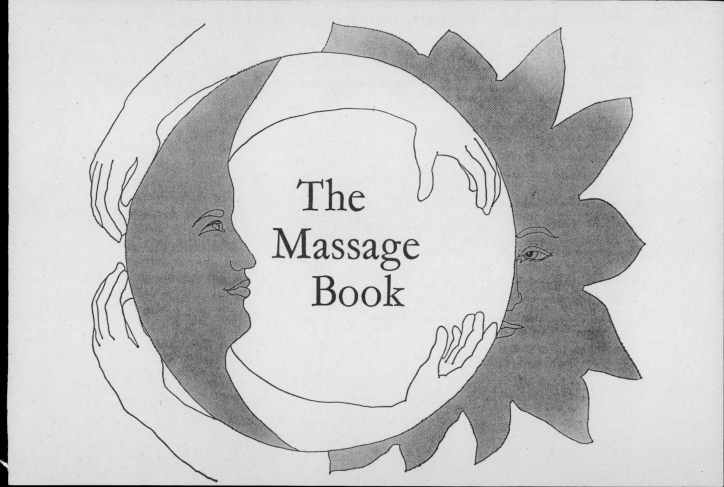

The
Massage
Book

Penguin Books Ltd, Harmondsworth, Middlesex, England
Penguin Books, 625 Madison Avenue, New York, New York 10022, U.S.A.
Penguin Books Australia Ltd, Ringwood, Victoria, Australia
Penguin Books Canada Ltd, 2801 John Street, Markham, Ontario, Canada L3R 1B4
Penguin Books (N.Z.) Ltd, 182–190 Wairau Road, Auckland 10, New Zealand

Published in the United States by
Random House Inc. and The Bookworks 1972
First published in Great Britain by Wildwood House 1973
Published in Penguin Books 1974
Reprinted 1976, 1977, 1978, 1979, 1980, 1981, 1982

Printed in Great Britain by
Fletcher & Son Ltd, Norwich

The illustrator wishes to acknowledge the use of copyright material from
Art Students' Anatomy by Edmond J. Farris, Dover Publications Inc., New York,
which appears on pages 205–15; reprinted through permission of the publisher

Contents

Why massage

Massage is for your mate, your family and your friends. It is for grandmothers and babies, for pets, for those you love and, if you are up to it, for those you hate. To do massage is physically to help someone, to take care of them. It is for anyone with whom you feel prepared to share an act of physical caring.

Contrary to myth, massage is a healing art and not an advanced sexual technique. Naturally, when practised by lovers, it can be a beautiful extension of sexuality. The flowing peace and aliveness it so easily brings to the body can be channelled, if both parties desire things so, in that direction. But this is merely one of the many possibilities that massage holds out to us.

The core of massage lies in its unique way of communicating without words. In itself this is not unusual; by touching and hugging, for example, we often let those around us know that we like them, or that we sympathize with them, or that we believe in their worth. Massage, however, can transpose this kind of message into a new and different key. When receiving a good massage a person usually falls into a mental–physical state difficult to describe. It is like entering a special room until now locked and hidden away; a room the very existence of which is likely to be familiar only to those who practise some form of daily meditation. By itself this state is a gift. However, he who is giving the massage need not stop there. The more he can tune in to his friend's heightened awareness, the more he can convey something of his own inner self and experience as well. The least touch becomes a statement, like drawing with a fine pen on sensitive paper. Trust, empathy and respect, to say nothing of a sheer sense of mutual physical existence, for this moment can be expressed with a fullness never matched by words.

In its essence massage is something simple. It

makes us more whole, more fully ourselves. Your hands have the power to give this to others. Learn to trust that power and you will quickly find out better than anyone can tell you what massage is all about.

How to use this book

I have written this book with two ends in mind: to tell you how to do massage, and to explain a little of what I see as its meaning and purpose.

The first third of the book contains a lot of practical information which you will want to know before you begin: the nature of massage oils, how to do massage on the floor as opposed to doing it on a massage table and the like. If you have never done massage before, I strongly suggest that you read through these chapters before tackling the later parts of the book. In particular take a good look at 'How to use your hands'. Even if you already know some massage I would recommend at least a glance at this chapter.

In the middle third of the book you will find instructions on how to give, stroke by stroke and body part by body part, a long and thorough complete massage. The type described is one of many possible variations of what has come to be known as Esalen-style massage. This approach to massage, developed in recent years at Esalen Institute growth centre in Big Sur and San Francisco, is in turn a variation of a European tradition over a century old, commonly called Swedish massage. Many of the techniques I teach in my own workshops for Esalen are included in this section.

The type, the illustrations and the physical design of this book have been planned in order to make it as convenient as possible for you to have it open at your side when you want to try doing some massage with a friend. However, before you start be sure to read over both the short introduction to the instruction section and the particular descriptions of whatever strokes you wish to try out. I would also advise you to start small; don't try to learn more than half a dozen strokes or so at one sitting. Finally, whenever you get

9

a chance, have the strokes you are attempting to learn done to you as well.

Don't worry, incidentally, if as you thumb through this book the strokes in the instruction section look difficult to you. In actual practice they are much easier than they look to be on paper. Numerous people who originally knew no massage have tested portions of this book before it was printed. All found little difficulty in learning the strokes once they actually tried them.

The final third of the book is designed to help you develop your own personal massage style. To this end I have included a series of more advanced technical suggestions, some brief information about other types and traditions of massage, and, most importantly, some comments about the meaning of massage and how an understanding of this meaning can aid you in doing better work with your hands. Read this part of the book whenever you like, but I suspect that it won't make a great deal of sense until after you have become fairly familiar with the material presented in the instruction section. Master a few basic techniques first.

Then, with a glance at a few of the guideposts in the last part of this book, by all means go on from there.

Oils and powders

The only really good way to do massage is with oil. Your hands cannot apply pressure and at the same time move smoothly over the surface of the skin without some kind of lubricating agent. Oil fulfils this function better than anything else.

The two kinds of oil most commonly used for massage are vegetable oil and mineral oil. As far as lubrication goes they are equally satisfactory. Mineral oil is used in almost all professional studios because it is the cheaper of the two. My own preference, however, is very much for vegetable oil.

My reasons, I admit, are based largely upon intuition and hearsay. Ever since the widespread realization that natural foods are more healthful for us there has arisen a massive underground lore concerning, among other things, the care and treatment of the skin; one especially frequent claim is that vegetable oil is good for your skin and mineral oil is bad for it. Why?

Well, answers one person, vegetable oil is easily absorbed by the skin whereas mineral oil tends to clog the pores. And, responds another, vegetable oil adds vitamins to the skin whereas mineral oil if anything destroys certain ones. And so forth. Whether any or all such reasons are true, I don't really know; nor, so far, have I come across any solid scientific research pointing one way or the other. Yet my own bones seem to vibrate with the same general message, and until I see proof to the contrary I intend to keep on massaging and getting massaged with vegetable oil.

Given that you are using a vegetable oil, what particular vegetable it happens to come from does not, I suspect, greatly matter. Everyone does seem to have his own favourite; at the moment I find myself in an almond oil phase. In the past, however, I have used olive oil, safflower oil, avocado oil and numerous others; and all with equal satisfaction. Safflower oil, which is certainly as good as any of the others, has the advantage of being relatively inexpensive, and both safflower oil and olive oil have the further advantage of being available at almost any grocery store. Most other vegetable oils you can find on the shelves of a good health food store. All of them, incidentally, can be mixed in any combination with other oils.

Baby oil? If this is all you have around you can get by with it. It is quite difficult to use, however, because it soaks so quickly into the skin that during a massage new applications become necessary every few minutes. Hand lotions are even less satisfactory for the same reason.

Whatever oil you use, mineral, vegetable or other, it is more than likely to be neutral or worse in odour. If so, be sure to add something to it that will give it a pleasant scent. Musk is one of my own favourites; several drops added to a cup of oil will usually do nicely. Concentrated clove oil, cinnamon oil and lemon oil work well and can be bought at some drugstores. Today many head shops carry a wide variety of imported scented oils. Frangipani, a concentrated oil imported from India, is an especially popular one.

Once I even found a concentrated chocolate oil. This didn't work out so well, as I kept getting hungry in the middle of the massage.

A nice idea is to keep a variety of mixed oils with different scents on hand, and then to let whomever you massage choose the one he or she prefers. Picking a favourite oil usually makes a person a little more immediately receptive to being massaged with it.

Keep your oils, once mixed and scented, in plastic bottles that are not easily upset and that have narrow openings, i.e., an eighth of an inch or smaller. Any store that has cosmetic supplies is a good place to look for bottles of this kind. Many shampoos and hand lotions also come in them.

What about powders? Well, they work. Not as well as oils do: you have to apply them more often, and they don't cut down the friction between your hands and your friend's skin nearly as effectively. But there may be times when you will want to use a powder. Like when you want to massage a friend who can't stand the feel of oil against his or her skin (it happens). Or when you have run out of oil. Or just for a change.

Any talcum powder will do. Use it just as you would an oil.

And what about using nothing at all, besides your own hands? Of course you can do this. But it makes a decent massage much more difficult to give. Most of the strokes that will be described in this book can't be done without oil or powder. A few can, however, as you will see. You can always do massage, no matter what is or isn't lying around to do it with.

In the meantime lay in a good stock of oils and powders.

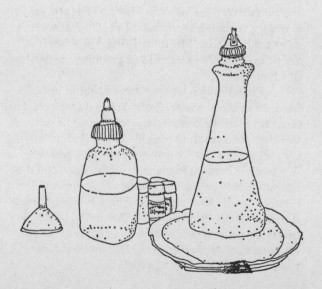

Working on the floor

The easiest way to do massage is on a massage table. But don't worry – if you don't have a table you can give a great massage working on the floor. It's a little more trouble and a little more tiring. Go about it in the right way, however, and you can cut these hassles to a minimum.

First, though, let me warn you about beds. Sleep on beds, do whatever else you want on beds, but don't try to do serious massage on them. The reason is that they are too soft to provide the kind of underlying support you need when you want to apply pressure. Try to press hard on someone lying on a bed and the only thing that happens is that he disappears into the mattress. Water beds are an exception because of their firm and exactly fitted support. Ordinarily, however, a bed is the worst possible place you could choose for giving a massage. Either get a table, or find ways to make yourself comfortable on the floor.

The main thing when working on the floor is to make sure that you have sufficient padding. A foam pad 1 or 2 inches thick works well. However, it ought to be both longer and wider than the amount of space that actually will be occupied by your friend: it should be 7 feet × 4 feet or even bigger. The reason for this is that you, who are to give the massage, will also need padding. Some strokes, for example, will require you to kneel next to your friend, and if you don't have something under your knees at these times you will end up needing a massage much more than your friend ever did.

If you have a foam pad too short or narrow to sit or kneel on beside your friend, then try to supplement it with whatever additional padding you can find.

Two or three sleeping bags can also be used. Even some thick blankets will help. Unzip the sleeping bags and spread them out to double width. Then pile up whatever bags and/or blankets you are using, as shown in the illustration.

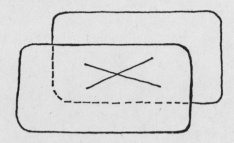

A single mattress taken from a bed and placed directly on the floor will also work, although its height from the floor makes it rather inconvenient to use. The thinner the mattress, the better.

Whatever padding you are using – foam, sleeping bags, blankets or whatever – cover it with a clean sheet before your friend lies down on it for his or her massage.

One minor problem that arises when working on the floor is that sooner or later you are going to knock over an oil bottle and spill some oil. If you are using a bottle with a sufficiently narrow opening, the amount of oil that will actually seep out will be very little. All the same, you may wish to take precautions against staining your rug, your sleeping bag, etc. The best preventive measure I have found is to purchase a large durable plastic sheet at a hardware store. Put the plastic sheet on top of whatever you want to protect, and then a bed sheet on top of the whole works. Also, the first time you use the plastic sheet take some tape and make an 'X' on the side that is up. Then when you fold the sheet to put it away make sure the 'up' side gets folded against itself without ever coming into contact with the opposite side. This will keep you from someday putting the oily side of the sheet down on top of whatever you are trying to protect.

The actual massage techniques used while working on the floor differ very little from those used while working on a table. Where some specific stroke needs to be done in a different way I will mention it in the instruction section. However, I will add here two pieces of advice of a more general nature. One is always to give a somewhat shorter massage when working on the floor than you might if you were working on a table. This will keep you from getting tired out. The other is to bend your own back as little as possible while giving a massage. What this really means is, pay attention to where and how you are sitting or kneeling, taking every care to provide for your own comfort the whole while. That way you will give your friend a better massage, and will yourself enjoy giving it infinitely more.

A last remark. Nothing so enhances massage done on the floor as a fire in a near-by fireplace.

Tables

Why a table? Its most important advantage is that it eliminates some bending and stooping as you work. This means that if you are giving a long massage your own back is less likely to get tired. A table also makes it easy for you to change your position with respect to the person you are massaging – from head to leg, from one side to the other side, etc. – without a break in the flow of your massage. Finally, it puts certain body parts (the sole of the foot, for example) more directly within the reach of your hands.

If you find that you are beginning to do a lot of massage, sooner or later you will probably want a table. In this case your options are three. You may find that some table which you already have around will, with perhaps a few modifications, serve well enough. Or you can buy one. Or you can build one.

The first requirement of a table is, naturally, that it be big enough for whomever you are going to massage to lie down on it, and sturdy enough to keep him or her there. Ideally the length and width should be about the same as that of your friend's body when he is lying flat with his arms close alongside his body; a professional massage table is usually 6 feet × 2 feet, for example. However, if the only table you have available is either much too long or, as is more likely, much too wide, you can make do with it. What this means is that instead of just lying in one place while you do all the moving around, your friend will have to shift his or her position from time to time during a massage. A disadvantage, but hardly a disaster.

Height is equally important. Too low, and you will have to stoop; too high, and you won't get the leverage you need. Traditional massage lore gives two measures for the right height of a table. One is that it should be roughly as high from the floor as the top of your thighs. The other is that if you stand straight with your shoulders level you should be able to extend one arm straight down with the hand at a right angle (i.e., so that the hand is parallel to the floor), and have the palm of your hand just graze the surface of the table. Of these two measures I find the second more accurate, and find more accurate still the simple test of trying out the table by doing a little massage. For a man or woman of average size, 29 to 31 inches (including padding) is the right height range.

Sturdiness must also be considered. A table should be sturdy enough not only for your friend to stay in place on it, but also for him or her not to worry about staying in place on it. If a table shakes and creaks with every stroke you can't very well expect your friend to relax on it.

Whatever the size and shape of the table you use, you must place some kind of padding on top for your friend to lie on. A one-inch foam pad is best. A sleeping bag will also work. The idea is to use something thick enough for whomever you massage to feel comfortable, yet thin enough for him or her not to bounce up and down under the varying pressure of your hands.

If you can't find a table that comes somewhat close to meeting these requirements, then the next step is either to build or to buy. Building a table can be fairly easy or fairly difficult, depending on how good you are with tools and how elaborate a table you decide to make.

The simplest and cheapest way to build your own massage table is to make two small sawhorses 28 inches or so high and 24 inches wide. (Any carpenter can also build them for you at little cost.) Then buy a piece of $\frac{3}{4}$-inch plywood cut 2 feet × 6 feet and a foam pad to match, and you are in business.

If you want to try something more elaborate, a friend of mine recently made a superb table that is both sturdy and easy to move and to store; it folds up into a neat package about 2 feet × 3 feet × 5 inches. Here is how you can build one too.

First assemble these materials:

2 sheets of $\frac{1}{2}$-inch plywood 24 × 36 inches
3 sheets of $\frac{1}{2}$-inch plywood 22 × 12 inches
4 1 × 4 inch pine or fir boards 36 inches long
4 1 × 4 inch pine or fir boards 22$\frac{1}{2}$ inches long

6 2 × 2 inch boards 29 inches long
1 24-inch continuous hinge
5 Stanley locking table leg braces #446¼ (be sure also
to get instructions on how to place them)
2 handles
6 3-inch strap hinges and screws
2 suitcase latches
8 brass corners
nails (1½-inch finishing nails without heads are best.
Bigger nails will split the wood.)
a strong glue.

(Note: these dimensions are for a table that will stand
30½ inches high including a 1-inch foam pad on top.
If you want your table either higher or lower, just vary
the length of the six 2 × 2 inch legs accordingly.)
    Then construct the table as follows:

(1) Cut the plywood and the boards for the frame and
legs to size.
(2) Build the frames, gluing and nailing the corners.
(Make rabbit joints if you feel ambitious.)
(3) Attach the tops and frames, gluing and nailing

them. (If you still feel ambitious you can also 'set
in' the top.)
(4) Hinge the legs to the undersides of the tops, gluing
and nailing the crossbraces.
(5) Attach the brackets. This is a tricky business, so try
to follow the directions that come with them as
closely as you can. You will have to play with them
a little to find the exact placement spot.
(6) Hinge the two halves of the table together.
(7) Attach the catches, handles and corners.
(8) Stain or varnish.
Put a 1-inch foam pad loose on top when you use the
table.

If you want to buy a table there are some
excellent ones on the market. Their chief advantage is
that they are lightweight and portable: most of them
are made of aluminium covered on the outside with
either leather or naugahyde, and can be folded
up into what looks like an overgrown attaché case.
Their chief drawback is their price, usually in the
neighbourhood of £70. The best place to find or
order one is at a large medical-supplies house. Be sure

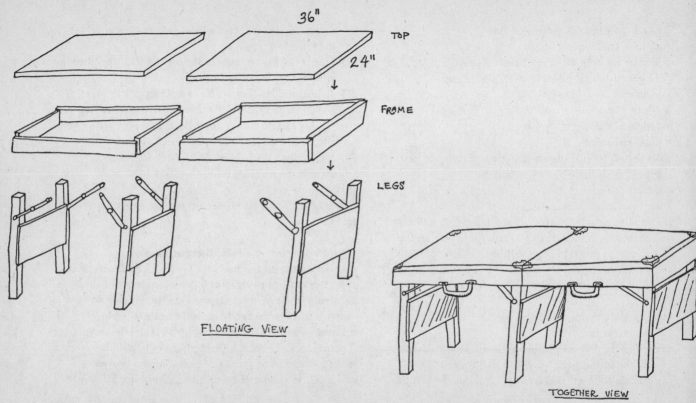

36"

TOP

24"

FRAME

LEGS

FLOATING VIEW

TOGETHER VIEW

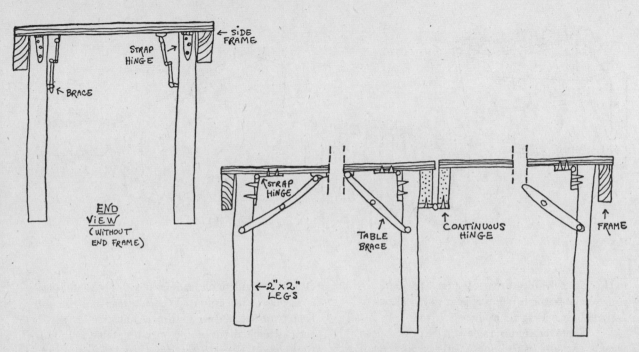

← SIDE FRAME

STRAP HINGE

← BRACE

END VIEW
(WITHOUT END FRAME)

STRAP HINGE

TABLE BRACE

←2"x2" LEGS

CONTINUOUS HINGE

FRAME →

CUT-AWAY VIEW OF TABLE (FROM SIDE, IF SLICED IN HALF)

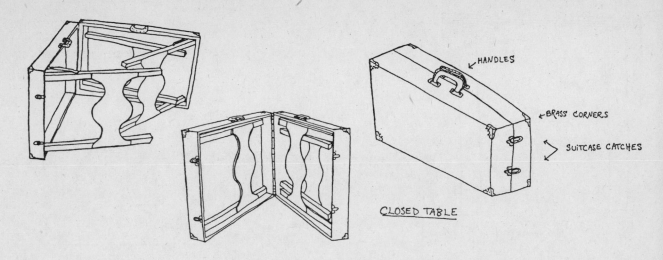

HANDLES

BRASS CORNERS

SUITCASE CATCHES

<u>CLOSED TABLE</u>

to check out the measurements first, as some commercial portable tables appear to have been designed for massaging midgets.

Whatever kind of table you use, put a clean sheet over it and its padding when you are actually about to give a massage. A white sheet on a narrow table has, incidentally, a definite set of psychological overtones; use a coloured sheet instead and you will keep your friend from getting a funny feeling that he or she is stretched out on the operating table waiting for the surgeon. Even better, buy a large piece of brightly coloured terrycloth at a fabrics store.

Getting things ready

Careful preparations and the right setting can make a good massage even better. Your friend will feel more comfortable, and you will too.

In choosing a place to give a massage the first thing to look for is solitude and quiet. A person receiving a massage enters a universe where the sense of touch alone is important; for this reason any outside noise and bustle can be extremely disconcerting.

The next thing to consider is warmth. Nothing destroys an otherwise good massage more quickly than physical coldness. The problem is the oil; a person with massage oil on his skin becomes easily chilled. The temperature in the room in which you give the massage should be about 70° F or slightly over, and the room should be without draughts. Heat the room up before you begin; err, if in doubt, on the side of making it too warm. It is much easier to keep your friend feeling

comfortable from the start than it is to warm him or her up once chilled.

For the same reason it is a good practice to keep a spare sheet on hand. Then, if during the massage your friend should begin to feel cold, you can use the sheet to cover the parts of his body you are not working on at the moment.

Make sure ahead of time that the oil is mixed and scented, that is in a convenient container, that you have more than enough for a massage and that it is warm. Warm means room temperature or close to it. If the oil is much cooler than this, warm it a little first before a fire or heater.

Arrange your table or your mat on the floor so that there is sufficient room for you to work on all four sides.

Don't use any kind of bright lighting that will

fall directly on your friend's face. Even with his lids closed this will cause him to tense the muscles surrounding his eyes. In particular never use direct overhead lighting.

The question of music is a tricky one. Although I think that massaging to music can be a helpful exercise (how and why I will discuss in a later chapter), I strongly recommend that as a general rule you do not play music while giving a massage. I love music, don't get me wrong, and it certainly adds a pleasant relaxing atmosphere to a massage room, but I find at the same time that music tends to siphon off the deeper currents of a good massage experience. It is like trying to meditate to music: however beautiful it may be in itself, the music casts its own veil over everything you are feeling. On the other hand I must in all fairness admit that I know excellent masseurs and masseuses who like to both give and receive massages in this way. So I guess you will have to experiment and decide for yourself.

Check your own hands before giving a massage. The most important thing is to make sure your fingernails are short – the shorter, the better. I trim mine down as far as my scissors can reach before a massage.

Also wash your hands. Any grit or stickiness will make itself instantly felt.

And warm them if they are cold. Rub them briskly together for several minutes, or, if they are extremely cold, let them bask a little before a fire or heater.

If you have long hair tie it back so that it stays out of your eyes.

If you plan to stay dressed, wear loose clothing, so that you can move around easily; and dress as lightly as possible, since you will be working in a warm room. I might add that doing massage in the nude is extremely pleasant as long as no one on either side is uptight about it.

Both masseur or masseuse and massagee tend to get thirsty during a long massage, and a little water to drink can be a nice thing to have on hand. Even better, when the massage is over let your friend first rest for as long as he wishes with his eyes closed, and then when he opens his eyes offer him a glass of cold fruit juice.

Finally, if you ever have the chance to do massage outdoors, in the sun and surrounded by nature . . . need I say more?

What to tell your friend

There are a few basic things one should know before receiving a massage. If you are the one who is going to give the massage, you will probably want to tell your friend something along the lines of the following comments.

The best way to receive a massage is in the nude. Even a minimal amount of clothing, e.g., underwear or a swimming suit, will get in the way of whoever is giving the massage, will require him or her to leave certain important muscle groups unmassaged, and will deny you what is perhaps the single most pleasant sensation of a complete massage, that of the total wholeness and connectedness of your body. If, however, to remove all your clothes would make you feel extremely nervous, then leave something on. The main thing, after all, is that you enjoy your massage. But do take off whatever you comfortably can.

Also remove rings, bracelets, necklaces, earrings, glasses and anything in your hair. And most important of all (so that your eyes can be massaged), contact lenses.

Whoever is giving you the massage will tell you whether first to lie down on your stomach or on your back. Either way, make sure that the top of your head is roughly even with the end of the table or the padding on which you are lying. Rest your arms at your sides.

Once you feel settled in place close your eyes. Then focus your attention on your breathing; this will almost immediately bring you more in touch with your entire body. Breathe either through the nose or the mouth. Let your breath get as long and smooth as it wants to be without, however, forcing it to do so, and let it flow as deep towards or into the pelvis as it can go. Try to sink yourself more and more into the present moment, letting thoughts drift out of your mind as easily as they have drifted in.

From this point on your job is simply to let yourself be completely taken care of. Don't try to 'help' with the massage in any way. When it is time for your arm to be lifted, let it be lifted for you. When your head has to be turned to one side, let the turning be done by your friend. I repeat: don't try to 'help' in any way; this can only cause a break in the relaxing flow of the massage. Instead keep your body as limp as you can manage, so that even when a limb is being lifted it would fall instantly to the table or floor if whoever was holding onto it were to let go. One exception: when lying on your stomach, turn your own head from one side to the other any time you feel your neck becoming stiff.

From the moment that you first feel the friend who is giving you the massage make physical contact with your body, try to turn your complete attention to his or her touch. This doesn't mean in any way to analyse it, or to try to figure out what particular technique he or she may be using. On the contrary, simply tune in to the quality of his or her touch the way you might listen to the sound of someone's voice without paying any attention to the meaning of the words.

At the same time continue to keep in touch with your breath throughout the massage. If you want, you can even imagine that your exhalation is flowing to whatever part of your body your friend is working on.

The less said during a massage, the better; during so direct an encounter with your own body, words can only be a distraction. Do feel free to speak up, however, if something that your friend is doing is physically hurting you; or if you feel cold; or if for any other reason you feel uncomfortable. Also, if any time during the massage you should feel a sigh within you, just let it out with the exhalation of your breath.

Finally, when the massage is over you needn't get up immediately. Lie still with your eyes closed; let yourself absorb whatever you are feeling a few minutes longer.

Applying oil

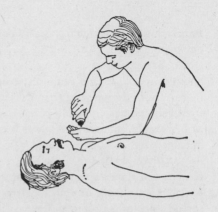

Applying the oil to your friend's body is a simple matter, but there are a few tricks to it worth knowing.

First of all, never pour oil directly from the bottle on to your friend's skin: for many people this is an extremely disagreeable sensation. Put the oil first on your own hands and from there on to your friend's body.

For the same reason be sure that the hand (your own) into which you are pouring the oil is a little to one side of your friend's body, and not directly above it. Then if you should spill a few drops of oil, as does sometimes happen, they won't fall on your friend.

Don't try to pour more than about three quarters of a teaspoon of oil into your hands at one time. Apply this first, and then pour more if you need it.

If the oil is at all cool, warm it in your hands by rubbing them briskly together.

Apply oil only to the part or parts of the body on which you are immediately about to work. Otherwise you will find that your friend's skin has absorbed a part of the oil before you get a chance to use it.

Apply the oil with both palms. Use any kind of simple stroking movement that you want, but make certain that it is both gentle and at the same time very definite and steady. This is especially important the first time you apply oil at the beginning of a massage. It will immediately help your friend to relax if the first impression of your touch is one of confidence and sureness.

Systematically cover the entire area that you are about to massage. Don't miss any corners.

Don't drown your friend's body in oil. Your friend should have no extra puddles of oil visible on his or her skin. About two teaspoons is enough for the average-sized back, for example.

If you do find that you have put on too much oil, you can always remove some of the excess with the backs of your hands or your forearms. Or you can spread some of the oil to another part of your friend's body.

A hairy chest – or leg or back – does require extra oil. Otherwise you will pull the hairs as you move you hands over the surface of the skin.

Be careful where you put down your oil bottle after pouring some oil. If you are working on the floor, try to find a place where it will be easy to find next time you need it and where you won't kick it over. If working on a table, try if possible not to put it anywhere on the table itself: sooner or later this results either in your knocking it over, or in your cramping your movements in order to keep from knocking it over. Much the easier way is to establish one or two convenient near-by places for the bottle before ever beginning the massage.

Here's a problem. One general rule of massage is that once you have first made contact with your friend's body you should try always to have at least one hand touching him or her until the massage is finished. But, as you can see, this presents a difficulty when you are ready to apply more oil: how do you hold your hand to one side of your friend's body when pouring the oil and yet keep physically in contact? The answer is to rest your elbow or a part of your forearm lightly against your friend's body while holding your hands to the side. This feels clumsy the first time you try it, but becomes easy and natural with practice.

One last hint. It took me several years of stumbling around massage tables to wake up to the fact that using two oil bottles instead of one, and placing one somewhere near one end of the table and one somewhere near the other end, can save a lot of steps and acrobatic stretching.

How to use your hands

Knowing how to be at one with your hands is the core of massage, the one real technique. The more massage you do, the more this knowledge will open itself to you. Hands are subtle, however, and getting acquainted with them takes time. I am still learning about mine. It is hardly an unpleasant task, but I know now it will never come to an end.

What I am going to suggest is just a beginning. I strongly recommend that before giving your first massage you read through these comments and try out the experiments mentioned at their end. But be patient, and don't expect to master everything overnight.

Here are some hints.

Apply pressure when you do massage. Once you actually have learned some strokes, the amount of pressure you will use will vary according to the particular stroke and the part of the body on which it is being used. But some pressure is almost always necessary. It has been my experience that many people first learning massage are nervous, consciously or unconsciously, about the possibility of hurting someone with their hands, and as a result they tend to apply almost no pressure. Don't worry; your friends aren't that fragile. Pressure feels good, as you will see when you yourself are being massaged. Learn to experiment with different pressures. Remember, whenever you are afraid you may be pressing too hard you can always check this out with your friend.

Relax your hands. Keep them as loose and flexible as possible while you are moving them. This is difficult – probably more difficult than it sounds to you – for two reasons. One is that to relax a limb while you are in the act of using it is a lot harder than to relax it while it is lying still. The other is that almost all of us, without being aware of it, carry a great deal of chronic tension in our hands. There are ways of getting rid of this kind of tension; doing massage is itself one excellent way, and in a later part of this book I will mention others. These ways do take time: months often, and sometimes even years. You can start in at once, however, merely by paying attention to your hands and by trying to relax them, even if only a degree or so, whenever they feel to you stiff or tight.

Mould your hands to fit the contours over which they are passing. Although certain techniques require, as you will see, that only a specific part of the hands be used, most massage strokes depend for their effectiveness upon your ability to keep your entire palm and fingers always in contact with the person you are massaging. For example, where possible don't let either the heel of the hand or the ends of the fingers slip into the air as you move from one part of the body to another. When you glide your hand over the hip, shape it exactly to fit the hip. When you move it from the chest to the arm curve it so that it wraps evenly and smoothly around the shoulder as it passes. Think of the way the water of a stream shapes itself to fit the rocks and hollows in its path.

Maintain an evenness of speed and pressure. Try to eliminate trembling, jerkiness and unnecessary stops and starts. Make any change of either speed or pressure a gradual one, never increasing or decreasing either too suddenly. Let the movement of your hands be as flowing and smooth as possible.

Don't, however, be afraid to vary both speed and pressure. Rhythm is an essential ingredient of massage. You can use different speeds and different pressures without sacrificing the steadiness of your movements. Variety in massage is a lot like variety in music: changes in tempo help avoid rhythmic monotony.

Explore and define the underlying structure of the body of the person you are massaging. (This is a matter of sensitivity, and is something completely apart from the study of formal anatomy; for some remarks about the latter you may refer to a later chapter of the book.) Make your hand constantly question, make it 'listen' to the tissue and bone beneath. Tune in to the texture of the deeper strata of the muscles. Is it thick or thin? Tight or loose? Formless or distinct? Where you encounter bone try to outline its shape. Think of your hands as telling your friend, 'This is your hip,' 'These are the tiny bones of your wrist,' 'This is the way your knee is shaped.' To articulate your friend's body for him or her in this fashion is one of the most important aspects of a massage. The more precisely you achieve this, the more your friend's pleasure in his or her massage will take on a deep, almost magical quality.

Use your weight rather than your muscles to apply pressure. It is a fiction that you have to be physically powerful to do massage. Whenever you want extra pressure, get it by leaning the weight of your upper body into your hands rather than by straining with the muscles in your arms and wrists. Straining with your muscles will only give you stiff hands, a less flowing quality of movement and a tired back.

Once you have made contact with your friend's body, try never to break it until the massage that you are giving or the exercise you are doing is completely finished. Many people, when being massaged, experience any interruption of physical contact as psychologically a little disconcerting. Even when you have to put on more oil keep at least a forearm or an elbow touching some part of your friend's body. Remember that your friend, lying still with his eyes closed, will have entered a universe of touch whose one reality is the contact of your hand.

Do massage with your entire body, not just with your hands. By this I don't mean that you should climb on to the table and roll all over your friend, but that your hands will be most alive when their movement is an extension of a more general movement coming from the rest of the body. This movement of the body need not be great; at times it may be so slight that an observer would scarcely be aware of it. Visible or not, however, you yourself should be able to feel it present as a sort of core from which the more exact movements of your hands are emerging. In some respects the experience of giving a massage is like that of dancing. As with dance, the more total the involvement of the body, the better the massage.

Pay attention to how you are standing, sitting or kneeling. When working at a table I like to stand whenever possible with my feet apart, my knees bent and turned out and my back straight. When you first try it this stance will feel awkward to you, but its advantages will soon become apparent. Having your feet apart (a couple of feet, when necessary even farther) permits you to easily swing your entire body up and down the length of the table merely by shifting your weight from one foot to the other. Also, lowering yourself by bending at the knees rather than bending your back forwards eliminates a tremendous amount of

potential strain and fatigue in your lower back. And working with a straight rather than a bent back frees your arms and hands for movements that are more controlled and relaxed.

When you are working on the floor the way in which you sit or kneel is largely dictated by the part of the body you are working on, the particular stroke you wish to use, and the like. However, because working on the floor requires more bending of your own back and is therefore more tiring, you must remain all the more aware of the position of your own body. Try when you

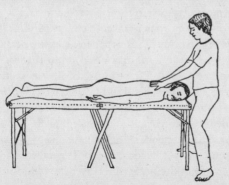

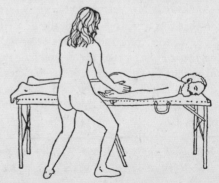

sit or kneel to keep your own back straight whenever possible. Also make sure, as I have already stressed, that you have some kind of padding under yourself as well as under your friend. In other words, take care of yourself all you can. The attention you give to your own comfort will be translated to your friend as increased grace and precision in the movement of your hands.

Remember always that you are massaging a person and not an intricate muscle-and-bone machine. Muscle and bone we are, but person too; and we are person throughout every physical cubic inch of us. Your friend is his or her body, as you are yours. Stay aware of this at all times, and keep your hands aware of it; it will have a direct and critical influence on the quality of your touch. About all this there is of course much more to say, and I will discuss these things further in a later chapter.

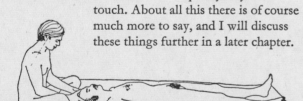

In order to make these suggestions more concrete here is an experiment that you might try. Have a friend lie down on his (or her) stomach and apply oil to the entire back side of his body. Then put the palms of both your hands against his skin, and start moving them. Don't worry at all about whether they are doing some or another orthodox massage stroke; just move them up and down your friend's body however you wish. Explore how present, how 'right there' it is possible for you to feel in your hands. Have your eyes sometimes open, sometimes closed. From time to time experiment with some of what has been suggested above. Try out different pressures, different speeds and any other changes in quality that suggest themselves to you. Be as spontaneous as you can; let your hands do most of the thinking. At the same time stay alert to exactly what is happening.

Try this for five minutes, ten minutes or whatever feels good to you, but do it for only as long as you enjoy doing it.

Come back to this exercise as often as you like; it can always teach you something new. These are fundamentals of which our 'mastery' is always only partial.

Introduction to the strokes

Time now to get down to the nitty-gritty of technique. In the section that follows you will find descriptions and illustrations of approximately eighty different massage strokes. Before you start in, however, here are a few necessary bits and pieces of information about how this part of the book has been arranged, about the use of the strokes themselves, and, in case you have never done any massage before, about the best way to go about learning.

The order in which these strokes are presented is not important. If you were to use all of them in sequence, you would end up having given a friend a complete body massage of about an hour and a half in length – a massage that would have started with his or her head, then have worked progressively down the front of the body to the feet, and then (your friend having turned over) up the other side of the body ending on the back. Or, if you were to use only those strokes which I have marked with a star,* you would give a shorter massage covering the same territory and taking about half the amount of time. The more you experiment, however, the more you will find other, equally good ways to select and combine these various strokes. They are the fundamentals from which your personal massage style will naturally develop.

The particular strokes marked with a star * are in no way 'better' than the ones not so marked. They merely represent one example of how a short massage can be put together out of the material offered below.

The instructions below have in a sense been written for someone who is right-handed. That is, it is the right rather than the left hand which is favoured whenever there is a choice. If you are left-handed, all you have to do is to substitute your left for your right hand in any instances that seem appropriate.

I also generally speak as if you are doing

massage on a table: 'move to the foot end of the table', etc. In almost all cases, however, what you do if you are working on the floor is exactly the same. Whenever a stroke must be done differently on the floor I have included alternative instructions.

At certain points you will notice that your friend's arm, leg or head must be lifted or moved. Make sure that you yourself do all the lifting or moving, and that your friend in no way helps out. If he does try to help, or, as sometimes happens, if he slightly stiffens the limb in resistance, just call his attention to it and ask him to relax the limb in question as much as possible.

Learn to make your transitions between strokes seem like a part of the strokes themselves. Even to divide a massage into separate 'strokes', as I have done below, is in a certain sense arbitrary. Massage at its best makes use of specific techniques, but only by weaving them into a continuous flowing movement that remains always inventive and spontaneous. Let your hands find a natural way to glide from one stroke into another; your friend should never be able to tell exactly where the one has ended and the other begun. Ideally, in fact,

his or her experience of your entire massage should be like that of a single unbroken stroke winding its way all over his or her body.

Remember also, as has already been mentioned, to break physical contact as seldom as possible during a massage. Once you have begun, try always to have at least one hand touching your friend until the massage is completed.

Massage is basically non-verbal and is best done in silence. While you are first making yourself acquainted with techniques, you will of course need to talk with whomever you are massaging in order to find out how he or she is feeling as you work. Other than this, try to focus all your attention on your sense of touch.

If you are learning massage for the first time it is important to go about it in the right way. Here are a few suggestions. My experience is that they can make a big difference to how quickly and easily you learn.

First, a warning! *Don't try to learn too much at one time.* A half dozen strokes or less are plenty for one session. In the beginning you may find massage quite tiring to do. Very soon, as you learn correctly how to move and position your own body, it will become much less so. But do start with small doses and work up from there!

When you are ready to start in, read over the entire description of a stroke before attempting to do it. An extra reading beforehand of all the strokes you plan to learn at one time will help even more.

Once you do get together with a friend to try out some of the strokes, make sure that your friend gives you as much feedback as possible. Find out what feels good, what bad, what so-so; what feels too light or too heavy; what too fast or too slow; and anything else you want to know. Ask often, and encourage your friend to speak up whenever he or she feels like it. This information will prove invaluable to you.

Experiment especially with different amounts of pressure. Try a stroke lightly, then with more pressure, and then with more pressure still. And ask for feedback at each step.

Don't worry if a stroke at first seems clumsy or awkward to do. Usually if you check out with your friend he or she will have a very different feeling about it.

Finally, whenever possible have the strokes which you are trying to learn done to yourself. You will never really be able to tell how a stroke 'works' until you have felt it on your own body. I might add that the nicest way of all to learn massage is with a friend who also wants to learn. That way, you can try out several strokes at a time and he or she can do them on you in turn. This will immediately provide both of you with an 'inside' understanding of what you are doing.

Have a good time!

The Strokes

Head and neck

When I give a complete massage the head is one of my favourite places to begin.

As I have said, the sequence of the different parts of the body that will be followed in these instructions is largely arbitrary. And in a later section of the book I will tell you more specifically about other possible sequences, and why, depending on circumstances, you might want to follow one or another of them.

For now, however, let me say that it is difficult to go wrong in starting out with the head.

The main reason for this is, it seems to me, that having one's head worked on feels like both one of the safest and one of the most startling parts of a good massage. Safest because, in our nervousness about being touched (and we all have at least a residue of this, especially at the very beginning of a massage), it is in the extremities of the body – the head, the hands and the feet – that we least feel the force of our culture's strong taboos against physical contact. And startling because, although the head is the part of the body with which, sadly, we tend most to identify ourselves, it is also one of the parts from which – just as sadly – we feel physically most disconnected. To discover, through massage, that the head belongs to the physical body is a surprise, like awakening from sleep. As a result, by doing his or her head right at the beginning you will provide the friend you are massaging with a good initiation into the deeper and more subtle side of the experience to come.

So let's start.

Stand or kneel so that you are facing the top of your friend's head. Apply a little oil to your fingers, but do not spread the oil on the face prior to beginning. The actual surface of the face is so small that it requires little oil: with the few drops on your fingers you are ready to begin.

The most natural order in which to massage the different parts of the head is first to do the face, starting at the top of the forehead and working systematically down to the chin; then to the ears; the neck; and finally the scalp.

Remember, a star * marking a stroke means not that it is better than any of the others, but that it is a part of the short massage as described on page 35.

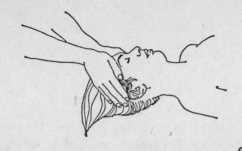

I ⋆ Before anything else I like to hold my palms lightly against my friend's forehead for a few moments. Cover the forehead with the heels of your hands, letting the fingers extend down the temples. Apply no pressure. Pause as long as seems right and comfortable to you: a few seconds, half a minute, whatever. Centre yourself. Let your friend grow accustomed to your touch.

2 ★ Now begin massaging you friend's forehead with the balls of your thumbs. First mentally divide the forehead into horizontal strips about a half an inch wide. Then, starting with your thumbs at the centre of the forehead just below the hairline, glide both thumbs at once in either direction outwards along the topmost strip. Press moderately: use about the pressure it takes to stick a stamp on an envelope. Continue all the way to the temples, a surprisingly sensitive place, and end there by moving your thumbs in a single circle about

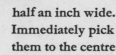

half an inch wide. Immediately pick up your thumbs, return them to the centre of the forehead, and begin the next strip down, again moving your thumbs from the centre outwards. Then, working progressively downwards, do each of the others in turn, ending with a strip running just above your friend's eyebrows. Remember to conclude each strip with another small circle on the temples – a flourish not strictly necessary, but your friend will feel it's very 'right'.

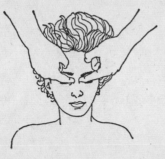

3 ＊ The next stroke is for the rim of the eye sockets. With the tips of both forefingers press first against the boney rims of the two eye sockets right where they connect with the nose. Press quite hard for about one full second. Then lift your forefingers, move them about a third of an inch along the upper half of each rim, and press again. Pressing in this fashion is good for the sinuses, and in this particular spot it also feels better to most people than a rubbing movement.

Continue in this fashion, moving about a third of an inch each time you press, until you have reached the outermost point of each eye socket (i.e., the point farthest from the nose). Then return to the point nearest the nose and begin again, this time working the length of the lower half of the rim.

4 Now the eyes themselves.

Did you remember to make sure before starting that your friend was not wearing contact lenses ? If not, ask about them now.

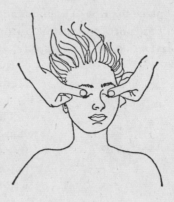

Lightly run the balls of your thumbs straight across your friend's closed eyelids. Start right beside the nose and move outwards. Go very slowly and use a minimum of pressure, just enough that you can feel the eyeball move ever so slightly as your thumb passes over it.

Do this three times, moving your thumbs in the same direction and lifting to return them to the starting point each time.

5 ★ Now place the tips of the forefinger and middle finger on each hand just to either side of the nose, and just below the point on the rim of the eye socket where you started the last stroke. Pressing firmly, draw the tips of these fingers in a path around the

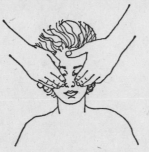

lower edges of the cheekbones, across the cheeks in the direction of the ears and then back up to the temples for a final circle.

The lower edges of the cheekbones, in case you aren't sure of your geography at this point, lie roughly on a line with the bottom of the nose. If you press firmly and pay attention to the feel of the stroke, however, your fingers will have no difficulty in finding the right place to go. Do this stroke at least twice. The second time you might want to linger a while on the edges of the cheekbones immediately below and to the sides of the nose, working the muscles beneath by making tiny circles with your fingertips. Let each fingertip move in a circle a quarter of an inch wide or smaller, pressing hard without lifting. Dig in. Don't hurry. This minute area is a focal point for tension in the face, and a little extra work here goes a long way.

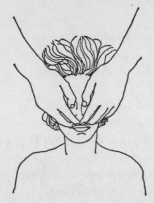

6 ★ Finish the lower half of the face with a series of horizontal strokes like those you did on the forehead. First use the forefinger and the middle fingers of both hands. Place the tips of these fingers at the centre of the face between the nose and the mouth. Stroke outwards on to the cheeks and then up to the temples, ending with the usual circle.

Next do a series of three strokes in the same way between the mouth and the tip of the chin. Start each time at the centre and end on the temples.

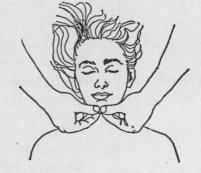

Then lightly grasp the tip of the chin between the tips of the thumb and forefinger of each hand. Follow the edges of the jaw until you have almost reached the ears, and then glide the forefingers (and the middle fingers, too, if you wish) into a last small circle on the temples.

If your friend has a beard, simply go firmly right over it using the same strokes.

This completes the face. Now slide your fingers gently to the ears.

7

Ears seem to me one of the most intriguing parts of the body. I love having mine massaged. Here are a lot of ways to work on them. Use all or any part of this according to your own judgement.

For your first trial run I suggest that you do just one ear at a time. Soon, however, you will find yourself able to do both at once without difficulty.

First run the tips of your fingers several times up and down the back of the ear where it connects with the rest of the head. Move gently and smoothly.

Follow this by gently running the length of your forefinger several times back and forth in the 'V' formed by the topmost part of the ear and the skull directly adjacent. Then lightly pinch the outer edge of the ear and the ear lobe between the thumb and forefinger. Start at the lobe right next to the skull and work around, moving your thumb and forefinger about a third of an inch between pinches.

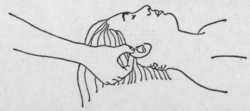

48

Next, with the tip of the forefinger lightly trace the natural hollows of the inside of the ear. Work from the circumference towards the centre. Stop just short of actually closing off the ear channel.

If so far you have been doing just one ear, now do the same steps on the other.

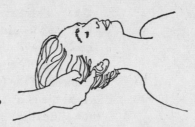

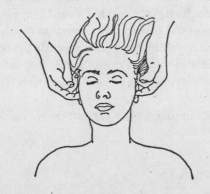

Finally, for the *coup de grace*, tell your friend to listen to the sound inside his head. And then, moving with extreme slowness and gentleness, close both his ear channels with the tips of your forefingers. (Be sure to close both sides at once: nothing will happen if one ear is closed alone.) Keep them closed for about fifteen to thirty seconds. Although some people don't care for this many enjoy a brief but pleasant journey.

49

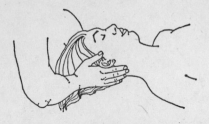

(FROM THE SIDE)

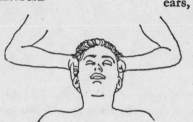

8 This next stroke will feel both odd and awkward as you do it. It is perfectly safe, however, and to your friend will feel extremely good. Lightly cover your friend's face with both palms, heels of the hands on the forehead and fingertips near the chin. Let your hands rest in place a moment; then slide them gently down, going over and past the ears, until the little fingers of both hands are against the table. Next begin pressing with both hands as if you were trying to push them together. Make sure your hands are below and in no way pressing on the ears. Crouch slightly and hold your elbows straight out to the side in order to get as much leverage as possible. Start with a gentle pressure and gradually increase it until (unless you are a person of unusual strength) you reach a point at which you are pressing as hard as you can. Then decrease the pressure just as gradually.

After you have released the pressure, hold your hands in place a few seconds more before going on to the next stroke.

Time now to move to the neck.

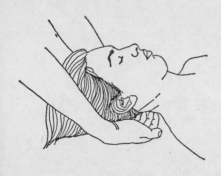

9 Bring both hands palms up under your friend's neck. Then, curving your fingers a little, rapidly drum with the fingertips against the neck. Keep the backs of your hands on the table. Press fairly hard, as if playing a piano. Work up and down the neck, and as far onto the back itself (it won't be very far) in the immediate area of the spine as you can comfortably reach.

10 ★ Next put your hands under the back of your friend's head and gently lift it a little. Then turn it slowly to the left until it rests easily in your left hand. If you sense that your friend is resisting you, or that he is trying to 'help', ask him to relax his head as if he were letting it drop to the table. If after this he still has trouble letting go his head, you may be able to help by gently raising and lowering the head a few more times.

    Now slowly rotate the heel of your right hand against the top of your friend's shoulder while

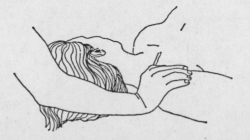

bringing your fingers down the side of the shoulder,
under the shoulder, and on to the back. Keep your
fingers moving across the top of the back
towards the spine; and then, just before
reaching the spine, on to the back of the
neck.

Continue up the back of the neck
until your fingertips near your friend's
hairline. Then turn your hand about ninety degrees so that your fingers are
pointing more upwards (i.e., so that they are perpendicular to the neck itself) and, pressing
more lightly, come back down the side of
the neck.

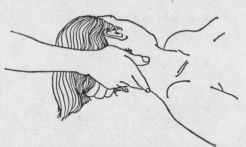

Then, moving from the base of the neck, cross
the topmost part of the chest straight to the
shoulder. From there you can go right into
the same stroke again without stopping.
Repeat three or four times.

The next two strokes are also done with
the head tilted to the side. I prefer to do all
three on one side before turning the head and
repeating them on the other.

II With the head still tilted to the left, move the fingers of the right hand in slow circles about an inch wide against the back of the neck. Press firmly. Work up the back of the neck to the hairline. Then, pressing more gently, do circles down the side of the neck, working all the way from just below the ear to the collar-bone. Repeat.

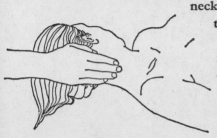
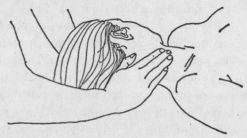

I2 Holding your friend's head still turned to the left, find the boney horizontal ridge where the neck meets the back of the skull with the fingertips of your right hand.

Now move your fingertips in tiny circles just below this ridge. Press firmly. You will feel a sort of furrow stretching horizontally across the neck; follow this furrow with your fingertips.

Check in with your friend if you have trouble locating the right place. This is a nice stroke, and he will know at once when you have found the spot.

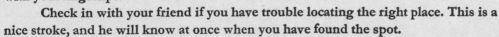

13 End your work on the neck by lifting your
friend's head as far forward as it will go. Use
both hands. Move very slowly.

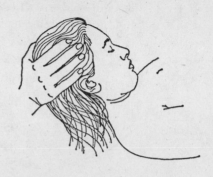

You will feel resistance either soon before or
soon after his chin has touched his chest. Stop for a moment
when you have reached this point. Then gently nudge his
head about an inch farther forwards. Bring the head back to
the same point, and then push forwards once or twice again.
If a gentle push isn't enough, then don't push at all.

Again move slowly as you bring the head back down.

14 ★ All that's left now is the scalp.
Again lift the head and turn it to the left. Making your
right hand into the shape of a claw, work the scalp on the
right side of the head with your fingertips. Press hard, moving
your hand in tiny circles. Try to press hard enough that
you are moving the skin itself over the bone rather than
simply sliding your fingertips back and forth across the
surface of the skin. Work systematically (for example,
in several wide rows up and down the head) so that
you cover the entire right side of the scalp. Repeat on the other side.

Chest and stomach

Spread oil on the chest, the stomach, the sides of the torso and the shoulders.

I★ Begin the chest and stomach with what I will call the main stroke. Because it covers large areas of body surface easily and quickly, this is one of the most effective strokes in massage. With slight variations it can be done on the chest and stomach, the arm, the front of the leg, the back of the leg and the back.

Stand above your friend's head. (If working on the floor, kneel above the head with your knees to either side of the head.) Place your hands with palms down in the middle of the chest. Have the heels of your hands resting just below the collar-bone, your fingers pointing towards the feet, and your thumbs lightly touching each other. Now glide both hands slowly forwards, pressing firmly on the chest and then more lightly on the stomach. Keep your hands together

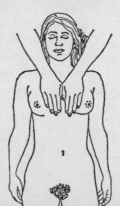
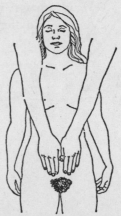

until you reach the lower half of the stomach; then separate them,
moving both hands straight to the sides.

Bring both hands over and down the hips all the way to the table.
As soon as your hands touch the table, begin to
pull them along the sides of the torso in the
direction of the shoulders. Pull firmly, using your
strength; at this point the stroke should feel to
you as if you were actually about to tug your friend several
inches down the table.

Just before reaching the armpits pull your hands – heels of the hands still
moving first – up on to the topmost part of the chest. Then, pivoting
each hand on its heel, swing the fingertips from the
sides to the centre of the chest. By gliding the
hands forwards, and straightening them and bringing
the thumbs together as you move, you can go from
here straight into another round of the same stroke
without breaking the flow of your movement.

Two reminders that will help make this stroke feel just right. First, be steady. Move at an even and confident pace. Second, remember to mould your hands so that they exactly fit the contours they are passing over. Let your hands tune in to your friend's shape as if you were moulding his or her body out of clay.

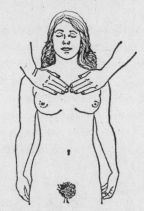

Here is an interesting variation. After pulling your hands back on to the upper chest, send them over and down the sides of the shoulder instead of pivoting them towards the middle of the chest. Continue without a break right under the shoulders and on to the topmost part of the back, slipping your fingers between the table and the back. As soon as your fingers have reached a point right beside – but not directly upon – the spine itself, slide your hands gently over the trapezius muscles (the muscles curving from the neck to the shoulders) and back on to the upper chest.

Another variation, more interesting still. Go down
the sides of the shoulders and on to the back as before.
Again stop just short of the spine. This time, however, pull
your hands lightly on to the back of the neck and then between
the back of the head and the surface of the table. Keep your
hands moving towards yourself until your fingers are completely
clear of the head. Don't lift the head up; keep
the backs of your hands against the table in

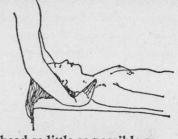

order to disturb the head as little as possible as
you slip your hands from beneath. Once you have
broken contact return your palms immediately to
your friend's chest.

Do the main stroke from three to six times on the
chest and stomach, with or without variations. Occasionally I also repeat it between other strokes
on the chest and stomach; sometimes I even return to it after having gone on to massage other
parts of the body. Returning every once in a while to a major stroke like this one gives a massage
a certain pleasing unity. For both your friend on the table and yourself it can have much the same
effect as the repetition of a basic theme in a piece of music.

2 Run the tips of the thumb and forefinger of both hands several times along the collar-bone. Have the thumb on one side of the bone and the forefinger on the other. Move your hands first towards each other and then away from each other. Press lightly.

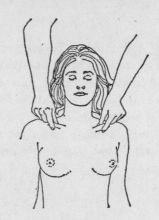

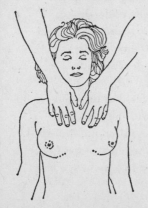

3 * Work the upper chest with the fingertips of both hands. Press firmly, moving the fingertips in tiny circles. Start next to the collar-bone and work systematically so that you cover the entire upper half of the chest. Omit the breasts for a woman, however, as this stroke does not feel good here.

4 ★ Professional masseurs usually do not massage a woman's breasts. Most women I know consider this both prudish and condescending. If your friend is a woman, here is a good stroke for the breasts and the muscles supporting them.

Cup both hands over the breasts. Very gently rotate the breasts as far as you can easily and move them in three full circles moving to the right, and then in another three circles moving to the left.

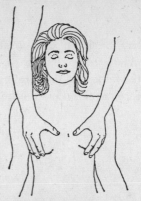

5 Now make both hands into fists. Starting at the middle of the chest just below the collar-bone, slide the knuckles of both fists outwards across the chest and then down the sides of the torso to the table. Press lightly. Follow the ribs. Try, if you can, to let individual knuckles glide between individual ribs.

Do successive horizontal strips in this fashion until you have covered the entire rib cage. Stop short of the stomach. Remember to go lightly: hard pressure will make this stroke feel terrible. If your friend is a woman, when you get to the central portion of the rib cage do just the two inches or so of ribs between the breasts.

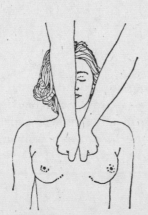

6 ★ This stroke is called pulling, and it is done along the sides of the torso.

Move around to one side of the table and reach across to the opposite side of your friend's torso. With your fingers pointing straight down pull each hand alternately straight up from the table. With each stroke begin pulling with one hand just before the other is about to finish so that there is no break between 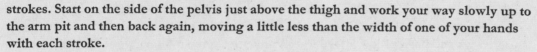 strokes. Start on the side of the pelvis just above the thigh and work your way slowly up to the arm pit and then back again, moving a little less than the width of one of your hands with each stroke.

　　　Once up the side and then down again is enough. Cross to the other side of the table and repeat on your friend's other side.

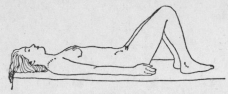

7 ★ Move now to the stomach. Walk around to your friend's right side if you aren't there already, making sure to keep one hand in contact as you move. The various organs in the stomach area will be less constricted – and hence what you do on the stomach will feel better – if your friend has his knees in the air while you are working directly on the stomach. There are two ways of going about this. The first is simply to place your friend's legs in the right position and then let him balance there himself; by sliding his foot back and forth a little you will quickly find a natural point at which the legs almost balance themselves. The second way is to raise the legs and put a pillow folded in half underneath them for support. I usually do it the first way simply because I don't like to hassle with a pillow in the middle of a massage. The second way, however, does have the slight advantage that your friend doesn't have to siphon off even a fraction of his energy in order to keep his legs in place. Now stand at your friend's right side and begin slow full circles on the stomach using the palm of your left hand. Move clockwise – most

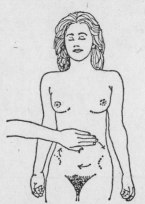

important on the stomach, as the colon is coiled clockwise. With each circle
pass first just below the ribs, then a little on to the left side of the torso at the waist, then
just above the pelvic bone, and then a little on to the right side of the torso at the waist.

After one complete circle you can add the right hand. Keep the left hand moving
steadily in the same fashion; after it has passed from the lower to the upper half of the
stomach, however, add the right hand for about a half of a circle running from hip to hip
alongside the pelvic bone. As soon as the right hand has reached the right hip, remove it
and position it in the air near the left hip so that it can repeat the same crescent movement
after the left hand has made another round. Work out the timing so that whenever the right
hand is actually massaging, it is at a point on the circle directly opposite to the left hand.

Do a half dozen continuous circles with your left hand, adding a partial circle with
the right each time.

8 Awkward as this one may seem at first, in the long run it will be a lot easier for you to do than for me to describe.

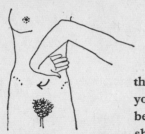

Place the back of your right hand – that's right, the back of the hand – flat against the centre of your friend's stomach. Have your wrist bent at a ninety-degree angle; your fingertips should be pointing towards you and your forearm should stick straight into the air with the elbow pointing away from you.

Now start rotating your hand clockwise. After you have completed about a quarter of a circle start gradually turning your hand over on to its palm at the same time; this will also necessarily bring your elbow closer to the level of the table. Keep on rotating and keep on turning, however; so that by the time the circle has been completed, your hand has again been turned on to its back and your elbow raised to a position directly above your hand.

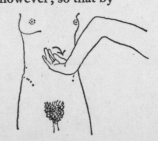

Make half a dozen circles. The feel of this stroke should

be flowing and steady and slow. Don't wander about the stomach; keep it right at the centre. If your friend's knees have been raised you may gently return his legs to the table.

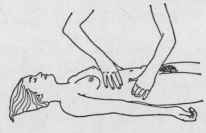

9 Now knead the sides of the torso in the vicinity of the waistline.
Kneading is not difficult. Reach across to the side opposite you. With each stroke of your hands gently squeeze the loose flesh at the waistline between your thumb and fingers; grasp as much as you can comfortably hold on to and then let it slowly slip from between your fingers. Also move your hands a little with each stroke, left hand going to the right and right hand going to the left. If you alternate hands, beginning a new stroke with one hand slightly before finishing a stroke with the other, you will find yourself falling into a slow, lazy, natural rhythm in which the hands are always in motion.
After a few rounds in this fashion you can introduce a change into the stroke. Change your kneading

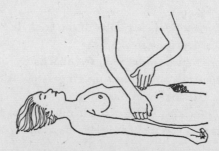

into simple stroking, and instead of moving your hands horizontally (i.e., parallel to the table) along the sides of the torso, begin sliding your fingers under your friend's back right at the waist and drawing your hand vertically up the side of the torso and an inch or two on to the stomach. Follow the waistline and press slightly with the fingertips. Start each stroke from points progressively farther under the back, and start the last two or three from just beside the spine itself.

The shift from the first to the second version of this stroke need not be abrupt. Try doing three or four rounds running horizontally from hip to ribs and back; and then gradually make your strokes more and more vertical until you end with one or two rounds running along the waistline itself.

Then around to the opposite side of the table and do the same on your friend's other side.

IO

This last stroke is actually for the back, but it feels nicest when done immediately after the previous stroke.

Reach both hands under your friend's back, one from one side and one from the other, right at the waistline. Palms up, fingers pointing towards each other. Bring the fingertips just to either side of the spine.

Now, keeping the backs of the hands against the table, press the fingertips of both hands as hard as you can just to either side of the spine. Press hard enough to actually raise the middle of your friend's body a tiny bit into the air. Press for about one full second and release. Then again for a second and release. Then again. After the third time or so, slide your hands, still pressing with the fingertips but pressing much more lightly now, out from under the back and, again following the waistline, on to the stomach. As with the previous stroke, articulate the waistline as you go.

If you are working on the floor, here is – at last – one place where you have an advantage over someone working on a table. After (or even instead of) pressing your fingertips next to the spine, squat so that you are straddling your friend's body, lace your fingers together behind the spine itself, and lift the middle of your friend's body several inches off the floor. Then slide your hands along the waistline, pressing slightly with the fingertips, as you let your friend down again. For your friend, the sensation of being lifted will give this stroke an especially pleasant feeling.

Don't bother with this variation, however, if you are working on a table. Because you are forced to reach from the side it's both more tiring for your own back and more difficult to do correctly.

Whichever version of this stroke you are using, a nice way to finish is to keep following the waistline with your fingertips until your hands meet at the centre of the stomach. Go more lightly while crossing the stomach itself. Once your hands meet, you can then find some graceful way to glide them to wherever you plan next to work.

The arm

Arrange your friend's right arm at his side with the palm turned down against the table. Spread oil on the arm and shoulder.

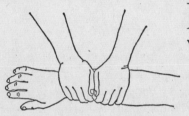

I   *   Begin with a variation of the main stroke. Place both your hands palms down across your friend's wrist, cupping them so that they cover the sides as well as the top of the wrist. Have your hands side by side, with thumbs touching.

Pressing firmly, glide both hands together up the arm. Separate them only when you reach the top of the arm, sending the left hand over the top of the shoulder and the right down the inside of the arm just short of the armpit.

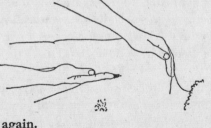

Now pull both hands back down the arm, starting with your left hand on the outside and your right on the inside. Press more lightly. Once you reach the wrist you have two options. One is simply to slide your left hand around on to the top of the wrist so that both hands are in position to begin the same stroke again.

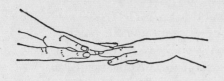

The other, if you feel like something with more of a flourish, is to slide both hands down the length of your friend's hand and right off his or her fingertips. Let your right hand slide along the top of the hand and your left hand the bottom.

Press more lightly on the hand, and be extra delicate and precise as you leave the fingertips. Immediately afterwards move your hands into position for your next stroke so that your friend experiences as little a break in contact as possible.

2 ★ This stroke is called draining.
Raise your friend's forearm so that it is standing upright with the elbow still against the table. Now make a ring around your friend's wrist with the thumbs and forefingers of both your hands; tilt your hands away from you so that your palms are facing up as you hold the wrist. Have your thumbs against the inside of the wrist, and have both thumbs touching each other.

Now, squeezing lightly with your thumbs and forefingers, slide both hands slowly down the length of the forearm as if you were 'draining' it. When you reach the crook of the elbow slide both hands back up again, still keeping your thumbs and forefingers in contact with the skin but now applying no pressure at all. Repeat several times.

Why, you may ask, do we use pressure going down but not coming up? The answer is that the veins, which lie closer to the surface of the skin than the arteries, are more immediately affected by external pressure. Hence when we 'massage towards the heart', as a traditional bit of massage lore puts it, we are giving an extra push to the blood circulating through the veins towards the heart. For many of the other strokes I am describing to you this traditional rule does not greatly matter. When draining the forearm, however, a little experimentation will soon convince you that your friend will be happiest when you apply pressure going down – but not up as well.

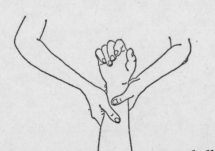

3 ★ Keep your friend's forearm in the same upright position.

Placing the fingers of both hands against the back of your friend's wrist for leverage, begin massaging the inside of his wrist with the balls of your thumbs. Use your thumbs alternately, and send each stroke downwards and out towards one or the other side of the wrist. Gradually work your hands downwards until you have covered all the muscles lying along the inside of the forearm.

4 A quick treat in passing for the elbow.
First, with your friend's forearm still upright,
make a loose fist with one hand and lightly massage the
crook of his arm – the inside part of the elbow area –
with your knuckles. This is a tender area, so be gentle.

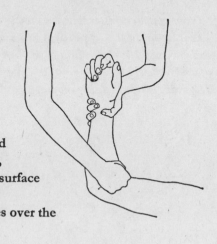

Next, lift the upper arm a little
off the table with one hand, and,
using the tips of the thumb and
fingers of your other hand,
massage the boney surface
of the elbow itself.
Work in tiny circles over the
entire elbow.

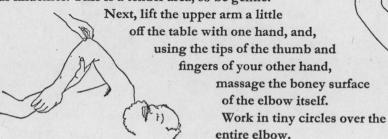

5 ⋆ Now repeat strokes 2 and 3 on the upper arm. You will find
that keeping the upper arm in a steady vertical
position can be a bit of a problem, however. One solution
is to place his hand on your own left shoulder and to press your
cheek against it much as if you were holding a violin
in place.
A second is to bend
his arm at the elbow
and to let the
forearm dangle across his
body at about the level
of the neck. If you use this position take care not to
slap the forearm against his chin while you are working
on the upper arm. Taking your pick of these two
positions, first drain the upper arm and then work the
exposed muscles with your thumbs just as you did for the
forearm.

6 Next hold the entire arm straight upright. With your right hand grasp the wrist; with your left push horizontally against the elbow to keep the arm from bending in the middle. Now, keeping it vertical and unbending, bob the arm lightly up and down in its socket. Press down and then immediately release the pressure a half dozen times or so in quick succession.

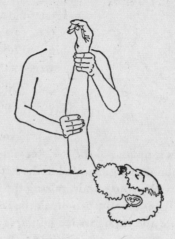

7 Your friend's arm is still standing straight upright, right? Now toss it from side to side. Lower the arm first to the right (i.e., towards your friend's hip), still holding the wrist with your right hand and the elbow with your left.

Then lightly toss it up and to the left, keeping your hands in contact. As soon as it starts to fall to the left (i.e., towards your friend's head), switch your hands, raising the left hand to the wrist and lowering the right to the elbow, so that you now can break the fall with your left hand. Let the arm fall almost to the table and then toss it again, this time to the right.

Switch hands again as it is falling to the right, and you are ready to repeat the entire sequence.

If your friend's arm feels stiff, and does not fall naturally and easily, remind him to let go of it.

Toss the arm three times back and forth.

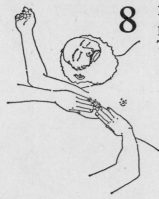

8 For a last good-bye to the arm here is an especially nice stroke made popular by Molly Day Schackman.

Toss the right arm one more time (see the previous stroke, in case you have been following a different sequence) to the left, catch it, and then let it rest in place, the upper arm on the table beside the head and the forearm partially resting in the air. Meanwhile place both your palms lightly against your friend's armpit area, with the fingers of either hand pointing towards the other.

Now begin spreading your hands to the sides, leading with the heels of the hands. Start with a light pressure. Send the right hand down the side of the torso and the left along the upper arm. As soon as they have passed the armpit itself turn both hands so that they are vertical with respect to the table; while turning them keep them moving apart at the same pace.

At the same time lightly grasp the arm with your left hand, fingers on top of the arm and thumb below, and curve your right hand a little so that the full palm presses against the side of the torso as it passes.

Keep both hands in this position as you continue moving them apart. Increase the pressure slightly. Stop when your right hand reaches your friend's hip and your left reaches his wrist.

Now, keeping your hands in place, hold more tightly and stretch the arm and the hip away from each other. Hold this stretch for about one full second, and then release, breaking contact just long enough to bring your hands back to your friend's armpit.

Repeat the entire stroke one more time. A moment or so after breaking contact the second time, return both hands to the arm itself and gently put it back into place at your friend's side.

I prefer to massage both the right arm and hand before going on to the left arm and hand. If you have just finished your friend's right arm, you may wish to go on to the following section on the hand before moving over to his or her left arm and hand.

The hand

The hand requires very little oil. What you have left on your own hands after massaging the arm will be more than sufficient.

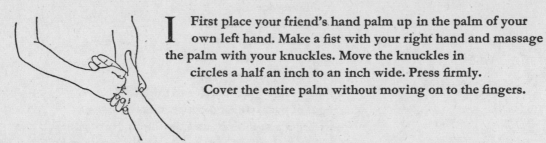

I First place your friend's hand palm up in the palm of your own left hand. Make a fist with your right hand and massage the palm with your knuckles. Move the knuckles in circles a half an inch to an inch wide. Press firmly.

Cover the entire palm without moving on to the fingers.

2 ★ Next go over the same area using the tips of your
thumbs. Hold the back of the hand with your fingers
and press hard with the thumbs, moving them also in small circles.
This time, however, continue up over the heel of the hand and,
pressing more gently, an inch or so on to the inside of the wrist.

Want to try something more elaborate? Do
this stroke on the palm (but not
the wrist) while holding your
friend's hand
as follows.
Have your
friend's hand palm up.
Place the little
finger of your left hand
between his forefinger and
middle finger; the fourth and middle
finger of your left hand between his
forefinger and thumb; and the forefinger of your left hand
on the other side of his thumb. At the same time place
the little finger of your right hand between his middle

and fourth fingers; the fourth finger of your right hand between his fourth and little fingers; and the middle finger and forefinger of your right hand on the other side of his little finger.

Got that?

Now push all your fingers as far on to the back of his hand as you can. Then push your fingers hard *against* the back of his hand. See what this does? If you are pushing correctly you will have bent his fingers back so that the entire surface of his palm is stretched taut as a drum. And now, keeping his fingers bent back, begin working the palm with the tips of your thumbs. Press hard, and go patiently into every tiniest nook and cranny. As you will find out the first time it is done to you, this stroke is more than worth the extra effort.

3 ★ Now work the back of the hand with the tips of your thumbs. Be thorough. Go also an inch on to the wrist, paying particular attention to all the tiny bones your thumbs will find there.

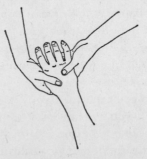

4 For this stroke you will have to follow some anatomical guidelines.

Hold your friend's hand palm down in your own left hand, and for a moment study the back of his hand. Notice the small raised cords, just under the surface of the skin, that appear to run from the base of the wrist to the first knuckle of each finger. These are actually the tendons that are used to extend the fingers. (If you have difficulty locating them try looking at the back of your own hand by itself while stretching your fingers as far out and back as they will reach. This will raise the tendons and make them more visible.)

Now, thinking of these tendons as ridges and of the spaces in between as valleys, slowly run the tip of your thumb down each valley in turn. Go all the way from the base of the wrist to the little flap of skin between each successive pair of fingers. Use enough pressure for your friend to be able to feel each valley as perfectly distinct; use a little less, however, as soon as you reach the flap of skin between the fingers. Do each valley one time, using your right thumb for the two valleys nearest the right side of the hand and your left thumb for the two valleys nearest the left.

Here is a flourish you can add, if you feel so moved, each time your thumb reaches the little flap of skin between two fingers. Press the underside of the flap with the tip of your forefinger as your thumb begins to press from above, by this means giving a gentle pinch to the skin as your thumb and forefinger slide off it. It will make a nice stroke feel even nicer.

5 Although a little difficult at first, this stroke is quite simple once you get the knack of it.

Hold your friend's hand palm down with both your hands. Have the heels of your hand pressing against the middle of the back of his hand, and the tips of your fingers pressing against the middle of the palm underneath. Have the heels of your hands touching each other, and the corresponding fingers of both hands also touching one another.

Now begin pressing very hard upwards with your fingertips and downwards with the heels of your hands. At the same time begin very slowly sliding the heels of your hands from the middle of the hand to both edges. Stop when the heels of your hands are at the edges of your friend's hand.

Do this stroke three times.

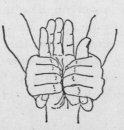

(from Beneath)

6 ★ Now do the fingers themselves.

Hold your friend's hand palm up in your left hand. With your own thumb and forefinger lightly grasp his thumb where it joins with the rest of his hand. Now slide your thumb and forefinger slowly from base to top of the thumb, twisting your hand from side to side in a corkscrew motion at the same time. Pull a little as you go. End by going right off the tip of the thumb into the air.

Do each finger once in the same way.

7 ★ Here is a nice way to finish your work on the hand.

For a minute hold your friend's hand sandwiched between both of yours. Make contact with as much of its surface as you can. Be still, go inside yourself, and concentrate on your own breathing. Then focus your attention back on to your friend's hand and try to let the energy of your breath seep from your own hands into that of your friend.

This pause need not be long – thirty seconds is fine. Afterwards you will find yourself refreshed, and your friend will have opened himself a little more to what is yet to come.

Front of the leg

See that your friend's feet are a foot or so apart. Apply oil to the entirety of the front and sides of the right leg.

I * For the main stroke on the leg, it is important to stand or kneel in exactly the right place. If you are using a table stand near your friend's right foreleg and turn forty-five degrees towards the opposite end of the table; in other words you should be roughly facing the pelvic region of your friend's body. Have your weight on your right foot and place your left foot a couple of feet towards the head of the table.

    If you are working on the floor kneel alongside your friend's foreleg. Be facing in the direction of your friend's head; have your knees approximately parallel to his or her knees.

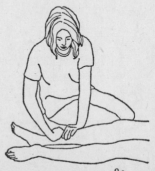

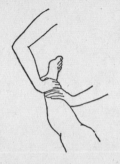

Now place your right hand across your friend's ankle with fingertips facing your side of the table. Place your left hand just in front of the right with fingertips facing the opposite side of the table. (If you are working on the left leg the right hand goes in front of the left hand.) Both hands should be cupped, with fingers together; the thumb of the left hand should be resting against the little finger of the right.

Now glide both hands from one end of the leg to the other. The movement should be slow and steady. Go lightly over the knee but elsewhere use plenty of pressure; this can be most easily done by leaning slightly over the leg and thus using the natural effect of your own weight rather than an increased muscular effort. If you are standing, transfer your weight from your right to your left foot as you move. If kneeling, you may, if you wish, raise yourself slightly upwards and forwards in order to keep the upper part of your own body directly above your hands as long as possible.

The trickiest part of the stroke comes when
you reach the top of your friend's leg.
Here the hands divide and go their separate
ways. The left hand continues upwards until
the fingertips find the hip bone. It
then follows the line of the hip all the
way down to the table; as it does so,

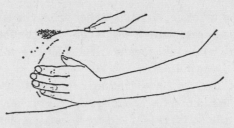

the fingertips with a slight extra pressure outline the curve of the
bone itself.

      Then, once the fingertips have actually made contact with the
table, the left hand begins to move along the side of the leg back
towards the foot.

      At the same time the right hand moves more slowly

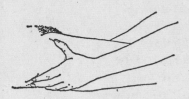

down the inside of the thigh. There is a natural crease in the skin between the
pelvis and the inside of the thigh; the fingertips should follow this crease,
making a detour around a male's genitals where necessary, straight down
to the table. At this point the right hand is also ready to head back towards
the foot. Now as you gradually transfer your weight back on to your
right foot, pull both hands along the sides of the legs all the way to the
ankle. Keep the fingertips on both sides moving against or just above the
surface of the table. Use less pressure than going up; however, let your friend
feel a definite pull as your hands move down.
When you move your hands into place to repeat the stroke

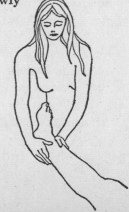

be sure to end up with the left hand higher up on the foreleg than the right. Otherwise the hands will be in each other's way when it is time for them to divide. For the same reason, when you later move to your friend's left leg you must there place your right hand higher up than your left.

I find that there are two secrets to making this stroke feel exactly right. The first is to articulate the hip bone as carefully and as precisely as possible with the left hand. For your friend this will feel as if you are drawing a picture of his body's structure at this point, a sensation which most people find particularly pleasant. The second secret is to pace the movement of the two hands, after they have divided at the top of the leg, so that they end up parallel to one another when they begin their downward journey back towards the calf. This means that the inside hand must move considerably more slowly than the outside one. You can, of course, just move it at the same speed and then let it rest in place until the left catches up. The stroke feels nicest, however, if you can somehow work it out so that both hands stay constantly in motion.

A nice variation: move the hands up the leg as before, but coming down use just your fingertips and make the pressure as light as possible – as if you were stroking the skin with feathers. This feels exquisite, as I urge you to verify the next time you are the lucky one on the table.

Repeat the main stroke three or more times. I like also to include it now and then between some of the other strokes that I use on the front of the leg.

2 For the next stroke, place the palm of your left hand flat against the outer side of your friend's foreleg. Have the hand halfway between the ankle and the knee, with the fingertips pointing towards the knee. Now, looking at the inner side of your friend's foreleg, picture this side as divided into three parallel strips running from ankle to knee. Place your right hand at the ankle end of the topmost strip with fingertips pointing towards the knee.

Then, holding the left hand in place, slowly glide the right hand along this topmost strip until the fingertips are just short of the knee. Then bring it back to the ankle, leading now with the heel of the hand, without any change in the speed or pressure of your stroke. The left hand stays in place the whole time. However, it exerts pressure in opposition to the moving right hand so that the muscles of the foreleg are gently squeezed between.

After covering the first strip once both forwards and backwards, do the next two strips in succession. Then place the right hand flat against the inner side of the foreleg, and with the left hand do three strips in exactly the same fashion on the outer side.

Next move to the thigh (or, if you prefer, to our next stroke for the knee and then to the thigh) and follow the same sequence. However, since the thigh is wider you will here have to do four or more strips on each side. On the inner side let each strip run from a point parallel to the knee to the crease in the skin between thigh and pelvis. The strips on the outer side should also begin at a point parallel to the knee, but should go on to include the hip as well; let the fingertips of the left hand make contact with the edge of the hip bone each time before returning.

3 ⋆ Now the knee! This is one of my favourites. Your
friend may well discover for the first time
what a pleasure it can be to have a knee.
Although it looks complicated, the stroke is
fairly simple. First I am going to break it down
for you into halves. Begin by placing the crossed
tips of both thumbs against the lower edge of the kneecap.

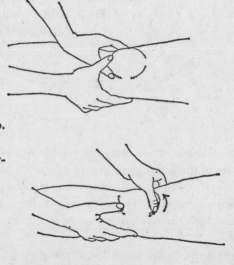

Next with the tip of the left thumb circle the edge of the kneecap. Move to the right (in other words, counter-clockwise), and make a complete circle. You will find a small furrow between the edge of the kneecap and the bone underneath; press the tip of the thumb into this furrow with a light but steady pressure. Then do the same thing with the right thumb, this time starting to the left, or clockwise.

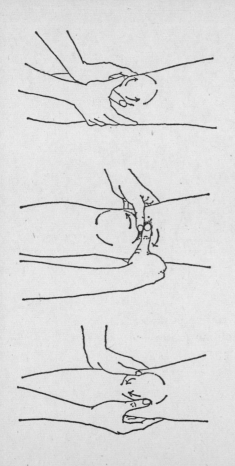

Now for the actual stroke, merely move both thumbs at once exactly as you moved them separately. First bring them up either side, then let them cross at the top, and then finish by bringing each thumb down the side opposite that from which it started. At the bottom of the kneecap cross them again and you are ready to begin another circle. Do three or more slow circles without lifting your thumbs or stopping. Afterwards drum lightly all over the top of the kneecap for several seconds with the fingertips of both hands. Finish by gently rubbing the sides of the knee with the fingers of both hands at once. Make half a dozen or so wide circles on either side of the knee.

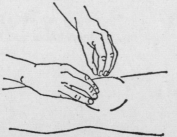

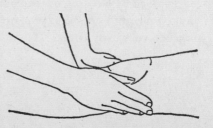

4 For the next two strokes your
friend's leg must be raised
so that the knee rests in the air.
Lift with your left hand from
beneath the knee while with your
right hand you slide the foot
until it is parallel to the knee
of the opposite leg;
the knee should
be high enough
for the leg to be
almost able to
balance in place.
Next, if working
on a table, anchor the
leg in place by backing up and sitting so that you gently pin your friend's toes under
your own right buttock. If you are working on the floor, kneel and hold his foot
between your own knees.

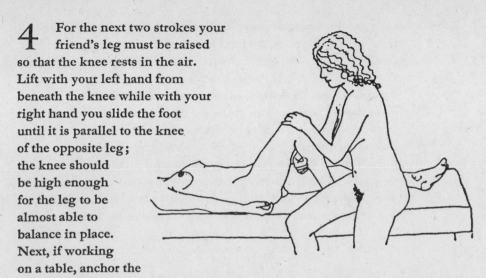

Now, lightly clenching your right fist, reach under the leg from the right and with the inside of your forearm massage the calf muscles on the underside of your friend's foreleg. Starting with the inside of your wrist at the base of the calf, work in long narrow circles going first from left to right. As you come up the left (from where you are facing) side of the calf, keep sliding your forearm to the left so that by the time you have made it to the top of the calf you have almost reached the crook of your elbow.

Coming down again on the right side, slide your forearm back to the right until the inside of your wrist is once more against the base of your friend's calf.

Circle two more times in the same direction, then another three times in the opposite direction. Give this stroke your best attention: it is also one of everybody's favourites.

5 This one is called 'rolling' the thigh. Leave your friend's leg in the same raised position that you used for the previous stroke.

Place your palms on either side of the thigh just below the knee, your fingers extended outwards. Now vigorously move both hands back and forth, moving the left hand forwards (i.e., in the direction of its own fingertips) while the right hand moves back (i.e., in the direction of its own heel), and vice versa; and at the same time slowly work both hands down the length of the thigh. Continue down the thigh almost to the pelvis, and then return upwards with the same motion. Repeat the entire stroke one more time.

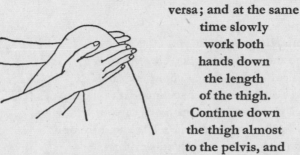

As with the arm and hand, I like to massage both the right leg and the right foot before going on to the left leg and foot. If you wish to do the same, follow your work on the right leg by going on to the next section for the foot.

The foot

If any single part of the body deserves your best attention it is the foot.

Psychologically it is the point at which we experience our connection with the ground that supports us. It is where we feel, if and when we are lucky enough to do so, that we are 'rooted'.

From a bone and muscle point of view, moreover, it is an unusually delicate and complicated piece of equipment. If you could strip off your skin you would find twenty-six separate bones making up the skeletal machinery of one foot alone.

But what counts most for those of us doing massage is the role the foot plays within the nervous system of the body. In the sole of the foot are concentrated literally tens of thousands of nerve endings, and the opposite ends of these nerves are located all over the rest of the body.

Thus the foot is a 'map' of the entire body. No muscle, no gland, no organ whether internal or external is without a set of nerves whose opposite ends are anchored in the foot. And what does this mean? Simply that when we massage the foot we stimulate and affect all the rest of the body as well: So critical, in fact, are these groups of nervous correspondences between the foot and everything else in the body, that an important means of medical diagnosis and healing through foot massage, commonly called 'zone therapy' by practitioners, has been built entirely upon it. I will have more to say about zone therapy in a later section. Enough for now that you be aware that while massaging the foot you are giving an extra 'shadow massage' to the rest of the body as well. So do good work – a little here goes a long way.

The strokes for the foot are much like those for the hand. Also like the hand, the foot requires little oil. Whatever you have on your hands after massaging the leg will most likely be enough.

I First make a fist with your right hand. Steady the foot with your left hand, and with the knuckles of your right hand massage the sole. Move your knuckles in small circles; press hard. Be sure to cover the entire sole, including the bottom of the heel.

2 ★ Next go over the sole with the thumbs of both hands. Hold the foot in place with your fingers and work both thumbs at once in small circles. Again cover the entire sole. Go slow. Be thorough. Remember those thousands of nerves connecting the foot with the rest of the body.

If you are working on the floor you will find this one of the more awkward strokes of the massage. One thing to do that can help: sit cross-legged facing in the direction of your friend's head and rest the foot or the back of the ankle on your own knee or leg. Another way: prop the foot up on a thick cushion or pillow.

3 ★ Next work the top of the foot, using your thumbs in the same way. Again be vigorous and be thorough; don't let any tiny patches escape unmassaged. When you reach the lower half of the foot – in other words when you near the ankle and the heel – you will find it easier to use the tips of your fingers. Circle the ankle bone itself – the round bony protuberance about an inch wide on either side of the ankle – several times with your fingertips, doing both sides at once.

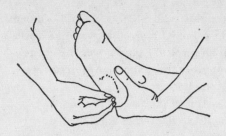

4 When you finally reach the lower end of the heel, gently lift the foot from beneath the ankle with the left hand and work the bottommost edge of the heel with the tips of the fingers and thumb of the right hand. Press hard.

5 Next look at the top of your friend's foot and find, just as you did for the hand, the long thin tendons running from the base of the ankle to each toe. Run the tip of your thumb, pressing firmly, down each of the valleys that lie in between these tendons. Start at the base of the ankle and end at the tiny flap of skin between the toes. As for the hand, you may, if you wish, gently squeeze this flap of skin by pressing the tip of your forefinger against its underside as your thumb passes over its top. Do each valley one time.

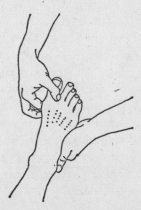

6 Next squeeze the foot just as you did the hand. Grasp the foot with both hands, heels of the hands against the top of the foot and fingertips pressing into the middle of the sole. Have the heels of your hands touching each other, and the corresponding fingers of both hands also touching one another.

Now begin pressing very hard downwards on to the top of the foot with the heels of your hands and upwards into the sole with your fingertips. At the same time very slowly let the heels of your hands slip from the middle of the foot out to either edge. Stop right at either edge.

Do three times.

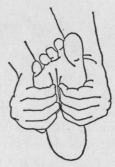

(from Beneath)

7 ★ Now the toes themselves. With your left hand hold the foot steady; with the thumb and forefinger of your right hand grasp the base of the big toe. Then gently pull, twisting from side to side in a corkscrew motion, until your thumb and forefinger slide off the tip of the toe. Do each toe in turn.

8 ★ Finish the foot just as you did the hand. Clasp the foot between your hands, one palm along the sole and the other along the length of the top, and for a moment allow yourself to be still. Centre yourself and become aware of your breathing. Imagine that you're sending your breath into your hands, allowing the energy that circulates in your own body to mingle with that of your friend's.

Back of the leg

If you are following the sequence I have used in describing the strokes, it is time to have your friend turn over on to his stomach. Remember to keep one hand in contact as he moves. Have him lie with his head turned to whichever side he wishes, and remind him to turn his head to the other side whenever his neck feels tired.

Spread oil on your friend's right leg, buttock and hip.

I * Begin with the main stroke. The version for the back of the leg is almost exactly like the one for the front of the leg. Place your friend's feet a foot or so apart. Stand beside your friend's right foot. Place your left hand across the back of the ankle with fingertips pointing towards yourself, and your right hand just above with fingertips pointing towards the opposite side of the table. Pressing firmly, move both hands together up the leg; go more lightly, however, over the back of the knee. Remember to transfer your weight from your left to your right foot as you move.

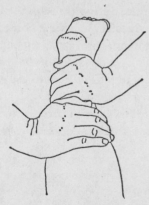

Separate your hands at the top of the thigh just
as you did on the front of the leg. Send the right
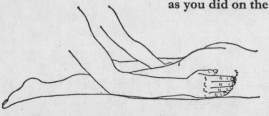 hand over the top of the buttock until
the fingertips locate the hip bone. Glide
the hand down the hip to the table,
firmly articulating the curve of the bone,
and then bring it along side of the leg back
towards the foot.

At the same time move the left hand more slowly down the inside of the thigh. Try
to work out the timing (as with the front of the leg, this will take a little practice) so that the
left hand arrives at the lowest point it can comfortably reach on the inside of the thigh just
as the right hand, coming off the hip, passes into a position directly parallel to it. Then pull
both hands along the sides of the leg all the way back to the ankle. As your hands near
the ankle, try to return them to the starting position of the stroke without a break in the
flow of your movement.

Repeat this stroke three or more times, and return to it as often as you like
between the strokes to follow.

2 Remember the 'Indian burn' when you were a kid? Here is a version of the Indian burn that feels as good as the old one felt bad. In massage we call it 'wringing'.

Cup both hands and place them, with fingertips pointing away from you, side by side across the base of your friend's calf. Have the underside of the fingers and as much of the palms as possible in contact with the leg.

Now let's first look at the stroke in slow motion. Move your left hand away from you and down, maintaining full contact with the leg, until the fingertips reach the table. At the same time move your right hand towards you and down, until the heel of the hand also reaches the table.

Next move both hands all the way in the reverse direction, ending with the heel of the left hand and the fingertips of the right against the table. Then move both hands back to the opposite position. And so forth.

Now speed up this movement and you have 'wringing'. Keep both hands crossing rapidly back and forth, and at the same time work them together slowly up the length of the leg. The crossing movement, though light in pressure, should be as fast and vigorous as you can make it without sacrificing definiteness. Keep the hands always crossing in directions opposite to each other, and keep the thumbs always brushing against each other.

Continue the stroke all the way to the top of the leg and back down again. One time up and back is enough.

3 Next we 'drain' the leg just as we earlier 'drained' the arm.

Place your palms against either side of the foreleg right at the ankle. Have as much of the palms as possible in contact with the leg, with fingers either touching or pointing towards the table on a slant of about forty-five 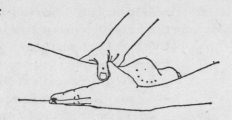 degrees. Across the base of the calf place both thumbs, pointing in opposite directions and touching each other.

Now slowly glide both hands up the foreleg, squeezing gently with palms and thumbs alike. Stop just before you reach the knee and then, moving at the same slow pace but this time with no pressure, glide the hands back down the length of the foreleg. The thumbs remain touching each other throughout the movement.

Go up and back three times, applying pressure each time during the upward movement only. Then move to the thigh and, starting just above the knee, do the same stroke three more times. As you near the pelvis the width of your friend's thigh will probably force your thumbs apart. Simply bring them together again on the way back down.

4 * Next use the balls of your thumbs to massage the thick muscles of the calf. Press firmly, moving your thumbs away from you in short, alternating strokes. Cover all the back of the foreleg.

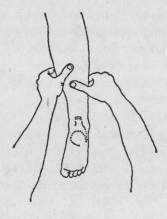

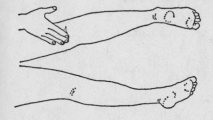

5 With the fingers of one hand lightly massage the slightly hollow area in back of the knee. Work your fingers in small, gentle circles.

6 ★ Next comes 'pulling' on the inside of the thigh. Beginning on the inside of the thigh just past the knee, pull your hands upwards in slow alternating vertical strokes. Keep the palms in contact with the skin, and the fingers pointing toward the table. Begin each new stroke just as you are finishing the previous one. Keep the pressure gentle, and the rhythm slow and steady.

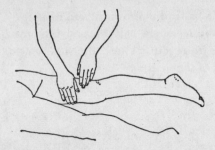

Start each stroke a little higher up the leg (i.e., farther from the knee), until you reach a point just short of the pelvis. Then slowly work back down towards the knee in the same fashion.

If your friend had his or her way you would probably keep doing this stroke all afternoon, but twice up and back is sufficient.

7 Next try 'raking'. This is a good stroke almost anywhere, but I particularly like to use it on the back of the leg, the buttocks and the back itself.

Hold each hand with the fingers spread apart and slightly curved. Stiffen the fingers a little. Each hand should now look like a claw.

Now begin working down the length of the leg with short alternating strokes. Begin at the top of the leg or, if you want, on the buttock itself. Keep both hands in the claw position, and use only the fingertips for actual contact. Work rapidly and with a very firm pressure, making each stroke about six inches long.

Go systematically down the entire leg, trying to cover as much as you can of the sides as well as the back of the leg. Work downwards only; for some reason this stroke doesn't feel good when done in the opposite direction.

As soon as you have reached the ankle, start again from the top of the leg and repeat one more time.

8 Finish by lifting the foreleg and bending it back towards the buttock. Find the point at which the foreleg resists being pushed back, and then, *gently* nudging it an inch or two farther, bounce it several times in this position. Push the heel of the foot against the buttock if you can do so without straining. Then lower the leg slowly back to the table.

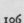

The buttocks

The buttocks are the easiest part of the body to massage. Not the least of reasons for this fact is that here almost anything you do feels good.

I ★   Begin by kneading the flesh of either buttock exactly as if you were preparing bread for the oven. Lift the flesh and squeeze it between the thumb and the other fingers. Knead rhythmically, alternating hands. First cover one buttock thoroughly and then go on to the other. Moving from one to the other side of the table isn't necessary: you can knead either buttock from where you stand.

2 For the next stroke consider the buttocks to go all the way from the waistline to the tops of the thighs.

Stand at your friend's left side. Hold the middle three fingers of your right hand (or your left if you are left-handed) tightly together so that the tips form a triangle with the middle finger on top, and place these three fingertips at a point just below your friend's waistline and just to the right of his spine. Pressing firmly, begin working your fingertips in circles a half an inch wide or smaller, and at the same time slowly move your hand towards the opposite side of the table. Continue to make circles in this fashion, following an imaginary strip running straight across and then down the side of the buttock (or what in this case you might call the lower back) until your fingers reach the table. Then with almost no pressure slide the fingertips in a straight line back up the same strip. Continue working across and down the side of the buttock in strips of this kind. Let each strip begin about an inch farther down the buttock; start each one just beside the spine, or, once you have run out of spine, just above the groove between the buttocks; each time slide back up the same strip once your fingers have reached the table. Work all the way down the right buttock and then cross to the other side of the table and do the same for the left.

3 The next stroke is not difficult, but finding the exact spot to do it can be a little tricky.

With the fingertips of one hand lightly probe the flesh roughly an inch to the side of the centre of the buttock. What you are looking for is a slight hollow or indentation between two large folds of muscle, the Gluteus medius and the Gluteus maximus. Usually it is more readily felt with the fingers than seen with the eyes. If you can't find it, don't worry. Either your friend is a freak, or you may simply need a little more practice. In either case just go ahead with the stroke at any point that looks to you like it ought to have been the proper spot. It will still feel reasonably pleasant.

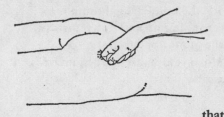

Now double up one forefinger, press its second knuckle into this hollow, and slowly turn your hand as far as you can in either direction. Turn three times each way and then stop. That much feels quite pleasant, but more may make your friend imagine that he is being bolted to the table.

This stroke of course should be repeated on the other buttock. I prefer, however, to go on and do the following stroke on the same buttock, and then to cross over and repeat both on the other.

4 If you never found that hollow, here's your second chance. Back to the same spot, this time with the heel of your hand. Point the fingers up into the air and press the heel straight into the hollow. Now vibrate your hand as fast as you can; try to make your whole arm tremble and shake as if you were getting an electric shock.

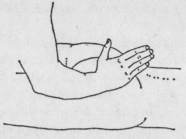

After ten seconds or so of vibrating your hand in place, start moving the heel of your hand over the rest of the buttock. Keep pressing, keep vibrating. In order to be systematic about covering the entire territory, I would suggest that you divide the buttock again into one-inch-wide strips. This time, however, think of the strips as running up and down instead of across the buttock. Start with the strip running next to the groove between the buttocks and end with the one bordering upon the table. Move your hand up (i.e., towards the head) one strip and down (i.e., towards the feet) the next.

5 * Now for the simplest stroke of our massage. Spread the fingers of your right hand as wide apart as you can, and then place your hand firmly against the lower slopes of both buttocks at once. Now shake your hand lightly but very quickly from side to side, shaking the buttocks beneath at the same time. Looks silly ? Just ask your friend how it feels.

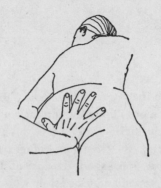

The back

According to the yogis of India and Tibet, our psychological and spiritual
condition is more dependent on the state of the spine than on any other part of
the body. I am inclined to believe this is correct for a number of reasons, not the
least of which is the deep sense of release most of us feel when the back is properly
and thoroughly massaged. Because of its importance as well as its size, I would
suggest that you spend more time working on the back than on any other single
part of the body.

Spread oil on the back, the shoulders and the sides of the torso. Also the buttocks if
you have not worked on them just previously.

I ★   Begin with the main stroke on the back.

One nice thing about the main stroke on the back is that it can be done in either direction.

If you are working on a table the easiest way to do it is from a standing position at the end of the table above your friend's head.

If you are working on the floor, however, you have two choices open to you. One is to sit or kneel just above your friend's head and to do the stroke exactly as described for working on a table. The other is to sit straddling your friend's thighs – a very comfortable position from which to work and to run the stroke in the reverse direction. If you want to do the latter, read through and try to understand the first way of doing it before attempting it in the opposite direction.

Here's the first way. Stand or sit above your friend's head. Place your palms on either side of the topmost part of the back with fingers pointing towards the spine. Have the tips of your fingers right beside, but not on, the spine itself; like many others for the back, this stroke feels much less pleasant if allowed to wander directly on to the spine.

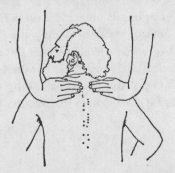

Now glide your hands down the entire length of the back. Maintain a firm pressure, leaning forward to use as much as possible of your own weight. Press extra hard with your fingertips. You will be able to feel a small furrow just to either side of the spine; let your fingertips press right into these furrows as they pass.

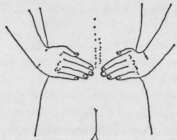

Separate the hands when you near the lower end of the spine, leading the hands over and down the sides of the hips until they touch the table. Then slowly pull both hands along the sides of the torso in the direction of the shoulders. Pull hard, almost hard enough to move your friend on the table. Just before reaching the armpits, glide your hands once more on to the topmost part of the back. Then pivot them, turning the fingers towards the spine, so that they are in place to repeat the entire stroke.

A good variation of this stroke is to take both hands all the way over the tops of the buttocks before pulling them back along the sides. In general it is a nice idea, when doing strokes for the back, to include the buttocks whenever you can.

If you are working on the floor and prefer to sit straddling your
friend's thighs, just start with your hands on
the lower back with fingertips pointing
towards the spine. Take your hands
straight up the back; separate them at the
top of the back, bringing them over the
shoulder blades and down to the table; and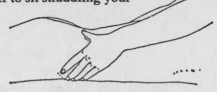
then pull them back down along the sides. And if you want to make it all feel even
better, let your fingertips outline the tops of the shoulder blades when your hands
separate at the top of the back. Use a little extra pressure with your fingertips and they
will pick up a natural curving groove that they can follow all the way from the spine to
the shoulders themselves.

Do the main stroke on the back from four to six times, repeating it whenever
you wish between other strokes as well.

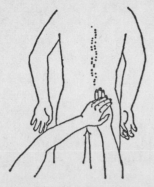

2 Now stand on either side of the table beside your friend's lower back. Or, if you are working on the floor and have decided to sit straddling your friend's thighs, you may continue from the same position.

Place your right hand on your friend's lower back just to the right of the spine. Have the fingertips of the hand right at the waistline and pointing towards the head. Then place your left hand palm down on top of your right. Now make a circle with both hands around the hip bone. Follow the waistline straight to the table, go several inches down the hip (i.e., towards the feet), cross up on to the top of the buttock, and from there go back to the waistline beside the spine. Lean your weight into your hands and use plenty of pressure.

Repeat this circle at least four times. Then do the same on the other side of the lower back, again starting at the waistline just beside the spine and this time circling your hands to the left.

This is an important stroke, by the way, since the lower back is a high tension area for almost everyone.

3 ★ Now work with your thumbs on the lower back. Using the balls of your thumbs, make short rapid alternating strokes moving away from you. Let both thumbs go over the same spot at least several times before moving on. Work close to the spine just below the waistline, in an area about the size of a large grapefruit.

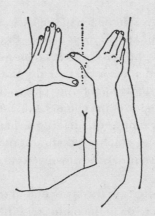

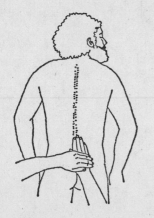

4 ★ The 'rocking horse'. One stroke that actually does go up and down the spine itself. Stand at your friend's left side. Place your right hand on your friend's spine, heel at the lower end of the spine and fingers pointing towards the head. Place your left hand on top of and across your right, fingers pointing towards the far side of the table.

Now slowly glide both hands straight up the spine. Keep the pressure moderate and steady.

As soon as you reach the top of the back, start
down again at the same speed. As you come down, however,
lift your right hand slightly so that it is no longer
touching the spine and at the same time dig the tips of your
right forefinger and middle finger into the two furrows that lie
immediately to either side of the spine. Glide both fingertips
straight down these two furrows, pressing as hard as you can. If
you bend both fingers as much as possible at the joints closest
to the tips, you will maximize the downward pressure at the
tips themselves.

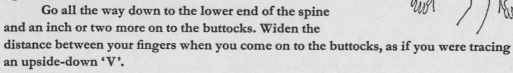

Go all the way down to the lower end of the spine
and an inch or two more on to the buttocks. Widen the
distance between your fingers when you come on to the buttocks, as if you were tracing
an upside-down 'V'.

The Anne Kent Rush variation of the rocking horse is one of the great strokes in massage. Go up the spine as usual. Take your left hand away from your right, however, as soon as you reach the top of the back. Then with the right hand begin coming down as before, digging the tips of the forefinger and the middle finger into the two furrows to either side of the spine. Only bring it just four inches or so down the spine and then take it away. Meanwhile do the same thing with the left hand, starting about an inch farther down from where the right hand started; begin pressing with the left forefinger and middle finger slightly before the right forefinger and middle finger have broken contact. Then begin stroking again with the right hand, this time starting an inch down from where the left hand started; and so on. Work this way down the full spine, overlapping your strokes and starting each a little lower on the spine. Your friend will experience this as waves flowing down his or her entire back.

Do the rocking horse two or three times.

5 Now do pulling along the sides of the torso, just as you did when you were working on the chest and stomach. Reach across the table and work the side opposite you. (If you are working on the floor and are straddling your friend's thighs, this stroke can be done from where you are sitting. Just lean a little to the right as you massage the left side of your friend's torso, and vice versa.)

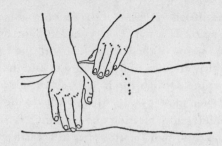

Start just above the thigh, and work up to the armpit and then back again. Pull each hand straight up from the table, keeping the fingers pointing downwards. Find a slow hand-over-hand rhythm, letting each new stroke begin just as the one before is about to finish.

Work once up and then down again on both sides of the torso.

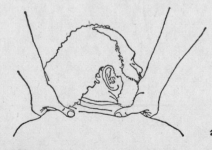

6 Now we move to the upper back, frequently another high tension area. Begin by kneading the muscles curving from your friend's neck onto his or her shoulders. Work the muscles gently between the thumb and fingers. Do both sides at once.

7 Next the shoulder blades.

    This is a great stroke, by the way, but is extremely awkward to do without a table. If you are working on the floor you may well want to skip this one and go straight on to the next stroke for the upper back.

    The first problem is to raise one of the blades so that the surrounding muscles are made more accessible. Standing at your friend's right side (if you are working on a table you may actually find it easier to kneel while doing this stroke), take his right hand and place it palm up in the middle of his back. Then lift his shoulder an inch or two from the table and slide your 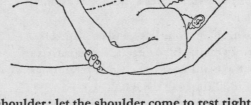 own right forearm, underside up, under the shoulder; let the shoulder come to rest right at the crook of your elbow; and then with your right hand clasp your friend's forearm (if you can't reach it, don't worry about it) near his elbow. Now the blade is raised and you are ready to go to work.

The key area to massage is the furrow running around three sides (top, side nearest the spine, and bottom) of the now raised blade. First run the fingertips of your left hand several times slowly back and forth along all three sides. Be firm: strong pressure feels good here.

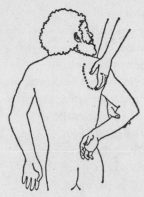

Next make tiny circles with your fingertips, again going several times along all three sides. Dig in, going very slowly and making your circles a quarter of an inch wide or even smaller.

Then, to finish, shape your left hand as if it were a claw, pressing firmly on the blade itself, try actually to move the skin over the blade in circles. Go several times to the right, then several times to the left. Then slide your hand lightly down the length of your friend's arm, put his hand and arm back on the table, and gently extract your own forearm from under his shoulder.

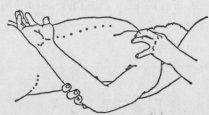

Do the same on the other side.

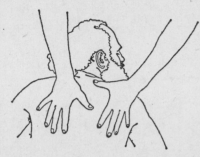

8 ★ Now use your thumbs on the upper back just as you did on the lower back. Stand above your friend's head. Move your thumbs away from you in short and rapid alternating strokes. Stay off both the spine and the shoulder blades themselves. Concentrate first on the muscles just above the blades, then on those lying between the blades and the spine.

9 The 'corkscrew'. Easy once you get the hang of it. Stand on either side of the table. Place your right hand on his right shoulder, left hand on his left. Have the fingers of both hands pointing towards the table.

Now slowly pull both hands, heels first, towards the spine. Press as you pull. When the hands are about to meet, swing each hand a hundred and eighty degrees around so that the fingers end up pointing in the opposite direction. Keep both hands moving at the same pace the whole time, left hand moving to the right and right hand to the left; your forearms will cross as your hands pass the spine.

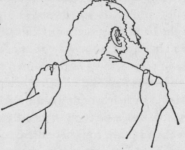

Continue moving the hands across the back until the fingertips of both hands have simultaneously reached the table. At the same time lead both hands a little lower down the back (i.e., in the direction of the feet), so that the right hand touches the table just below the left armpit, and the left hand just below the right armpit.

Start gliding your hands back again towards the spine the moment your fingers have made contact with the table. As before, begin by moving them heels first; then pivot them a hundred and eighty degrees in the middle of the back, uncrossing your forearms as you do so; and end by sending the right-hand fingers first to the table on the right side, and the left hand the same way on the left. Also, as before, bring them about three inches farther down the back.

Continue in this fashion, crossing and uncrossing your arms and moving a little lower down the back each time your hands go from one side to the other. Stop when your hands have reached a point roughly abreast of the lower end of the spine. Then head up the back again in the same way, ending with your hands once more on the shoulders.

Once down and back up again is enough.

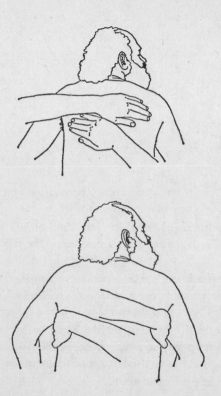

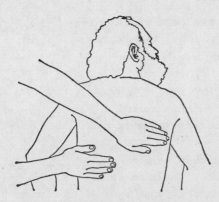

IO Here is the equivalent of 'wringing' (stroke 2 for the back of the leg) for the back.
Run your palms in speedy horizontal strips across the back. Pull your right hand towards yourself as you push your left hand away from yourself, and vice versa. Keep the hands moving constantly, rapidly and without ever leaving the surface of the skin; generate as much friction as you can. Keep off the sides of the torso – this would slow you down too much.
Starting at the top of the back, work gradually down the length of the spine and back up again.
Once down and back is sufficient; especially since this stroke, if you are doing it right, is tiring for you if continued very long.

II This one is more subtle than it looks.
Trace your friend's spine from neck to tail bone with the forefinger and middle finger of one hand. Start where the neck meets the base of the skull. Use the tips of the two fingers. Keep the pressure moderate and move very slowly, letting your fingers take in the particular texture of each vertebra in turn.
That's all.

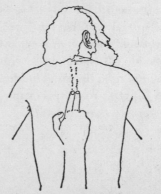

12 * Finish with this one.

Place the undersides of both your forearms straight across your friend's back halfway between the top of the back and the lower end of the buttocks. Have your forearms as close together as you can, and tilt your hands back so that the skin on the underside of your forearms is stretched a little.

Now slowly spread your forearms apart, pressing hard. Keep them moving at the same pace until one forearm has reached the top of the back and the other has crossed the buttocks. Then lift them off the surface of the skin, instantly return them to the middle of the back, and repeat the stroke.

After two passes over the spine itself, lean a little over the table, slant your forearms slightly downwards, and do the same stroke along the far side of the back. Then readjust your position and do the same along the near side of the back. Then, starting again at the centre but this time working at an angle, do the stroke diagonally so that one forearm ends at the shoulder nearer you and the other passes over the buttock on the opposite side. Then conclude with a second diagonal stroke, this time going to the far shoulder and the near buttock.

A superb stroke, this is an especially nice one for ending your work on the back.

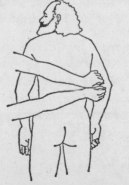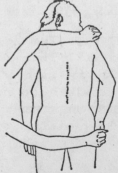

Full-length strokes

The best way to end a massage is with a few good strokes running up and down the full length of the body. Besides being fun for you to do, such strokes will leave your friend with a deeper awareness of his body as a connected whole.

I Do 'raking' as described earlier for stroke 7 on the back of the leg. This time work down the length of the back, over the buttocks, and continue all the way down one leg. Then again down the back, the buttocks and all the way down the other leg.

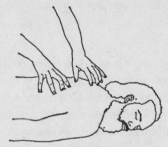

2 'Hacking', a stroke which feels better than its name sounds, was the one being done the last time you saw someone getting a massage in a Hollywood movie.

Drum the outer edges of the hands lightly, but as rapidly as possible, against the spine. Start at the top of the spine and work downwards; continue moving at the same pace all the way down one leg. Then work back up the length of the body, retracing the same path. Then repeat, this time going down and back up the other leg.

3 Now glide both hands up one leg as if you were going to do the main stroke for the back of the leg (see stroke 1 for the back of the leg). But this time don't divide the hands at the top of the leg. Instead, continue without a break right over the buttock and up one side of the back. Separate the hands and pivot them only when you have reached the top of the shoulder blade on the same side of the body. Then bring them heels first down the side and leg, all the way back to the ankle. Don't go on to the spine. Repeat once or twice more. Then go around the table and do the same on the other side.

4 This one is called the 'bear walk'. I have heard it claimed that to this day, in some of the most rural villages of Eastern Europe, for a few coins you can lie on the ground and have a trained bear administer the authentic version of this stroke.

Reach across the table and press one palm against the top three inches or so of the farther side of your friend's back. Have the heel of your hand just to the far side of his spine. Press very hard, leaning as much of your weight into your hand as you can. Next press your other hand right beside the first – in other words, immediately below it on your friend's back – again taking care to place the heel of your hand just to the far side of the spine. Then cross your first hand over and press it immediately below the second, and so on. Begin pressing with one hand just as you release the pressure of the other. Walk the bear all the way down the side of the back, over the buttock, and down the leg; and then (having crossed over to the other side of the table) up the other leg, the other buttock, and the other side of the back. Press as hard as you can each time. One exception: press much more lightly on the backs of the knees.

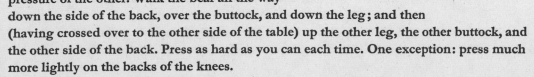

5 If you spread the thumb and forefinger of one hand as far apart as possible, the skin between the two becomes taut. This creates a versatile tool for massage. The next stroke is done entirely with these few inches of stretched skin. Stand at your friend's left side. Run the spread thumb and forefinger of your right hand all the way up the left leg, over the buttock, and up the left side of the back. Press hard, move rapidly, and use only the thumb, the forefinger and the 'V' of skin stretched between. Go lightly over the back of the knee.

As you near the top of the back begin bringing the left hand – thumb and forefinger spread in the same fashion – back down the same route. Then again up the full length of the body with the right hand, then again back down with the left, and so on.

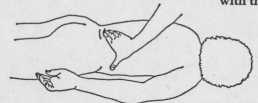

If your own feet are spread several feet apart (or, when working on the floor, if you spread your knees as far apart as you can), you can weave your entire body back and forth along with the movement of your hands. A lively and forceful stroke, this one can be particularly enjoyable to do. Go up and down a half a dozen times or so. Then, naturally, the same on the other side.

6 Now try the main stroke going up both legs at
once. Stand at one side of the table near your
friend's feet and stretch yourself a little over the
table. Place your right hand across the back of
your friend's right ankle, fingers pointing inwards;
and your left hand across the back of your
friend's left ankle, fingers also pointing inwards.

Go right up both legs, over the buttocks,
and up the back. Walk a little with the stroke
if necessary. Coming down, pull both hands
down the sides of the torso, over the hips, and
down the outer sides of the two legs. Keep the
movement even and steady, and try, if possible,
to exert an equal amount of pressure with both hands.

Go at least three times up and down.

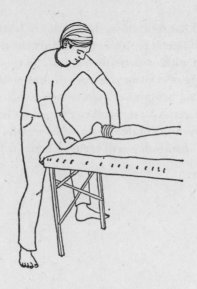

I might add that stroke 6 is one stroke that actually is a lot easier if you are
working on the floor. All you have to do is to kneel between your friend's legs and do
the entire stroke from there. If I am feeling dexterous and don't think I will unnerve
whomever I am massaging, once in a while I even climb up on to my massage table in
order to do this stroke at the right pace and with the right evenness of pressure.

7 * Using both hands at once, do a series of feather-light strokes straight down from the head and neck to the feet. Use only the tips of your fingers, and go as lightly as you can without actually leaving the surface of the skin.

For a change of texture you can also use your nails a few times. By curving your fingers a lot you can bring your nails into play no matter how short they are. Before you finish, however, for at least a moment go back to feather-light stroking with your fingertips.

Be soft, slow and subtle. By now your friend is likely to be so relaxed that your least touch will seem rich and full.

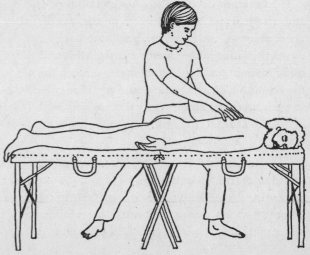

8 ★ The chief thing about the Last Stroke is to do it carefully. It always leaves a lingering impression.

One possibility: take a final feather-light stroke down the length of the body and precisely off both feet at once.

Another: glide your hands down your friend's arms, and then hold your palms lightly against his or her hands for a little while before breaking contact.

Another: have your friend turn over, massage his or her face once more, and then hold your palms lightly against his forehead for a little while. This is especially nice if you began the massage this way.

After you have taken your hands away do not disturb your friend for at least several minutes. Move quietly. Cover him with a sheet if you suspect that he might be cold. (Remember that a room feels about five degrees colder if your skin is oiled.) If you like to be still and inside yourself for a few moments after completing a massage, now is a good opportunity.

Other sequences

When you are giving a complete massage, in what order or sequence ought you to work on the different parts of the body? Ask five different masseurs or masseuses (a masseur is a man who does massage, a masseuse a woman) and you will get five different opinions. My own feeling, after much experimentation with different orders and combinations, is that there is no 'ought'. In fact the one recommendation I would make is that you vary the sequence which you follow as much as you can. Both for yourself, and for those of your subjects who have already had some experience with massage, this will go a long way towards keeping what you are doing from feeling habitual and stale.

What are the possibilities?

The first question is, where to start. I very much like beginning with the head, for reasons which I have mentioned in the instructions on how to massage the head. However, also among my favourite places to begin are the abdomen, since it is physically and psychologically the centre of the body; the feet, since they are the part of the body with which many of us are most out of touch; and the back.

Concerning the back there is a little more to say. One practice I do follow is always to begin with the back whenever the person I am about to massage seems nervous or uptight about the massage itself. Like the head, the hands and the feet, the back is a part of the body where almost everyone feels more safe in being touched. At the same time it provides a particularly large area that is ideally suited to a lot of good massage work. Start on the back, and you can go a long way toward relaxing someone who is nervous. After this, once it comes time to move elsewhere, he or she is likely to experience the other parts of his or her body as feeling much less vulnerable.

I also go straight to the back whenever the same

kind of problem occurs during the course of a massage. If the person I am massaging appears suddenly to have become nervous about being touched, I immediately leave the place I have been working and move to the back, having him turn over if necessary. After spending some time on the back I then return to the place I first was working. Almost always the situation has changed for the better.

Another practice I usually follow in determining the sequence of body parts is to move from one part to another which is immediately adjacent whenever possible. In other words, I massage the hand either just before or just after massaging the arm on the same side, etc. Somehow this seems to make more sense – it feels more 'right' – to the person being massaged. Nevertheless, this rule is no more strict than any other, and I myself frequently break it. For example, as an interesting change of pace (either for myself or for a subject who has already received a number of massages) I sometimes begin by massaging both feet and both hands before anything else.

A more obvious convenience, both to you and to the person being massaged, is for you to complete one side of the body before turning to the other. The most common exception: sometimes I like to end a massage by covering one or more parts of the body a second time. Suppose, for example, I have been roughly following the order outlined in the instruction section of this book. At the end I might ask my subject again to turn over on to his back and then once more massage his face – an especially nice way to close. Or I might finish with some additional full-length strokes on the front half of his body.

What about the order of the strokes themselves on any one part of the body? On the whole this is arbitrary; almost any order you follow will do. One nice touch, however, is to both begin and end with strokes that cover the entire body part being worked on – for example, on a leg both begin and end with the main stroke. Also, whenever you find it necessary to divide a body part into several smaller areas – for example, when using separate strokes for the foreleg, the knee and the thigh – it will feel best to your subject if you work systematically from area to adjacent area rather than moving around at random.

Finally, the very principle that you must

completely finish one part of the body before going on to another is itself arbitrary. It is true that most people, including most professionals, do massage in this way. But it is not the only way; and, as I am increasingly becoming convinced, it is not even necessarily the best way. I do think it is a good idea to work part by part in the orthodox fashion until you have become quite adept at doing massage. Once you feel ready for it, however, try giving an occasional massage in which you go from one to another body part with every other stroke or so. After a stroke on the leg, for example, move to a stroke to two on the stomach and chest, from there to the arm, then the neck, then back to the chest and so on. If done with the right smoothness and flow, a massage of this kind will not only keep your subject more sensitive and alert but also give him a more satisfying sense of his body as a connected whole. You will probably also find for yourself that it is more fun to do.

To sum up, the only 'right' order to follow while giving a massage is the one which feels the most fitting at the moment. Try never to do exactly the same massage twice.

Making up your own strokes

Making up your own strokes is not hard. The more massage you do, the easier it will become. Your hands, you will find, have tremendous imagination. The secret lies in learning ways to trigger this imagination.

The simplest and most direct method to go about discovering new strokes is every now and then during a massage to stop whatever you have been doing, suspend what you were planning and let your hands try out whatever they want. Ask your hands, not your head. Try to give them as much freedom as possible. They will often surprise you.

Other ways of experimenting can also give you new ideas. One good way is to try to transfer a stroke 'meant' for one part of the body on to another part. Sometimes this will work – usually with a lot of changes in the nature of the stroke – and sometimes not. But whether it works or not your hands are likely to discover something new in the process.

Another device is to try to find all the ways you can to massage more than one body part with a single continuous stroke. In other words, find or invent a stroke that includes, e.g., both the back of the leg and the lower back. The obvious way to start doing this is simply to combine two or more strokes that you have already learned. Later, as you get into this kind of thing, you will find yourself becoming more and more innovative.

It can be an additional help to experiment with different ways of moving your hands. Most of the strokes listed in the instruction section of this book are versions of what in classical massage jargon is called 'effleurage' – stroking with the full open palm. But a number of other ways of working with your hands can also be put to use on almost any part of the body. Try, for example:

* stroking with the balls of the thumbs (as shown in the instruction section for the inside of the wrist)
* moving the fingertips with deep pressure in tiny circles (as shown for the chest)
* kneading (as shown for the buttocks)
* raking (as shown for the back of the leg)
* stroking with the heels of the hands
* stroking with the undersides of closed fists
* drumming with the fingertips
* hacking (as shown as a full-length stroke)
* large sweeps and circles with the undersides of the forearms (as shown for the back)
* pressing lightly with the elbow (use the flat part of the elbow, not the tip)
* light slapping (best done with the hands cupped)

And you will find others.

Another good device is to seek out every way you can to let your hands articulate and define the muscular and skeletal systems of your subject's body. Let your hands say, 'Here this is, and this is how it is shaped' – a muscle group, a curve of a bone, or whatever. Many new ideas will come to you if you try exploring in this manner.

A further help along the same lines: learn some anatomy. As you have no doubt noticed, no knowledge of formal anatomy is required for using the strokes given in the instruction section of this book. But the more you learn about the underlying physiological structure of the body, the more you will be able to both refine the techniques presented here and develop new ones of your own. A good way to start is to make yourself thoroughly familiar with the charts in the chapter on anatomy in this book. After that you might try exploring a few textbooks on anatomy, or even taking a course or two on the subject.

New strokes are easy to find. The key is continual experimentation. After all, that's how massage came into being in the first place.

Body tension

What is tension? In the sense in which we are using the word here, it is a stiffness or tightening of the muscles and the connective tissue beyond the amount of tonus needed for normal healthy functioning. Its origin is mostly, and possibly entirely, emotional in nature, and the greater part of it is chronic, which is to say that it is with us at all times – even when we are sleeping. As such it is a constant drain (although often a subconscious one) upon our vitality. When it is released, we normally experience a surge of heightened energy.

Whenever you are about to massage a friend try to study the patterns of tension in his or her body before he or she climbs on to the massage table. This takes practice but once you have done a certain amount of massage you will be surprised how easy it can be to 'read' another person's body.

One important set of clues is to be found in the person's general physical posture.

For example:

Are your friend's shoulders too high? Hunched forward? Held rigidly back? Is either shoulder pulled up higher than the other? Is either pulled in closer to the neck, making that half of the torso appear smaller than the other half?

His head, looked at from the side – thrust forwards? Held back? Either is an indication of tension in the neck.

Does his face, or any part of it, appeared pinched and tight?

His back, looked at from the side – how wide or narrow is the 'S' of its curve? Wideness in the top part of the 'S' indicates tension in the shoulders and upper back; wideness in the lower part, tension in the pelvis and lower back.

Another set of clues can be found in the way your friend moves and uses his body. Is he naturally mobile and expressive, or does he tend to 'hold himself in'? Do some parts of his body appear vital and active, while other parts are left rigid and unused? Are his gestures easy and flowing, or more sharp and staccato? Does his face easily reflect the flow of his emotions, or does it appear constricted and immobile?

Once your friend is undressed and lying on the table you can learn still more.

For example, do all parts of his body appear to sink down into the table, or with some or all does he appear to hold himself a tiny bit up from it?

If he is lying on his back, do his feet lean a little outwards, or are they pointing rigidly upright? If the latter, look for tension in legs and hips.

Do his hips look tight, turned in?

Do his hands look as if he is about to make a fist with them?

Does his chest look tight and pulled in?

The colour of the skin provides another set of clues. Wherever it appears whiter and more faded, look in that area of the body for a greater amount of tension.

Take a look also at the movement of the breath in the body. If the breath is shallow and makes itself visible more in his chest than his abdomen, look for a lot of tension in the entire torso and the neck as well.

After you have looked with your eyes, the next step is to 'look' with your hands. This, of course, is most easily done during the massage itself. In the long run you will find that by touching another person you can tell even more about the patterns of muscular tension in his body than you can by looking at him.

What do your hands 'look' for? Here there is less that I can tell you. In a particularly tight area – especially in the upper back just above and beside the shoulder blades – your fingers are likely to find tiny lumps, anywhere from the size of a pea up, buried under the flesh; normally these are either deposits of waste matter or knottings of the connective tissue. In general, however, where someone's body is tense the flesh simply feels tight, feels stiff and resistant to your handling of it. Being able to sense this with any precision is a skill you will develop only by doing a lot of massage on a number of different people with different body types. Pay attention to the variations you find from person to person, and your hands will gradually get the knack of it.

Once you have located tension in a person's body, what do you do about it?

The first thing is to massage a much wider area than just that of the tension itself. The reason for this is that the place which either you or your subject have found is actually only the focal point of a larger, more diffused pattern of tension.

The next step is to do some good massage work directly on the focal point or points themselves. Use strokes with plenty of pressure: the best are those using either the tips of your fingers or the balls of your thumbs, as these concentrate the pressure of your hands in a much smaller area. Go slowly and systematically, tuning in all you can to any minute changes that may be taking place in the muscles and tissue on which you are working.

In some regions of the body – especially around the upper back, the shoulders and the neck – you will find that when you are working on a tense area even a moderate degree of pressure may cause your friend a small amount of pain. If so, tell your friend that this is a 'good hurt' and that he will immediately feel better when you stop. Don't, however, press extremely hard (i.e., with all or most of your body weight) on a place that hurts; not, that is, unless you have had either a lot of experience doing massage or the chance to study deep massage with a teacher. Extremely hard pressure can in fact be a useful tool for working on tension of this sort, but you must know exactly what you are doing when you use it.

The occasion is rare, but you will sometimes encounter a subject with a lot of body tension who will get up off your table and discover that he feels more tense after the massage than he did before! What has happened is this. In all of us tension exists in layers, and we frequently use a surface layer of tension to cut ourselves off from any awareness of the deeper layers beneath. A good massage may reduce much of this surface layer without, however, having been able to have as great an effect upon the other layers below. This means that the deeper layers may now make themselves fully felt for the first time. The person will actually have considerably less total tension but, having been made more aware of what is really going on in his body, he experiences more tension than before!

One more warning. Never neglect the rest of the body for the sake of one or two areas of higher tension. Do economize, cutting down on the amount of time you might have spent on one part of the body in order to spend more on a more tense part; but don't economize too much. The living tissue of the body is an interconnected whole, a single envelope whose various parts are much more dependent upon and responsive to one another than is commonly realized. For reducing tension, and for every other aspect of massage as well, the one rule before all others is: deal with the body as a whole.

Nervousness, discomfort and the tickles

Excessive nervousness, physical discomfort on the table and ticklishness can all set roadblocks in the path of a good massage. Sometimes these obstacles are insurmountable; usually, however, you can find ways to get around them. Here are a few remedies and countermeasures which you will want to have at hand.

Nervousness during a massage comes in many shapes and varieties. Most people who want a massage in the first place are not particularly afflicted by it. Some people are, however, and among these the most common reponse is nervousness about being nude.

Fortunately, this is fairly easy to deal with. One simple method is to place a towel over the buttocks when your friend is lying on his (or her) stomach, and over the genitals when he is lying on his back; a second towel can also be placed over a woman's breasts.

A sheet can be used instead of a towel, or in addition to it. This way only that particular body part actually being massaged need be exposed at any one time.

A third solution: have your friend wear either his or her underwear, or a swimming suit. Needless to to say this will drastically cut down on the number of strokes that you can do. However, nudity more than loses its value at that point at which it leaves a subject so tense that he or she cannot enjoy his or her massage.

The other form of nervousness during a massage is an excessive uneasiness about being touched. This fear, while overlapping with the fear of nudity, is different from it and comes from another place in the personality. It is also more difficult to deal with. It manifests itself sometimes as an extreme tightening and pulling in of the body as it is being touched, sometimes as a violent trembling and sometimes simply as an overt refusal to proceed any further with the massage.

If your friend reacts with this degree of

nervousness there is not a great deal that you can do. One possible step, which I have already mentioned in the chapter on sequences, is to leave whatever body part you have been working on and move to the back. Massage done on the back, more than any other single body part, often has an immediate calming effect.

Another approach that can sometimes help is to spend a few minutes working closely with your friend on his breathing. First ask him to feel the weight of his body against the table and leave him alone (i.e., don't touch him) for a minute or two while he does so. Then ask him to follow the movement of his breath within his body, to let his breath, without forcing it, become as long and natural as possible, and to let it flow as deep into his torso as he can manage. Then, after another minute or so has passed, place one of your hands lightly under the nape of his neck and the other on his stomach just below the rib cage. Watch his breath closely, and with the hand on his stomach begin pressing down slightly as he exhales and then releasing the pressure as he inhales. Don't take your hand away at any point; just alternately increase and decrease the pressure without breaking contact.

The idea is to get him to deepen his breath spontaneously. This you can 'suggest' to him with your hand. Each time he exhales, continue to press lightly downwards a fraction of a second after his exhalation appears to have stopped. And each time he inhales make the pressure of your hand so light that it almost – but not quite – breaks contact. Also, if you see his breath is beginning to get deeper, try moving your hand a little lower on the stomach. This will lead his breath lower into the pelvis and will help him to relax still further.

At this point you may find that your friend is accepting your touch more calmly and that you can safely resume the massage. If not, you can try more of the same a little while longer. Move your hands around to different places on his body – his head, his shoulders, his own hands – and in each place follow the same pattern for several breaths, pressing lightly with his exhalation and then releasing the pressure with his inhalation. But don't expect miracles. If your friend has a serious block against permitting himself to be touched, this kind of gentle non-verbal persuasion will be unlikely to overcome it.

I might add that there are numerous other emotions which are sometimes released when the body receives a good massage. Sadness, for example; your friend may at some point find himself inadvertently crying, or wanting to cry. When you are aware of this happening be sure to interrupt the massage temporarily and encourage your friend to cry for as long as he feels like it. Usually after a few minutes of crying he will want to begin the massage again – and will probably experience the rest of the massage, in fact, as unusually calming and soothing.

Another phenomenon along these lines, one a bit more unusual, is involuntary vibrating. A sudden trembling and shaking in the flesh that can go on without stopping for some minutes, it is caused by a quick release of body energy that previously had been dammed up in constricted muscles and tissue. Usually it occurs either in the region of the stomach or the thighs, or both. Unlike the more agitated and jerky trembling that can stem from nervousness at the beginning of a massage, vibrating is a highly beneficial physical and emotional release that should be considered a part of the massage itself. Encourage your friend to let it happen, to enjoy it and not be frightened by it and to let it spread, if possible, to other parts of his body. Keep one of your hands resting against his shoulder, the back of his neck or his head, and with the other slowly and very gently (i.e., with no pressure at all) continue to massage his body in the areas where the vibrating is taking place. Help him to keep it going – the longer it continues, the greater the release within his body. After it subsides he will feel a wonderful mixture of calm and aliveness that will most likely stay with him for several days.

Physical discomfort while a subject is lying on the massage table must be taken care of or the massage will be practically useless. Generally there are only two possible solutions: change how a subject is lying or change what he is lying on. For example, a pregnant woman (who stands to gain even more than the usual physical benefits from a massage, by the way), who cannot lie on her stomach can lie on her side while you massage her back. Or, if someone lying on his stomach feels a lot of pain in his neck when he turns it to one side, a pillow placed lengthwise under both the head and the top of the chest will enable him to turn it less, or even not at all. Other problems can be handled in similar ways – pillows can often be a great help in these matters.

And then there are the tickles, the bane of massage. Normally you will run into them when massaging the soles of the feet, sometimes also on the stomach and the sides of the torso, and occasionally in other quite unpredictable places. The one solution is heavy pressure. Press hard enough – sometimes so hard that you are one step short of causing pain to the person being massaged – and the tickles will usually evaporate. If not, then make one quick stroke over the entire area, admit defeat and move on.

Massaging to music and other exercises

Three simple exercises that will add more flow and confidence to your massage touch.

First, try massaging to music. I have already said that as a general rule I don't recommend playing music while you give a massage; while providing a surface pleasantness, on a deeper level it is often distracting to the person being massaged. Nevertheless, music can be an extremely valuable aid to improving your massage technique.

The idea is to make the rhythms of your strokes mesh with the rhythm of the music. Pick out a few favourite records, preferably ones having a wide variety of rhythms. Check with whomever you are going to massage to make sure that this will be okay for his or her ear, put on a record, and start in. Don't force your hands to match the music right away: just do the massage strokes that you are used to, and at the same time let yourself tune in to the music. Before long you will find your hands of their own accord trying out new patterns, and moving with a new steadiness. Be sure to experiment with other records as well. Each new rhythm will teach you some new subtlety.

Another exercise is to try 'dancing' your massage. This can be done with or without accompanying music. Have your friend lie stomach down on the table – this exercise loses much of its value when done on the floor, by the way – and spread oil over the exposed surface of his body from head to feet. Then start moving your hands up and down his body. Only this time don't concentrate on him at all, nor on your own hands; instead focus entirely on the rest of your body and its movements. Enjoy yourself: dance! Move and sway all you can (keep your hands in contact, however). Experiment with as many different rhythms and patterns as you can.

It will probably surprise you to discover how greatly your entire body can become involved in the movements of massage. Also, be sure afterwards to have your friend tell you how it all felt on his side. Since you were concentrating so strongly on your own pleasure rather than on his, what he has to say may provide you with a second surprise.

One last exercise, difficult but always rewarding. Give an entire massage in complete darkness. Do everything with the sense of touch alone, including finding the oil bottle and putting on oil. You will make some mistakes and have many clumsy moments, but I can't tell you how this will help to bring your hands alive.

A variation, even more difficult: have a friend arrange for you to be led in the dark to a waiting subject that you do not know, and have never encountered before. A hard test – but one that will teach you a great deal!

No matter how much massage you may happen to know, I strongly suggest that from time to time you repeat these exercises, along with any others like them that you may happen to discover. You will always find something new in them.

A ten-minute massage

It can be done.

Not in the same way as a full massage: ten minutes is ten minutes no matter what. But if you make every minute count you can leave someone feeling surprisingly nourished.

I normally approach ten minutes of massage in one of three ways.

One is to my usual style of massage on just one or perhaps two body parts. Ten minutes of work on the back, for example; or perhaps five on the head and five more on the feet. Back, head, neck and feet are usually the most effective places for a brief massage. If you are into trading massage with someone on a daily basis, then see to it that each part of the body gets massaged one day or another.

Another way is to cover the entire body, or close to it, by doing just one or two of your usual strokes on each part (the main stroke, for example).

This method I find a bit hectic to both give and receive, but I do use it occasionally. Try it and see what you think.

A third way is to use any or all of the full-length strokes that you know on either the front or the back of the body alone, or on both. This feels superb, and is an especially good method for providing a quick energy pick-up for someone who is tired. Particularly effective are ten minutes of raking (Full-length stroke 1) or ten minutes of working with the spread thumbs and forefingers of both hands (Full-length stroke 5). Work on the arms as well.

And thas't it. Except that the best information I have to give you in this regard is that for couples, or for anyone else sharing the same life and the same home, the ten-minute massage can open the door to something extraordinary: doing massage together every day. In other words, when a day happens along on

which you have the time and the inclination you trade a
full massage - and on all the other days you trade ten
minutes' worth. I know that even ten minutes every
day sounds hard - and if your life is a busy one it is hard
until you get the habit of it - yet I assure you that
nothing else in the world costing so little effort will as
effectively change, over the course of time, the mood
and tempo of your entire life. Give yourself the chance.
You won't regret it.

Two on one

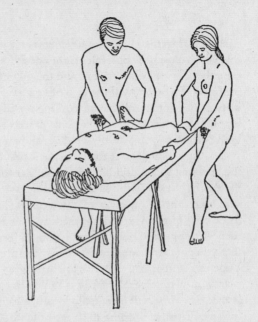

If you think being massaged by one person is great, wait until you try two.

Only it has to be done in the right way.

The keys to it are symmetry and tuning in. Each of the two persons doing the massage must tune in as fully to the other person doing it as to the person receiving it. Otherwise being massaged by two people feels just – well, interesting, the way maybe being massaged by an octopus would feel.

One good way to begin is with the main stroke on either the front or the back of the legs. The broad, easy sweep of this stroke will give the two of you who are doing the massage a good chance to pick up on each other's wavelengths.

You might start out by each taking one of your friend's feet, holding the foot with one hand against the sole and the other against the top of the foot. Then let your breath travel down your arms and into your hands

(imagine it if you can't feel it) as you let them rest in place for a moment. Next apply the oil and begin the main stroke. Each of you can take the leg on the same side as the foot which you were holding.

Once you have begun the main stroke, the

trick of it is to match your movements and your rhythm as closely as possible. Either decide ahead of time that one of you is to lead and the other follow – probably the best way if the two of you have not already had some practice in working together – or else try simply to keep your movements exactly parallel with neither of you leading, neither following.

Go up the legs at the same pace, first crossing the knees and then dividing your hands at the tops of the thighs at exactly the same moment. Try to make sure by means of any clues that you can catch hold of – (how each of you is standing, the way your hands on each side appear to press into the flesh of the leg, etc.) that you are using equal amounts of pressure. Go slow. Tune in. Your friend that you are massaging will sense exactly how much each of you is tuning in to him – and at the same time will be equally sensitive to how much the two of you are tuning in to each other.

This should give you the idea. In general it is easy to match your movements on the arms, hands, legs and feet: just do the same massage strokes together that you are accustomed to doing singly. On the chest, stomach, buttocks and back, however, the situation is different: here, although there are a few strokes which you can do together in the same fashion (I will explain some in a moment), the rest must be done by one person working on that particular part alone. The head and neck, of course, are best left to be massaged entirely by one person.

This means you have another decision to make (again, best to make it ahead of time). During those periods where one of you is working alone somewhere around the torso or the head, the other has two options: either to stand aside and wait, or to go to work on another area at the same time even though this means that the two of you are no longer working symmetrically.

Each has its advantages. If one of you stands aside and waits, this means that your friend being massaged need suffer no confusion, that he can concentrate without distraction on what is being done to him. If, on the other hand, you decide to work somewhere else at the same time, this has the advantage of preserving the uniqueness of a double massage – your friend doesn't suddenly lose half the 'touch energy' he was enjoying before.

As a rule I find that most people experience the second of these two solutions as a sensory overload and hence feel a little more comfortable with the first. There are others, however, who definitely prefer the second. You will simply have to choose for yourself, on the basis of both what the two of you feel like doing and what you feel your friend will most enjoy. One exception, by the way, to what I have just said: many people do seem to like having the head and the feet, the two poles of the body, massaged at the same time.

Fortunately there do exist a few good ways of working symmetrically, or close to it, on the front and back of the torso.

Pulling along the sides of the torso (stroke 4 in 'The Back'), can be done very effectively by both of you at once, both while your friend is lying on his back and while he is lying on his stomach. Stand on opposite sides of the table and reach across to the side of your friend's torso which is away from you. Have one of your arms between your partner's arms, and keep all four arms close together – touching or almost touching. Keep your strokes slow and steady, and make sure they are evenly matched.

Another superb stroke: one of you must stand at the head end of the table and do the main stroke on either the front or the back of the torso (stroke 1 in 'The Chest and Stomach'; stroke 1 in 'The Back'). The other stands at the foot end of the table and does the main stroke on both legs at once (as in stroke 6 in 'Full-length Strokes', without, however, going on to the back). The idea is to make all four hands move in the same direction at the same time. This means that one of you must wait and then begin just as the other is completing the first half of his stroke. In other words,

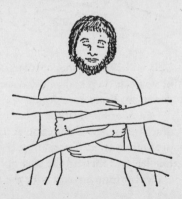

while one pair of hands is heading up the sides of the torso towards the shoulders, the other pair heads up the legs towards the hips; and vice versa.

Another stroke for the back and the buttocks: the Giant Hand. Lock all four hands together by entwining your fingers as shown in the illustration.

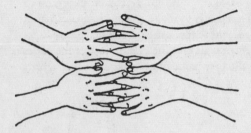

This will create a sort of oversized hand which the two of you can then make flow back and forth in every direction. Feels very good.

A number of the other full-length strokes described in the instruction sections can be done by two persons at once. Try raking; try the main stroke up one leg and then all the way up the back; try the bear walk; try long strokes with the stretched thumb and forefinger of one hand; try feather-light strokes.

Finally, letting all four hands 'roam' with no symmetry and no apparent pattern for a short period of time can be an excellent way to end a double massage. As I have said, many subjects will feel uncomfortable, as if split several ways at once, if you try this early in the massage. Coming later, however, it will feel much better. For one reason, your friend's body will now be more relaxed and open; for another, the strangeness of being touched by two people at the same time will have passed.

Do double massage from time to time. Besides being fun to do, it will leave you more versatile at massage in general. Double massage is a little like doing massage to music: tuning in to a partner's massage rhythm teaches you new possibilities for your own.

One last comment: doing double massage for a friend can be an especially fine experience for a couple. The act of mutually caring for a third person, plus the sensitivity to each other demanded at the same time, create a space in which a couple can experience their own closeness in a new and powerful way.

Self-massage

Being your own masseur is a little like being your own lover. It can be done, but somehow it just isn't the same thing.

There are several problems. Most obvious, I suppose, is that there are some areas of your body which you cannot reach. And others which you can, but not with the right dexterity and leverage.

This is actually the least of the difficulties, however. More important is that you can't fully relax. No one part of your body can completely relax while another part is busy at work; the body is too closely interconnected for that.

Also, your attention is split. When doing massage your attention must be on the activity of your hands; when receiving it you need to concentrate on letting go, on allowing yourself to be taken care of. Trying to do both at once means that you can really give yourself up to neither, and the massage done in this way can't help but remain superficial.

Most crucial of all, however, is that no communication and no exchange of energy can take place when you do massage on yourself. The expressive side of massage falls away, and what is left is something completely mechanical; a physical technique and nothing more.

Having said all this, let me now add what I think self-massage is in fact good for. First of all, if you are feeling tired and numb it can sometimes help bring your body awake. Second, a healthy physical relationship with yourself of this kind has its own psychological rewards. Learning to touch your own body is a good means of learning to accept it. Finally – and this is where, for anyone into massage, the real value of self-massage lies – it can show you a great deal about what feels good and what doesn't in massage. It can teach you about the hidden architecture of bone and muscle, about the effects of greater and lesser amounts of pressure and much more. You can use it as a valuable kind of exploration and feedback. The more you know about your own body, the more you will know about everyone else's.

I find that the best techniques for self-massage are kneading and squeezing, hard pressure with the fingertips, and slapping. Oil is not necessary. In fact it is next to useless; the type of strokes that require it cannot be done in self-massage because of insufficient leverage.

There is not a great deal that you need to be told in terms of specific directions. Simply press, poke and squeeze wherever you can – experiment and explore. Here are a few things which you might try.

Face and scalp Work either lying on your back or sitting up. On your back is a little better for your face, sitting up a little better for your scalp. For the face you can do most of what you do when massaging someone else; use your fingertips instead of your thumbs on the

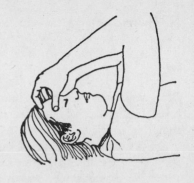

forehead, however. For the scalp, lots of vigorous rubbing with the fingertips.

Neck and upper back (*1*) Lie on your back. Press as hard as you can with your fingertips just to either side of the spine; wiggle your fingertips in place a little as you press. Start just below the spine as far under the back as you can reach. (You will probably not get much farther than a point about parallel with the tops of the shoulder blades.) Then do the same thing just

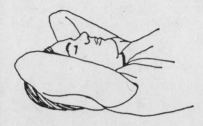

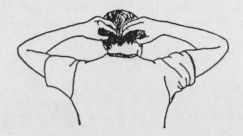

above the shoulder blades, working from the spine outwards to the shoulders.

Neck and upper back (2) Sit in a chair. First let your head (but only your head) hang as far forwards as possible. Then, pressing hard with your fingertips, make tiny circles just below the base of the skull; work from about two inches to one side of the spine to about two inches to the other side. Next, with your head again upright, let one arm and shoulder go as limp as possible. With the fingertips of the opposite

hand press hard just above the top of the shoulder blade; move your fingertips slightly as you press. Go slowly all the way across the top of the blade, starting at the shoulder and working towards the spine. Then go down the side of the blade closest to the spine as far as you can reach (it won't be very far).

Chest Knead and press with the fingertips while either sitting up or lying down.

Stomach Rub in a circle with one palm. Then gently press and knead with the fingertips.

Sides of the torso Knead and rub.

Lower and middle back This one is hard. Animals that rub against tree trunks probably have the best idea. The only effective thing I know to do is to stand and to press the tips of your thumbs as hard as you can just to

Legs (1) Sit on the ground or on a bed with the legs extended. Knead and press with the fingertips.

Legs (2) Lie on your back with your legs propped up against a wall or a piece of furniture. Lower one foot

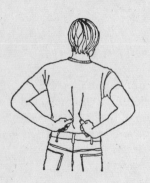 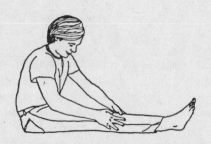 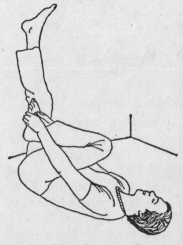

either side of your spine. Start an inch or two above the base of the spine; press each time for about five seconds and then move your thumbs up a half an inch or so and press again. Work your way up as high onto the middle back as you can reach.

so that it is just within reach. Working downwards from the foot, knead and squeeze the foot and the entire leg. Repeat as many times as you like, working downwards only. (This helps the veins to drain towards the heart.)

Buttocks Knead, either while standing or while lying on your stomach.

Feet Here you can do your best work, especially on the sole of the foot. Sit in a chair and rest one foot on the opposite thigh. At this angle you can work carefully and with plenty of pressure over the entire

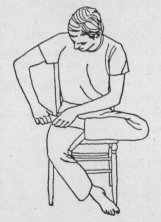

sole. Then with your fingers and thumbs work the rest of the foot. Don't forget the toes.

Everywhere Slap! Slap every square inch of the body that you can reach. Include the face, slapping more lightly. I find this more fun – and quicker – than any other form of self-massage.

So there you are. Let me add one more comment. To my mind, the real singular or one-person equivalent of massage is not self-masssge, but hatha yoga. If, despite my discouraging remarks, you find that self-massage does something magical for you, then you might explore whether yoga may not be able to do the same and much more.

Your animals too

By all means massage your animals. They will love it, and you will learn a few things. Born connoisseurs of massage, animals give feedback of an unmatched eloquence. Do the right thing and they will sprawl in a heap on the floor. Do the wrong thing and they will snap at you or paw your hands away.

The main rule when doing animal massage is to explore the bone structure. Here is an anatomical structure foreign to what you are used to working on; find out how it works, what its underlying shape is, and how you can adapt to it any of the massage techniques you are familiar with.

A few tips.

Pay particular attention to an animal's spine. Working up and down in the two furrows lying just to either side of the spine is almost always effective.

Don't neglect the base of the skull, an equally responsive place. It must be as high a tension area for animals as it is for humans, judging from the way they react to its being massaged.

Probe all around the shoulder blades. You can often go in quite deep between the blades and the spine. Always press gently at first, but don't be afraid gradually to try harder pressure. If an animal senses that you have just the right place, he will usually let you press surprisingly hard.

Individual animals seem to vary greatly when it comes to the stomach. Some don't want it touched at all. Others love having their stomachs lightly kneaded.

In general try to keep your touch consistently focused and definite. Animals tune in almost immediately, and if they feel that you know what you are doing they will start trusting you right away.

I'm pretty much a dog and cat man myself. I've never really gotten into horses and buffaloes, or for that matter mice and canaries, all of which I'm sure are whole massage worlds unto themselves.

No species is an island.

Massage for lovers

Bet you turned to this chapter right away, huh?

In that case, unless you are already well acquainted with massage, you may find it difficult to believe the first thing I have here to say: ordinary massage and erotic massage are two separate kinds of experience, and they lie many miles apart. The more massage you do and receive, the more you will come to appreciate this difference. One is sensual, the other sexual. One leaves the body feeling calm, the other leaves it feeling aroused.

Between your mate or lover and yourself an exchange of ordinary massage will always be a beautiful thing. For a couple, however, massage obviously offers other directions as well. To a greater degree than anything else I know of, massage can make sex both physically and psychologically more fulfilling. For a couple having difficulties with sexual intimacy, for example, it can add that critical element of mutual trust and relaxation which formerly was lacking from their physical relationship; I have known many couples who have made this discovery. And for the couple between whom sex is already mutually satisfying, massage can provide the means to an increased richness difficult to describe.

The key to erotic massage is not, as you might expect, a detailed massaging of the genitals. Naturally this can feel exquisite, and in itself it is fine as a part of sexual massage – but only as a part. The main focus of sexual massage should be something slightly different: the energizing and eroticization of the entire body. This experience alone can add to sex something completely new in quality, something more than a heightened intensity.

But how? The answer is that an erotic massage must proceed by stages. The boundaries between these stages hardly need to be exact, and they certainly don't have to be done in the order mentioned here. The important thing is merely that each stage be included, and that each receive its share of unhurried attention.

The first is simply that of ordinary massage. Give your partner a complete body massage of the kind described earlier in this book. Be as brief as you want, but make sure that every part of the body is thoroughly covered.

Next do feather-light stroking with the fingertips all over the body. I have already suggested that at the end of an ordinary massage you do a little of this (full-length stroke 6). For erotic massage, however, do much more: ten, twenty, any number of times more. This will greatly heighten the sexual sensitivity of your partner's body throughout its entire length. You don't even need to wait until you have finished the period of ordinary massage; you can include soft stroking at the same time, gradually increasing the amount as you go.

The next step is to concentrate more fully on those areas of the body which, other than and in addition to the genitals, carry a heightened sexual charge. These include primarily the pelvic region and the regions immediately joining – the stomach, the insides of the thighs, the buttocks, and the lower back – and the breasts. But also give some attention to the ears, the lips, the back of the neck, the palms, the insides of the elbows, the armpits, the soles of the feet, the big toe and the backs of the knees – all areas which respond easily to sexual vibrations. Do some additional ordinary massage work on these areas, returning to soft stroking whenever you wish.

Next comes the most important stage of all: connecting the genitals with the rest of the body. Here the idea is to do strokes which at some point lightly touch or graze the genitals, and which from there go immediately to other parts of the body. The effect this will have, especially coming after a period of full body soft stroking, will be to gradually transfer some of the higher sexual excitation usually associated with the genitals to the rest of the body as well.

The final stage is of course to focus your attention on your partner's genitals themselves. Pressing lightly with your fingertips, work slowly and with great care over the entire genital region. Cover each surface with tiny circles, outline the contours of each distinct part with one fingertip, and the like. Concentrate not on arousing your partner – this will happen by itself – but on making him or her feel that his or her genitals are a part of the body on a par with other parts, worthy of the same kind of attention and nurturing care.

What strokes and techniques should you use for erotic massage? For the most part you will find it easy to adapt those which you have already learned for ordinary massage. Just follow your own instincts and intuitions: when it comes to doing erotic massage with someone you love, the imagination is the most important organ which you have. Here are a few specific suggestions. (Note: much of this will probably make little sense unless you have already become familiar with the instruction section of this book.)

When doing feather-light stroking, move your hands so that your fingertips are barely brushing against your partner's skin. Work up and down the entire length of his or her body. Go sometimes slowly and sometimes a little faster; sometimes in straight lines and sometimes in waves, circles, spirals or whatever.

A good variation of feather-light stroking: use just the tip of one finger of one hand. Move it slowly all around the body. Though this looks more or less the same as using your entire hand, your partner will experience it as something distinctly different.

Here is a good additional stroke for either a man's or a woman's chest. Place the tips of both thumbs immediately next to and on opposite sides of one nipple. Pressing lightly, draw both thumb tips at the same time (but moving in opposite directions) directly outwards. Stop when you have reached the outer edges of the breast on a woman, or when the thumbs are about five inches apart on a man. Then return the thumbs to the nipple and, as if you were drawing the spokes of a wheel, do the same thing starting at points a fraction of an inch or so farther around. Continue in the same way, taking a total of about eight simultaneous strokes with both thumb tips to cover the entire breast.

For the feet: run one finger slowly all the way in and out between each pair of toes.

Try reversing your hands when doing the main stroke on the back of the leg – i.e., lead with your right hand instead of your left while massaging the left leg. Take both hands right over the top of the buttock before dividing them; then, as you take your outside hand (the left in this example) over the hip as usual, glide your inside hand lightly down between the buttocks and over any part of the genitals easily within reach before heading both hands back down the leg.

Work the fingertips of one hand in tiny circles around the tip of the coccyx (the tail bone). Use firm pressure, concentrating on the surrounding muscles rather than the bone itself. Then work more lightly down to the genitals and back, and then again more firmly around the coccyx.

Leading with the heel of the hand, bring one hand in a single steady motion up from the genitals, between the buttocks, up the spine and, turning the hand sideways now, on to the back of the neck. Let this hand rest on the back of the neck and repeat the same thing with the other hand; take the first away a little before you reach the neck with the second. Continue like this, alternating hands each time and having one hand always resting against the back of the neck while the other is moving.

Make tiny circles with the fingertips of one hand up and down the groove between the pelvis and the inside of the thigh on each side. Work slowly, and use plenty of pressure. Go several times all the way up and down on each side. Then, much more lightly, go briefly on to the genitals. Then, pressing the same as before, again between the pelvis and the thigh.

Move the tip of one forefinger in a tiny circle at the centre of the top of your partner's head. Move the tip of the other forefinger in a tiny circle on the perineum – a spot about the size of a coin between the rectum and the genitals. Press moderately. Keep both fingers moving slowly in unison for a minute or longer.

For the vagina itself, try placing the tips of both thumbs on the perineum (cf. the previous stroke) with one thumb tip directly above the other.

Pressing lightly, move both thumb tips together straight upwards to the top of the vaginal inner lips. Then separate the thumbs, one going to the right and one to the left; pressing more firmly, bring them down between the inner and the outer lips all the way to the perineum. Continue the same circular movement without stopping.

For the penis, place the tips of both forefingers against the perineum. Separate the forefingers, moving one to the right and one to the left, and follow the edges of the scrotum to the base of the penis. Continue without a break directly on to the penis, bringing the tips of the forefingers together again at the base of the underside (the side that is exposed when the penis is erect). Glide both forefingers together straight up the length of the penis, going over and down to the opposite side of the head. Then, pressing just below the lower ridge of the head (the coronal ridge), separate the fingers again and, following the ridge around, bring them both back on to the underside of the penis. Then, with the fingertips once more together, go back down the penis and around the scrotum all the way back to the perineum. Repeat without stopping.

Go on from here however you wish. Without hurry!

One last suggestion for couples. Do erotic massage together whenever you feel like it, but try if you have time to share frequent sessions of ordinary massage as well. In other words, try to expand your relationship within the world of touch in as many directions as possible. I guarantee that this will help to enrich your relationship in other dimensions as well.

Getting deeper into it: some directions

Perhaps by now you have mastered most of the strokes listed in the instruction section of this book. Perhaps you have also gone on, as was suggested in some later chapters, to explore other ways of using these techniques, and have had the satisfaction of seeing emerge from your experiments the beginnings of a massage style uniquely your own.

If so, you may feel that you have learned enough. And in a sense I could only agree with you. Give yourself a bit more practice along the same lines, and you will soon be doing massage as well as the average professional masseur or masseuse.

Perhaps, however, despite having come this far, you feel that you are not yet prepared to stop; that massage still holds something more for you, something deeper. In that case you are ready for the next step.

From this point on, getting deeper into massage means, in my opinion, that you must follow a single road: that of getting deeper into your own body.

Wherever in this book I have spoken of doing massage with your hands, this has been a convenient fiction. Massage is done (whether well or poorly) with the entire body; with its particular style, its gestures and its degree of aliveness; with the living sum of all one's attitudes towards and about it.

Nevertheless most of us are, in actual fact, largely cut off from the body; ordinarily we are in contact with only a fraction of its inner richness. And it is exactly about this that you must do something. Change the manner and degree to which you are aware of your own body, and you will radically change the way you do massage – and much else besides! Far more than we tend to realize, the very feel and texture of our lives is shaped by the way we live and experience our bodies. For myself, I know that many of the things that have made my massage better have made my life better as well.

How does one go about increasing his awareness of his own body? There are many ways, fortunately. I have mine; you will have yours. What I want to share with you here are some hints which, I feel, have a particular relevance to massage.

Let's look first at a few ideas about the body. Take them on a purely intellectual level, and, far from helping, they will only get in your way. Take them, however, as signposts for feeling, as ideas to be lived – and you may discover in them a key to many things within yourself.

You are your body. Today this is a truism in much of psychology and philosophy; another familiar way of putting it is that mind and body are one and the same. Our emotions, our outer perceptions, our spiritual life, and even our conceptual understanding of the world around us all begin and end within this intimate shadowy mass which is our being. Our body, its possibilities of movement, and its relation to gravity and the earth are the background from which everything else must emerge. To come to terms with this on a real emotional level is perhaps the most important kind of self-encounter a person can have. As Alexander Lowen puts it: 'When the ego roots itself in the body, an individual gains insight into himself. The deeper the roots, the deeper the insight.'

Yet, consciously or unconsciously, we tend still to resist the notion that we literally are our bodies. The ideas and suggestions that follow, while dependent upon this primary idea, perhaps at the same time can offer a means of coming more to grips with it.

The sense of touch is as important a contact with reality as the sense of sight. For centuries in our Western culture we have allowed the world as encountered by sight almost totally to dominate the world as encountered by touch. Learning to live again in the world of touch is for us now like travelling to a new and very strange country.

The place to begin is not just at the massage table, but also during the course of your daily life. Learn to dwell on the weight and texture of an object you pick up; on the feel and balance of your body where it presses against the chair you sit in, or the ground you walk on; on whatever you feel happening each time your body and the world make contact. Learn also to respond with your entire body, letting the feel of an object in your fingers, or of the sole of your foot against the floor, echo and reverberate everywhere within you.

Two books with a number of practical exercises that can help you to explore your sense of touch are Bernard Gunther's *Sense Relaxation Below Your Mind* (Macdonald), and Frederick Perls, Ralph F. Hefferline and Paul Goodman's *Gestalt Therapy* (Penguin Books).

Be patient, and respect the newness of what you are trying to do. Imagine yourself as a being from another planet trying to enjoy the realities of this one through a sense-form that you have never had to use before.

Your body tends constantly to express itself. It does so in many different ways and on many different levels.

Probably no other discovery has had a greater impact upon the human potential movement. Because we reveal through gesture, posture and movement so much more than we are fully aware of, the practice of 'reading' body language – unfolding the body's non-verbal messages and translating them into words – has become an important tool in gestalt therapy and the gestalt-oriented encounter group. (Take a look, for example, at Fritz Perls's highly readable *Gestalt Therapy Verbatim* (Bantam Books).

What this means for massage is, I think, that the quality of one's touch has an expressive range far wider than has ordinarily been thought to be the case. The body is permeated with a communicative force; and touching, no less than any other of its activities, takes place constantly within the field of this force.

Learn to 'listen' to your sense of touch (at all times, not just while doing massage) much the way you might listen to the sound of your own voice. Accept that you express yourself through touch – that in fact you can't help expressing yourself so – and tune in all you can to the ways in which you do so.

Even the objects in your hands or that your body otherwise comes into contact with – imagine yourself as greeting them, questioning them, talking to them through touch. Something like this does seem to happen on a primitive level, and with patience you can tune in to it. Learn to recognize your body as a flow of expressive interaction with both people and objects; as a web of mute speech endlessly being spun between yourself and the world.

Your body is a field of energy. Different traditions have called this energy by different names. In yoga it is the 'prana'. In Tai Chi Chuan, a form of moving meditation developed in China, it is the 'chi'; in Aikido, a Japanese form of awareness and self-defence, the 'ki'. Wilhelm Reich, coming to the same thing by a very different path, called it 'bio-electrical' and 'orgone' energy. Today most of the human potential movement, including Reich's most direct successors in bioenergetic therapy, has settled simply for 'energy'.

Although unalike in their methods, these different approaches have certain basic ideas in common about the nature and meaning of body energy. Central to all of them is the conviction that this energy can be directly experienced, that the whole point of becoming more deeply aware of the body is in fact to experience it and that many of the higher stages of personal growth are inseparable from increasingly enriched experiences of this sort.

What can the physicist, the chemist and the biologist tell us about the nature of this energy? So far, next to nothing. From a scientific point of view this energy has yet to be 'seen'. That is, no instrument has yet been found which can effectively locate and measure it. A small amount of research has been undertaken (e.g., bio-feedback experiments in this country, acupuncture research in France and Russia), but its results are of a highly tentative and preliminary nature.

This means that we are dealing with a scientific unknown. Even the language used to describe it is highly metaphorical and vague. And yet there is no question that this energy – this 'something' – can be felt from within. For centuries men have been charting some of its inward patterns and exploring ways to increase its flow. Anyone can be taught to feel it, to heighten it, to experience it more intensely and more subtly. And, I might add, beyond a certain point there is nothing else I know of that will so enrich your awareness of your body.

Here as before there is much that you can do by yourself. The main thing is, whenever you tune in to your body, to think of yourself not as a 'thing', but as a field of energy capable of experiencing its own inner dynamics. However, don't try to predict too closely what this will feel like, or what it would feel like if you were doing it 'correctly'. Just tune in, playing at the same time with the notions of 'energy' and 'field', and see what happens.

A few additional clues: one good way to start is to take frequent notice of what parts of your body seem most alive; and what parts seem least alive, or seem even not to be present.

Remember also that as a field of energy your body is a process; it is always in a state of flux. Pay careful attention to the aliveness or deadness of a single part, for example, and you will see that it never stays the same. Be aware also of any sensations of inner flow, warmth or tingling. The more subtle your attention, the greater number of minute changes you will experience taking place.

Whenever you have difficulty getting in touch with your body energy there are two devices that will almost always help. Once is to focus on your breath. Follow its rhythm, its changes and fluctuations, and the smoothness or jerkiness of its rise and fall; stay alert both to the breath itself and to any muscular movements or sensations accompanying it elsewhere in the body. The other is called 'centring'. The centre of your body is your abdomen; it is what in Japanese culture is called the *hara*. To centre yourself is to focus your attention on the central region of your abdomen and to let whatever you are doing – actions, feelings, seeing, speaking – unfold itself from this point. Focusing on the breath, and centring, can also be very effectively combined: follow the movement of your breath as before, but let each inhalation sink straight to the centre of your abdomen. Even better: imagine that your breath, passing through and on all sides around this centre point, is with each inhalation filling your entire body.

If you would like to try a small exercise that can help you to experience your breath in this manner, here is one of many developed by Magda Proskauer. Lie on your back. Let your body relax as fully as you can. Then with your breath do the following:

(1) Begin inhaling through the nose and exhaling out the mouth.

(2) Let your breath become as quiet, as smooth and as long as it wants to be without, however, forcing it in any manner.

(3) After each exhalation see if you can allow a pause to take place before inhaling again. Don't, however, do anything to actively 'hold' the breath out. Instead just don't do anything at all to bring it back in – in other words, let yourself wait until the breath comes back entirely of its own accord. (Don't worry, it will always come back!)

(4) Let each breath go straight to the abdomen. Don't worry about using the chest at all. Explore how much space you can feel within your abdomen, and to what extent you can feel each inhalation filling that space.

Next, if you would like to take this exercise a step further, add the following.

(1) Continue with the same breathing pattern – in the nose and out the mouth, pausing after the exhalation, and letting each inhalation go all the way to the abdomen.

(2) On every alternate breath, gently tighten your right buttock as you inhale. Make the movement as smooth as possible. Try to isolate the buttock muscles so that you are not flexing the muscles anywhere else in your body. At the same time send your inhalation right into the buttock itself.

(3) Release the buttock as you exhale, letting the buttock settle into the floor as much as it wants to go. Make this movement also as smooth as possible. At the same time imagine that your exhalation is going right out the buttock itself.

(4) Continue these two movements on every other breath. Rest, without moving, on the in-between breaths.

(5) After several minutes move to your left buttock and repeat.

(6) After doing the same on both sides, again let your breath simply filter down towards your abdomen, and

see what sense of inner space you now can feel in this portion of your body.

One last general clue: don't fall into the trap of trying to separate 'physical sensations' from 'emotional qualities'. To tune in to the energy which is your body is to feel neither just the one nor just the other, but the common root of both.

You don't have to stop here, however. By experimenting with the way of thinking and the activities suggested above you can learn many things. Nevertheless this represents only a beginning. As already mentioned, there are a number of more structured methods of heightening the awareness of one's own body. Some are Eastern disciplines having long traditions: meditation, yoga, Tai Chi Chuan and Aikido are several currently most popular. Others are more recent Western developments: for example, Proskauer breath techniques (a highly simplified example of which was just given above), group work in sensory awareness, and bioenergetic therapy.

If you want to develop as much skill and presence as possible in the practice of massage, I strongly recommend that you explore one or more of these approaches. Whichever you choose to try out, the very fact of your having some familiarity with massage will give you a head start. Among the various forms of 'body work' there is a great deal of overlap, and the practice of one tends strongly to reinforce the practice of any others.

You will discover for yourself which is most suited to your needs. All are of immense value in themselves, and all are helpful for massage as well.

However, among these various approaches there are two which, I am convinced, are especially valuable for massage: meditation and Tai Chi Chuan. I would like to say a little more about these in the next two chapters.

Meditation

Like massage, meditation is done with the entire body. This is not always explicitly recognized. The directions given the student of meditation usually emphasize what not to do: don't pursue thoughts; don't leave the present moment; don't move your body, etc. And this is only right, for the initial purpose of all meditation is to bring a temporary stop to the buzz and drone of our verbal thinking.

But what happens once our internal verbal chatter begins to quiet down? The answer is that eventually a lot happens; specifically what depending in part on the particular type of meditation being practised. Whatever the type, however, one of the most important effects will be a highly intensified awareness of the body. Internal verbal chatter is a defence against feeling the body. Remove some of this defence, and the field of energy that is the body can't help but make itself felt more strongly.

Whatever else happens – depending, as I have said, upon the particular type of meditation – is a development of this intensified body awareness. Once meditation is taken to a certain depth the body becomes like a rich music that can be played in any of a great variety of ways. There are some forms of meditation, for example, which lead simply to a sense of calmness and inner harmony; this calmness, however, remains thoroughly a physical one, a serenity that seeps through the body almost like a physical warmth. Other types explicitly make use of a focusing of attention on a single part of the body: for example, the abdomen or *hara*, or the 'third eye' centre in the forehead. A few of these latter types offer, if pursued far enough, what their practitioners feel is the most intense experience known to man: a sensation of one's body energy becoming fused with vaster energies of the cosmos.

Whatever the type of meditation practised,

for anyone into massage the side benefits are enormous. Make meditation a daily habit for a period of some months or more, and you will find yourself bringing to the massage table a sensitivity and inner focus which you would never have thought possible.

How can you learn? The best way is to find a good teacher. However, if the right teacher – right for you, no matter what he may seem to be for others – doesn't appear to be available, I would suggest exploring a few good books. Two helpful overviews of the different forms of meditation are Christmas Humphreys, *Concentration And Meditation* (Stuart & Watkins), and Claudio Naranjo and Robert E. Ornstein, *On The Psychology of Meditation* (Allen & Unwin).

A beautiful work on Zen meditation, invaluable for anyone beginning meditation whether he is specifically interested in Zen or not, is Yasutani's lectures in Philip Kapleau, ed., *Three Pillars of Zen* (Harper & Row).

Which kind should you try? This depends strictly on you, and what fits for you. There are any number of ways from which to pick. Depending on which you choose, for example, you may be instructed to keep your eyes open or closed; to breathe naturally or in a specific rhythm; to let your mind stay visually 'blank' or to concentrate on certain images; silently to repeat to yourself a word or phrase called a *mantra*, or to keep yourself from verbally concentrating on anything at all. My suggestion is that you experiment all you can. The important thing is to get started, and any style of meditation that helps you do that is for you a good style.

Any style is also excellent for massage. However, at this point I will share with you one piece of admittedly prejudiced advice. For reasons which I will explain in a later chapter, I think that any form of meditation which includes both some kind of active dwelling upon the breath, and some amount of concentration on the abdomen or *hara*, will have a few unique extra benefits for the practice of massage.

Zazen, for example, a style of meditation associated with the Eastern Zen tradition, includes both of these. So do some Yoga meditations which include focusing upon energy centres (usually called *chakras*) in the lower as well as the upper parts of the body. And there are others.

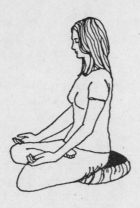

Here is a simple meditation with which you might experiment. It includes elements of both yoga and Zen traditions.

(1) Sit with your back comfortably straight. Sit cross-legged on a small firm cushion if you can do so without straining; if not, sit in a straight-backed chair with your knees a couple of feet apart.

(2) Breathe through the nose. Don't do anything to your breath, and don't change its rhythm in any way – with one exception. Do let yourself pause after each exhalation; try completely to suspend all activity on your part, and to let the breath come back in entirely of its own accord (i.e., the same as for the Proskauer breath exercise given at the end of the previous chapter).

(3) Also let each breath sink as low as you can and let it go into your abdomen. Don't force it to move lower; just be sure to let it go as low as it wants to go.

(4) Count your breaths. Count on each exhalation, going from one to ten and then start again at one. Repeat the same pattern for as long as you meditate.

(5) For the first five minutes or so focus all your attention on the centre of your abdomen, however vaguely or sharply you may feel yourself to be in touch with that centre. Then for the remainder of the period of meditation focus your attention at the middle of the forehead, on a point about half an inch above the bridge of the nose and about half an inch inside.

(6) Don't pursue thoughts. Try to let your mind become empty and still. Give all your attention to whichever point of the body you are concentrating on, and to the feel and flow of your breath.

(7) Give up all expectations. Try to be content with

whatever happens, even if for some time this means nothing at all.

(8) Don't try to meditate too long in the beginning. Ten minutes a day is fine. Gradually increase this amount when you feel ready. Begin each time by focusing for five minutes or so at the centre of the abdomen, and then move your attention to the middle of the forehead.

In general I find that, once a certain familiarity with the techniques and effects of meditation has been attained, elements of practice taken from different traditions can be very effectively combined. Say, for example, you have found a meditation that suits you well, but which does not include either centring (focusing on the abdomen) or dwelling upon the breath. You might then try either in some way combining these elements with your meditation itself (I would try this only if you have become fairly advanced in your practice), or else adding them during a short preliminary period at the beginning of your regular sitting. In short, experiment – it pays off.

Tai Chi Chuan

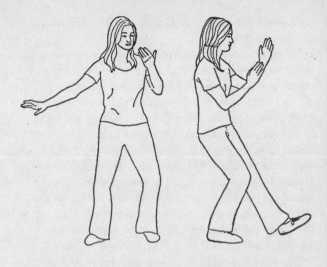

If the gods themselves were to give us something to make massage better, I suspect it would look a lot like Tai Chi Chuan. I am told that among the Chinese, who consider massage a high art, it is common for a masseur to take up the practice of Tai Chi as an integral part of his massage training. The reasons are not hard to understand.

Tai Chi is a form of moving meditation developed in China some generations ago. Based both upon the movements of animals and many traditional fighting movements, it consists of a series of slow, dance-like steps and gestures of the entire body. Depending on the particular school and the speed with which it's done, Tai Chi takes from about five to thirty minutes to perform, or, as the Chinese say, to 'play'. Although extremely beautiful from the point of view of the outside observer, the essence of Tai Chi lies not in its visual qualities but in the feel of it on the inside for the person who does it.

What makes it so fine for massage? Most obvious is the flowing quality of the movements of the hands. When doing Tai Chi the hands look like fish moving slowly through water. Yet every movement is absolutely precise and, despite its gracefulness, often performed with a great deal of hidden strength. This combination of smoothness and precision is also exactly what our hands need to acquire for doing massage.

Equally important for the massage are the stance and the movements of the rest of the body. Minute attention is given to balance and gravity, to centring and to the exact movements, internal and external, of the torso and legs in order to provide a base for the flowing gestures of the hands.

Finally, for the advanced student Tai Chi is unquestionably a form of meditation. Concentration is focused on the abdomen, attention is given to the breath, and energy is made to circulate throughout the body. As we will point out in more detail in the next chapter, these are inward activities which can be used with great benefit at the massage table as well.

I wish I could tell you an easy way to learn Tai Chi Chuan. Unfortunately, a trained instructor is necessary – without one you don't stand a chance of learning it correctly – and at the present moment decent teachers are few and far between. Teachers can be found at such places as growth centres.

This situation is improving, however, and in the near future will no doubt improve even more.

Wherever Tai Chi is available today, it is becoming immensely popular. Within a few years we will very likely see a new generation of teachers, and a far greater number of them, offering instruction in Tai Chi in many different parts of this country.

In the meantime all I can say is that if you are into massage, and if you ever do have the chance to learn some Tai Chi Chuan, take it. At least give it a try. Watch it being done, experiment with a few of the beginning movements, and see if Tai Chi speaks to you. If it does, I assure you that you are on your way to learning a lot more about massage.

The next step

Energy, meditation, Tai Chi, the body as self . . . what do they all mean when the time comes to actually give a friend a massage?

Largely a change of orientation. Up to this point while doing massage you most likely have been concentrating entirely on your friend and his or her needs. In itself this is good; certainly it is the fastest way to learn massage. The next step, however, is to learn to tune in to yourself at the same time. And this means, of course, tuning in to your body; into its mood and feel, its balance, its energy.

This is not an easy switch. In the beginning you will probably find it awkward. For a period of time, in fact, tuning in to yourself may even interfere with your ability to focus your attention on your friend. Don't worry, however; the change will come. And the more you let yourself follow a few of the paths suggested in the previous chapters, the faster it will come.

Also, don't let yourself be fooled by a false notion of the economics of attention. It's not true that you have only a fixed 'amount' of attention; giving some to yourself doesn't mean that you have to give less to your friend. At first it may well feel that way. Before long, however, you will find that your own body, more resonant and feeling within, will have become a better receiver of what lies without and that, far from giving your friend less attention, by tuning in to yourself you can give him more.

Beyond this there is not a great deal I can tell you; or need to. The following hints, however, may help you to get started.

Stay as much as you can in the present moment. Let outside thoughts distract you as little as possible. If you have undertaken meditation as a regular practice, try to be present to yourself now with the same fullness.

Stay aware of your breathing. While doing massage breathe always through the nose. Follow your breath; let it go as low as it can into your body, and, without forcing it in any way, let it become as long and smooth as possible.

Focus on the centre of your body – the internal centre of your abdomen or *hara*, however and wherever you feel it. Send your breath to this point if that helps you to stay aware of it. Think of yourself as doing massage from this place. Feel it as a source, a depth from which everything done with your hands can naturally emerge.

Don't programme too rigidly what you intend to do during a massage. Keep yourself fresh. Be clear about the order you want to use for working on the different parts of the body, also about what parts, if any, you suspect may require special attention. Beyond that, however (assuming that you by now are familiar with a sufficient amount of technique), rely upon your spontaneity and your sensitivity to what your hands are feeling rather than a detailed plan of action worked out in advance.

Be aware of the ground beneath you. Sense the floor beneath your feet, sense the support of the massage table as you gently press your friend against it, and sense your own balance between these points. Think of yourself as exploring with your friend his and your mutual connection with this supporting ground.

Be as alert as you can to the flow of energy in your own body. Try – in any way that feels natural, whether imagined or felt – to send energy to your friend with your hands, just as a healer does.

At the same time try to tune in to the flow of energy within your friend's body. This is extremely difficult at first, but with practice you will be surprised at how much your hands will be able to tell you. Don't have any preconceptions about what this will or won't feel like. Just tune in, and see what happens.

Remember that massage is always a form of non-verbal communication – but remember as well that the body tends naturally to express itself. This means that the communicative side of massage is not something external, something added; instead it is something already present and what we have to learn is how not to interfere with it. Massage is not Morse code: you don't need to worry about having a 'message' in mind before you begin.

Perhaps an analogy will help. Gestalt therapists often comment that the sound and the vocal mannerisms of a person's voice express far more than the actual content of what he is saying. The same applies to massage: although many attitudes and signals can be easily translated by using the hands, it is the quality itself of a person's touch which offers the greatest range of expression.

In other words, trust the body; let yourself be as fully rooted and present within it as possible; and communication will take care of itself.

In sum, massage is an act of celebration, an act in which the experience of the giver is as important as the experience of the receiver. Approach it as such, and you will learn from within yourself everything else about it which you might ever want to know.

Zone therapy

In Asia for many centuries physicians and healers have been using foot massage as an aid to the diagnosis and treatment of both major and minor health problems. In the West this form of treatment has become known as 'zone therapy'; and, more recently, 'reflexology'. Although largely ignored by the medical profession, it has come to gain a large underground reputation among practitioners of massage.

The principle is simple. For every important organ or muscle area in the trunk and head there is a tiny area that corresponds to it on one or both feet. To locate and treat a health problem affecting any of the upper part of the body you merely massage the corresponding area on the foot.

Sounds crazy? Of course it does to the Western ear – mine as well as yours. But I can only say that I have been experimenting with zone therapy on an informal basis for some time, as have a number of others with whom I am in contact, and I am convinced that there is a great deal to it. It is not a cure-all, and it is definitely no substitute for a visit to the doctor's surgery. But as a supplement to ordinary medical attention it can often provide a small but noticeable boost in health wherever it is needed.

Why does it work? There are a lot of theories. One frequently advanced is that it is the nervous system which is responsible: numerous nerves running from the foot to elsewhere in the body can cause a reflex action in any other appropriate body part, and this in turn, by stimulating circulation, can bring about a better nutritional intake and elimination of waste in the immediate neighbourhood of that same part. Another hypothesis – and my own suspicions are that the truth lies more in this direction – is that the connective tissue and the lymph system throughout the body are the vehicles for energy circuits of a nature as yet unanalysed by medical science, and that the right kind of massage work on the foot unblocks an energy flow that also affects the corresponding area of the body.

Whatever the reasons, however, zone therapy does seem to work. Here is how you can go about exploring it for yourself.

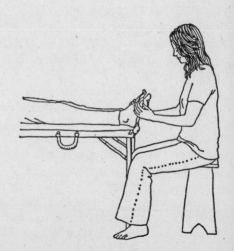

Arrange yourself and a friend so that the sole of his or her foot is easily accessible to you. If you are working on a massage table I find that the easiest way to do this is to have your friend lying on his back and to seat yourself on a stool so that you are facing the sole of his foot. Another way is to have your friend sit in a chair with one foot propped up on a low padded stool, and either to kneel or to sit on a small cushion facing him.

Next begin massaging the sole of his foot with the tips of your thumbs. Don't bother with oil. Press quite hard; use as much pressure as you would to push a thumbtack into a piece of wood. And, most essential, press everywhere. Work slowly and thoroughly over the entire sole. Then lift the foot slightly and work the sides of the heel all the way to the ankle bone. What you are looking for are any unusual concentrations of muscular constriction and, more importantly, any reactions of pain on the part of your friend. Stop when you find tightness or when your friend says 'Ouch!' Check the accompanying charts, determine what body part corresponds to the right or sore part of the foot, and let your friend know that he

has either a health problem or a strong potential for one in that particular part. Then, asking your friend to put up with a little more necessary hurt, continue to massage the same area on the foot with extra care and thoroughness.

Or, if you already know of some health condition that has been bothering your friend, you can go right to the corresponding area of the foot and begin working there.

Frequent short treatments, in the order of ten

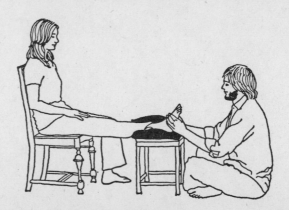

to twenty minutes once a day or once every two days, are best. Ideally you and your friend should continue with this programme both until his condition has improved and until he no longer feels the same sharp soreness as you massage his foot.

Connections on the top of both feet

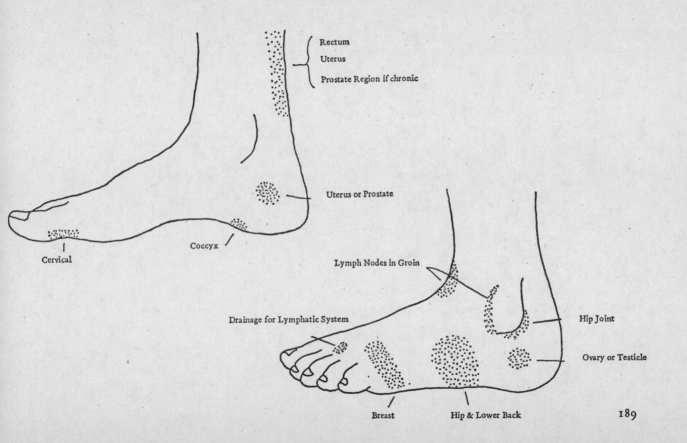

Rectum

Uterus

Prostate Region if chronic

Uterus or Prostate

Cervical

Coccyx

Lymph Nodes in Groin

Hip Joint

Drainage for Lymphatic System

Ovary or Testicle

Breast

Hip & Lower Back

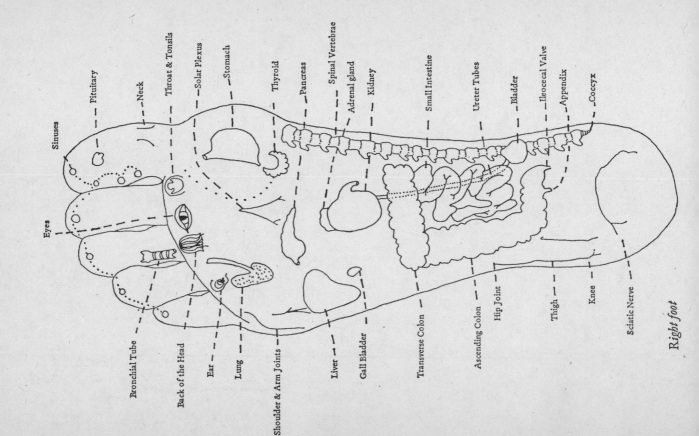

Sinuses

Pituitary

Neck

Throat & Tonsils

Solar Plexus

Stomach

Thyroid

Pancreas

Spinal Vertebrae

Adrenal gland

Kidney

Small Intestine

Ureter Tubes

Bladder

Ileoceoal Valve

Appendix

Coccyx

Eyes

Bronchial Tube

Back of the Head

Ear

Lung

Shoulder & Arm Joints

Liver

Gall Bladder

Transverse Colon

Ascending Colon

Hip Joint

Thigh

Knee

Sciatic Nerve

Right foot

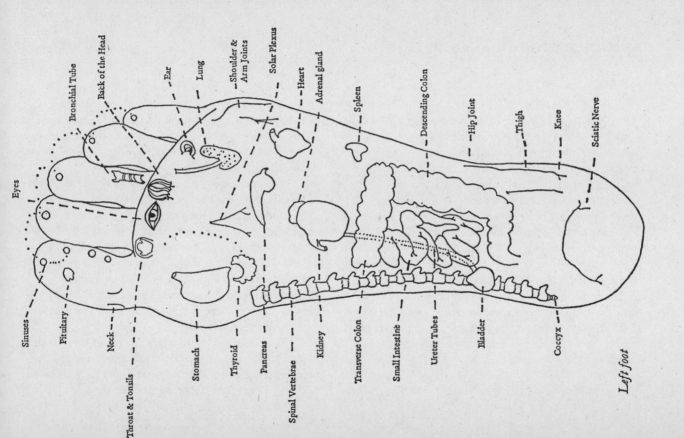

Eyes

Sinuses

Bronchial Tube

Back of the Head

Pituitary

Neck

Ear

Lung

Shoulder &
Arm Joints

Solar Plexus

Heart

Adrenal gland

Spleen

Descending Colon

Hip Joint

Thigh

Knee

Sciatic Nerve

Throat & Tonsils

Stomach

Thyroid

Pancreas

Spinal Vertebrae

Kidney

Transverse Colon

Small Intestine

Ureter Tubes

Bladder

Coccyx

Left foot

Other forms of massage

Once you have begun to make some progress with the type of massage described in this book you will naturally find yourself getting interested in other forms of massage as well. How many other forms actually exist? I've learned from experience not to try to answer this question. Every time I think I know, I find myself suddenly running across two or three totally different massage traditions the likes of which I have never before imagined, let alone heard of.

I want to pass on to you here a series of brief pictures of some of the more prominent among the different approaches to massage that I know. I have already told you about zone therapy. About the others I will limit myself to a more general description, and where I can, will tell you where you can go to find more specific information.

Reichian Massage. Strictly speaking there is no one form of Reichian massage. Wilhelm Reich, a breakaway disciple of Freud now newly famous as the grandfather of what has come to be known as bioenergetic therapy, while working with his patients did apparently use a number of techniques of direct physical contact. Many of these techniques have not only survived, having been handed down by a couple of generations of successors, they have been further extended and developed in several directions by those who have inherited them. What we have today is therefore really a family of related approaches, their two major similarities being their mutual descent from Reich himself and the more or less common goal towards which they are directed.

The chief purpose of Reichian massage – or of whatever we are going to label this general approach – is to assist the dissolution of what Reich called 'body armour'. Reich found that many individuals subconsciously use muscular constrictedness in various regions of the torso, neck and head as a defence against repressed emotions. By physically working on these areas along with a verbal analysis of the emotions involved, Reich sought to free the body to become a more sensitive and vital receptor of inner feelings.

One of the most common of these methods being used today is an extremely forceful palpitation of key areas of the torso and neck. The amount of massage given any one area varies widely from individual to individual; this must be determined by an analysis of his body and its expressive 'blocks'. Sharp jabs or pokes designed to stimulate certain reflexes are also sometimes used. So are lighter forms of stroking. In some cases these techniques are also coordinated with the cycle of the breath.

This style of massage is rarely practised by anyone other than a trained therapist. Normally it is made an integral part of a subject's ongoing therapy. Because of its power to release forms of emotional energy that can cause a tremendous immediate anxiety on the part of the subject experiencing them, it should be used only by someone whose professional background equips him to deal with such a therapeutic situation.

Rolfing. Also called Structural Integration, this is a method of deep massage developed over recent decades by Ida Rolf. Its major technique is the application of extremely heavy and concentrated pressure with one knuckle, or an elbow, or sometimes even the knuckles of a fist; often a single point on a subject's body is worked for several seconds at a time. Its purpose is to realign the muscular and connective tissue. Its results are dramatic: a complete reshaping of the body's physical posture.

A Rolfing 'treatment' consists ordinarily of ten sessions lasting an hour each. Usually the individual sessions are spaced a week or so apart.

The actual experience of being 'Rolfed' is worth mentioning. Usually it is a mixture of strong sensations – extremely painful, yet often exhilarating at the same time. The pain is manageable. It comes only in short bursts of two or three seconds' length, and stops immediately when the Rolfer's hand is taken away. It also usually has a curiously solid, almost reassuring quality to it; as opposed, say, to the freakish quality of pain in the dentist's chair. Along with the pain, moreover, often comes an intense and sometimes joyful excitement. One is being physically changed; one can sense muscles cramped for years finally loosening; often energy can be felt moving up and down the entire body.

Other strong emotions are frequently released during the course of the treatment. Sometimes intense childhood memories never before recalled also come to consciousness.

The physical effects of Rolfing are for the most part permanent. A number of subjects have also found that the deep changes in their posture introduced by Rolfing have led to equivalent psychological changes as well. More energy, a greater sense of well-being, and more directness in relating to others are some of the benefits most often cited.

Proskauer massage. A form of direct body treatment developed by Magda Proskauer, a pioneer in what has come to be known as breath therapy. An extremely subtle form of massage, it is closely tied to the rest of her work with the breath. The massage itself is timed to the cycle of the breath; a feather-light touch moving along certain muscle groups during the subject's exhalation is frequently used, for example. Designed to heighten the subject's awareness of, and trust in, his own breath, when done correctly it leaves one with the sensation of having been massaged from the inside by the breath itself.

Shiatsu. This is a Japanese form of massage done almost entirely with the balls of the thumbs. Of all the Asiatic styles of massage that I know, it is the most easily learned. Pressure is applied with the thumbs for several seconds at a time to any or all of hundreds of points located throughout the body. A complete massage usually covers every part of the body; when done for medical purposes, however, only certain combinations of points may be brought into play.

Shiatsu is tiring to do at first because of the sustained use of the thumbs. Even a tiny bit practised each day, however, quickly gives the thumbs the necessary strength and endurance.

Besides being an interesting form of massage in its own right, Shiatsu can serve as an extremely effective change of pace when combined with Western forms of massage. It also can be used for self-massage, since many of the points it makes use of can be massaged by a person himself.

Acupuncture. A traditional Chinese medical treatment. Based upon an elaborate theory of how energy manifests itself and circulates within the body, acupuncture is done by stimulating key combinations of very precise minute points scattered throughout the body.

As is commonly known, these points are usually stimulated by the insertion of slender metal needles up to a depth of about an inch and a half. Less well known, however, is that acupuncture is also sometimes administered as a form of massage, the necessary points being stimulated by pressure with a knuckle or thumb.

Relatively little of a concrete nature is known about acupuncture in this country, despite its recently having almost overnight become an object of fascination. In the West the most advanced scientific studies of its effects have been made in France, where for some time it has generated excitement within certain medical circles. On the basis of the dramatic and highly sophisticated medical cures acupuncture is reported consistently to achieve, one can't help but hope that a more sustained programme of research may someday bring about a sweeping transformation of our scientific understanding of the human body.

Polarity Therapy. This is the name given by Dr Randolph Stone to his own comprehensive integration of a number of massage and manipulation techniques which he has developed over the course of half a century.

Perhaps the easiest way to describe polarity therapy is that it looks like Rolfing and thinks like acupuncture. Like Rolfing, it makes frequent use of heavy concentrated pressure applied with a knuckle, thumb or elbow. Again like Rolfing, one of its functions is to bring about a realignment of the posture of the body.

Like acupuncture, however, the practice of polarity therapy rests upon an extremely detailed analysis of the nature of energy flow within the body. Much of this theory is derived from yogic and spiritual traditions in India. Dr Stone himself, a lifelong student of meditation, has spent many years in India, and is the director of a medical clinic there.

The professional worlds of massage

Perhaps by this time massage has come to interest you enough for the idea of doing it on a professional basis to look appealing. If so, what I have to say can, I'm afraid, only discourage you.

In the United States there are at least three distinct professional worlds of massage. They are very different from one another, and there is no getting around the fact that there exists little communication or understanding among them.

The world of massage most prominent in the public eye is that of the professional massage studio. Largely confined to big cities, their public image is about on a par with that of the dime-a-dance halls of a generation ago.

This notorious reputation is only partially deserved. In point of fact the studios vary widely among themselves. A few (in most cities a very small number, if any at all) are actually fronts for prostitution. Many others, although in fact offering strictly legitimate massage, seek by means of lurid advertising to capitalize upon this image. Unfortunately, even though their customers learn quickly enough what is and what isn't on the menu, this style of promotion serves only to reinforce in the public mind the same bastardized image of massage.

The atmosphere of most legitimate studios is at worst shabby, at best clinical. Although there exist some wonderful exceptions, the massage offered is usually of a strikingly low quality. In many cases the masseuses have received only a minimal amount of training, if any. In other cases they are more than competent, but tend to react to the tedium and the unpleasant vibrations in their working situation by giving an impersonal and mechanical massage.

Needless to say, I cannot recommend with much enthusiasm your looking for a job in a studio. As someone who enjoys doing massage (I assume this is one reason you would like to make it your work), you stand to be continually frustrated: the average client, thanks to the advertising he has been exposed to, will bring with him so many expectations along other lines that he will have a difficult time listening to what your hands really have to say. And as a woman (massage studios almost never employ men), or so I am told, you will find yourself repeatedly cast in an unpleasant and stereotyped role.

Going to other people's homes to do massage – doing 'outcalls', as it is called in the trade – is really an extension of the studio scene and presents most of the same difficulties. In many states a local business licence, usually available immediately upon payment of a small fee, is all that is legally required to do outcalls. Practically what it means is investing in a portable massage table (see the previous chapter on tables); arranging for transportation (a car is almost always necessary); advertising, either informally through friends and acquaintances or, as is usually necessary, through a local newspaper; and then waiting by the phone.

The advantages of doing outcalls are that you are your own boss, that you can usually expect to be paid more for the actual amount of time that you spend doing massage, and that over the course of time it can sometimes be a little easier to collect a regular clientele of the type with which you wish to work. For the most part, however, you will be subject to the same psychological unpleasantness that you would encounter in a studio, since here as elsewhere the distorted public image of massage acts as a kind of filter selecting who will call you and what his expectations are likely to be.

Men do outcalls as well as women. Most find themselves subject to many of the same hassles.

A quite different type of massage scene is to be found in the physical therapy room of most hospitals. Here massage is performed by trained physical therapists for strictly medical purposes. For the right person with the right credentials this can be a reasonable professional outlet for massage. For many, however, it suffers from several limitations.

First, you must be licensed as a physical therapist. Throughout most of the United States this means at least a year of full-time formal schooling leading to a degree in physical therapy. Second, as a physical therapist, you will discover that massage is only a part of what you will be expected to do; and when massage is prescribed, it will usually be only for extensive work on a single part of the body. Third, although free from the sexual ambiguities of the massage studio, the atmosphere of the hospital tends to be equally impersonal.

Some gymnasiums and health clubs also have massage rooms. Their atmosphere tends to be more like that of the hospital than anything else. No formal degree is ordinarily required.

Yet another world of massage is that of the growth movement. As I have already said, there are a number of growth centres, such as Esalen, where one can learn massage. A smaller number also have one or several masseurs or masseuses on hand in order to make massage available to members of workshops.

Comparatively speaking, those who hold such jobs tend to find them quite satisfying. One reason is that most of the people who come for workshops at a growth centre tune in quite easily to the value and meaning of massage. Another reason is that the atmosphere of a growth centre, where yoga, Tai Chi and other forms of 'body work' are also frequently taught, is often a stimulating one. Yet it is precisely these advantages, coupled with the tiny number of positions available, that make these jobs next to impossible to find. By all means try if you want; and good luck. But be prepared to be disappointed.

If, despite all this discouraging advice, you are still convinced that you want to do massage professionally, I do have one suggestion of a more positive nature: if you can't find the scene you want, then make your own. If the growth movement whets your appetite, for example, then find a growth centre that *doesn't* have a massage room and persuade them that they need one and need you to run it.

Or, if working in a studio appeals to you, start a small one of your own. Make the atmosphere as pleasant as you yourself would like it to be, keep your advertising tasteful, and put in a little effort to teaching those who come to you what massage is all about. Here in the Bay Area I have already seen one friend make this formula work beautifully. It can be done!

Anatomy

The more I teach massage, the more convinced I become that anyone learning massage for the first time is best off *not* studying formal anatomy until he has mastered some of the basic massage techniques. The reason for this is simple. In the beginning what you need to learn above all else is the art of tuning in with your hands, of being able to 'read', through the sense of touch alone, the overall feel and architecture of another person's body. Learning formal anatomy right from the start tends, I feel, to detract from, rather than hasten, the development of this sensitivity. Moreover, as I have stressed several times earlier, a knowledge of anatomy is in no way necessary for the learning of most basic techniques themselves.

Why then bother to study anatomy at all? For several very good reasons. Most important is that it will give you extra confidence. And, as I have mentioned, a knowledge of anatomy will help you to develop new massage techniques from those you have already learned. Also it can be of considerable help when dealing with certain problems – extreme tension concentrated in a particular muscular area, for example. Finally, it will satisfy some of your curiosity about how the human body really functions – and believe me, if you do a lot of massage, this is a subject that sooner or later will begin to fascinate you.

The following remarks and diagrams are designed merely to provide you with a brief overview. For more extensive discussions of anatomy see the bibliography in 'Some Reading'.

The skeleton. The bones themselves making up the skeleton have no 'feeling'. However, the nerve sheaths which encase them do, as does the connective tissue which attaches muscles to the bones. The bones also have important chemical and structural functions in the body. For massage, however, their main interest is their ability to serve as landmarks for muscle groups and areas of nerve sensation.

The long bones are always curved. These curves increase the elasticity of the bones, provide more attachment surface for muscles, and give special direction to certain portions of muscle.

There are approximately 206 separate bones in the human body. Make yourself familiar with some of the more important ones and you will be able to find your way around anywhere on the body.

The skull. The skull rests on top of the spine, directly upon the topmost spinal vertebra, which is called the Atlas. The skull is made of many smaller bones, including the cranium, which covers the brain, and the bones of the face. These bones are fused, however; for practical purposes you can consider them one piece, with the exception of the jaw.

The spine consists of twenty-four separate vertebrae extending from the base of the skull to the base of the lumbar region, plus the sacrum and the coccyx.

There are seven vertebrae in the neck (cervical vertebrae); twelve vertebrae in the upper portion of the back (dorsal), to which are attached the ribs; and five vertebrae in the lower back (lumbar). The sacrum and the coccyx consist at birth of separate and moveable vertebrae; however, over the course of time these vertebrae slowly fuse together until, usually by the time their owner has reached thirty years of age, they have become one immoveable bone. In general, up and down the entire spine, the lower the vertebrae the bigger in all dimensions it will be.

Each of those bumps which you can see along the spine is actually what is called a 'process', a spiny protective point sticking out of the main portion of the vertebra itself. With slight variations each vertebra is

Top view of vertebra   Side view of vertebra

shaped like the illustration above, having a cylindrical base with an enclosure behind for the spinal cord, and three bony processes, pointing to each side and directly backwards. If you press with your fingers you can usually feel all three processes.

Between the cylindrical sections of each pair of vertebrae rests a cartilage disc which cushions the vertebra during movement. Occasionally one of these discs can give a little to one side – the notorious 'slipped disc'.

The normal curve of the human spine is like so:

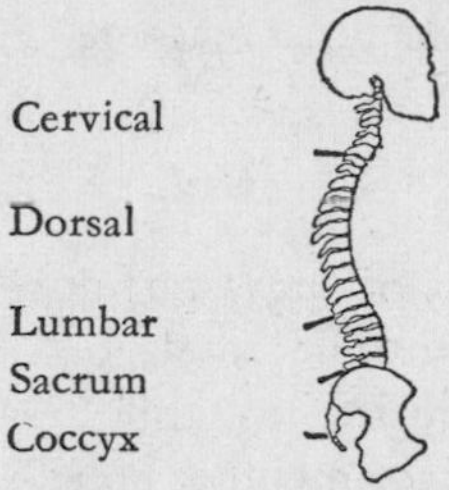

Cervical

Dorsal

Lumbar
Sacrum
Coccyx

The sternum is the hard flat ridge in the centre of the chest to which the ribs are attached in front.

The clavicles are the two narrow protruding bones at the very top of the chest. They extend from the top of the sternum to the shoulders.

The ribs, usually twelve in number, form the thorax and attach in back to the twelve thoracic vertebrae. In front, the top seven ribs are attached directly to the sternum. The next three are attached to the sternum indirectly by bands of cartilage so hard they they in turn feel like bone to the touch. The last two are called 'floating' ribs because they attach only to the vertebrae in back. The bottommost floating rib can present many surprises when you look for it with your fingers. Often you will find it in the 'right' position as shown in the diagram; sometimes, however, it slants downwards at a much sharper angle, in which case its lower tip is likely to show up buried in the muscles of the torso at a point not much higher than the hip.

The scapulae, or shoulder blades, are a particularly curious pair of bones from the point of view of massage. The first interesting item is their shape; note especially the acromian process, a sort of peninsula reaching up and to the side to connect with the clavicle at the shoulder. Note also the structural role which the scapula plays at the shoulder; the scapula and the clavicle alone form the entire architectural setting for the socket into which the humerus, the thick bone of the upper arm, is fitted. Finally, the clavicle is the *only* other bone to which the scapula is attached; although lying 'against' the ribs in back (some muscle and connective tissue actually lies between them), it is free to move over them an inch or more in every direction.

The arm. Notice that the upper arm consists of one bone whereas the forearm consists of two.

The hand consists of many tiny bones. The wrist alone contains eight.

The pelvis. The main thing about the pelvic girdle is that for all practical purposes it consists of one large basin-shaped bone. Each large hip bone consists originally of three bones which with maturation become fused, and both hip bones in turn become so tightly connected to the sacrum that the entire structure feels to the fingers like a single bone.

The greatest difference between the male and female skeleton is to be found in the pelvis. The female pelvic bones are wider apart, and also lighter and shorter. The male pelvic bones are broader, and have larger processes and ridges.

Because the pelvic structure is one large bone, movement of this area is achieved only by bending either the thigh joints or the spine itself where it meets the sacrum at the fifth lumbar vertebra. The immediate area surrounding the fifth lumbar is for this reason a foremost candidate for some good massage work on almost everyone.

The leg, like the arm, consists mainly of one large bone on top and two parallel bones below. The patella, or kneecap, is a small shield of bone buried in a large tendon and is not attached directly to any other bone. At the top of the femur, the huge bone of the thigh, note the greater trocanter sticking to the side. An important point of orientation for the observer, the visible bump produced by the greater trocanter is often mistakenly thought to be a part of the hip.

The foot, like the hand, is an intricate arrangement of numerous small bones.

The muscles, the intricate webbing of the body, are more than two hundred in number. They vary greatly in both size and shape. Some are smaller than your fingernail, others a good deal wider and longer than your entire hand. Some are cord-like, others are thick masses, and still others are flat sheets.

Surrounding each muscle is a fibrous sheath called connective tissue or fascia. Several layers of connective tissue also lie between the entire muscular system and the skin itself. The deepest layer of connective tissue actually constitutes a single continuous matrix, enclosing and even permeating the internal structure of each individual muscle.

Most muscles are attached in two or more places to two or more different bones; some, however, are attached at one or more points to the connective tissue adjoining other muscles. Movement in the body is made possible by entire groups of muscles working in unison, some relaxing at the same time that others contract.

In addition to studying the accompanying diagrams (drawn after Albinus) you might profitably spend some time with one or more good anatomical texts with pictures of individual muscles and muscle groups. I have included several in the bibliography in 'Some Reading'.

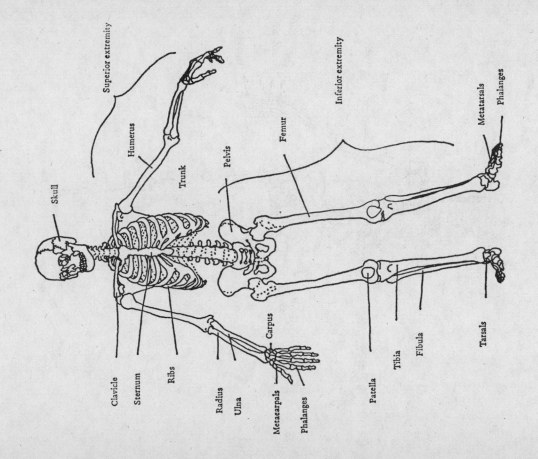

Superior extremity

Inferior extremity

Humerus

Femur

Pelvis

Trunk

Metatarsals

Phalanges

Skull

Clavicle

Sternum

Ribs

Radius

Ulna

Metacarpals

Phalanges

Carpus

Patella

Tibia

Fibula

Tarsals

Human skeleton, front view

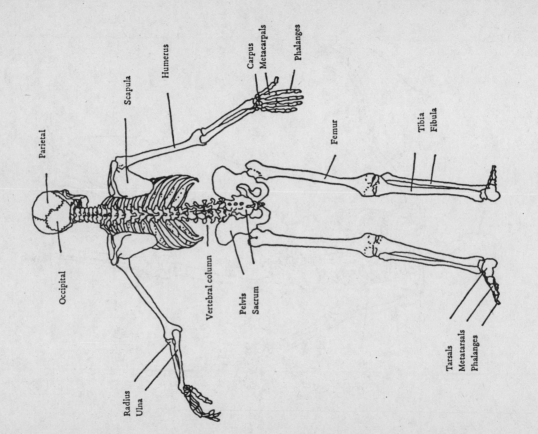

Parietal

Occipital

Scapula

Humerus

Carpus
Metacarpals

Phalanges

Vertebral column

Pelvis
Sacrum

Femur

Tibia
Fibula

Radius
Ulna

Tarsals
Metatarsals
Phalanges

Human skeleton, back view

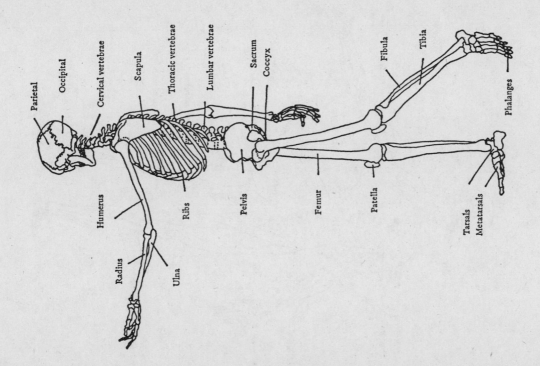

Parietal

Occipital

Cervical vertebrae

Scapula

Thoracic vertebrae

Lumbar vertebrae

Sacrum

Coccyx

Fibula

Tibia

Phalanges

Humerus

Ribs

Pelvis

Femur

Patella

Tarsals

Metatarsals

Radius

Ulna

Human skeleton, side view

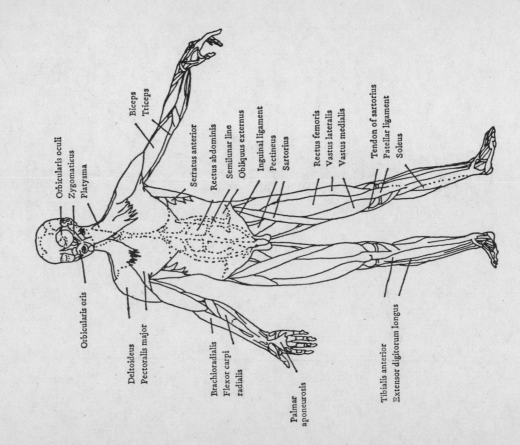

Orbicularis oculi
Zygomaticus
Platysma

Biceps
Triceps

Serratus anterior
Rectus abdominis
Semilunar line
Obliquus externus
Inguinal ligament
Pectineus
Sartorius

Rectus femoris
Vastus lateralis
Vastus medialis

Tendon of sartorius
Patellar ligament
Soleus

Orbicularis oris

Deltoideus
Pectoralis major

Brachioradialis
Flexor carpi
radialis

Palmar
aponeurosis

Tibialis anterior
Extensor digitorum longus

Muscles of human body, superficial layer, front view

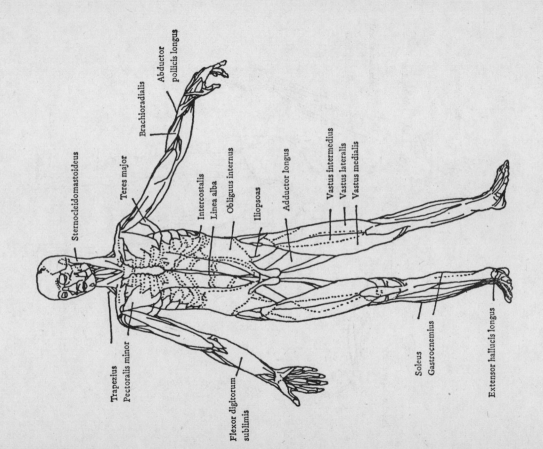

Abductor
pollicis longus

Brachioradialis

Sternocleidomastoideus

Teres major

Intercostalis

Linea alba

Obliguus internus

Iliopsoas

Adductor longus

Vastus intermedius

Vastus lateralis

Vastus medialis

Trapezius

Pectoralis minor

Flexor digitorum
sublimis

Soleus

Gastrocnemius

Extensor hallucis longus

Muscles of human body, deep layer, front view

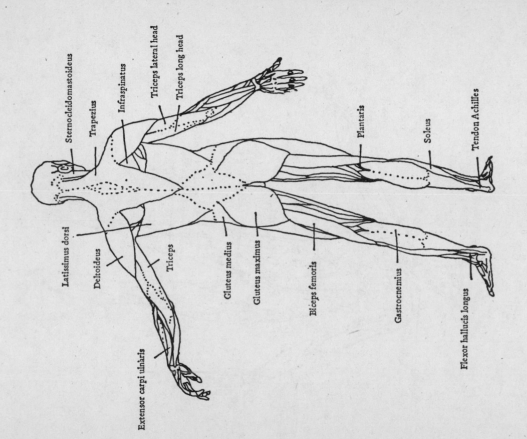

Sternocleidomastoideus

Trapezius

Infraspinatus

Triceps lateral head

Triceps long head

Plantaris

Soleus

Tendon Achilles

Latissimus dorsi

Deltoideus

Triceps

Gluteus medius

Gluteus maximus

Biceps femoris

Gastrocnemius

Flexor hallucis longus

Extensor carpi ulnaris

Muscles of human body, superficial layer, back view

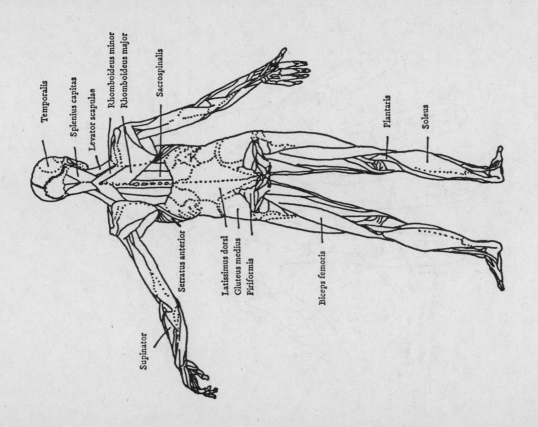

Temporalis

Splenius capitas

Levator scapulae

Rhomboideus minor
Rhomboideus major

Sacrospinalis

Plantaris

Soleus

Supinator

Serratus anterior

Latissimus dorsi
Gluteus medius
Piriformis

Biceps femoris

Muscles of human body, deep layer, back view

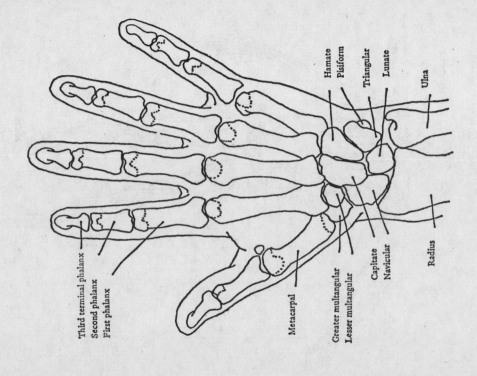

Third terminal phalanx
Second phalanx
First phalanx

Metacarpal

Greater multangular
Lesser multangular

Capitate
Navicular

Radius

Hamate
Pisiform

Triangular
Lunate

Ulna

Bones of the hand, palm view

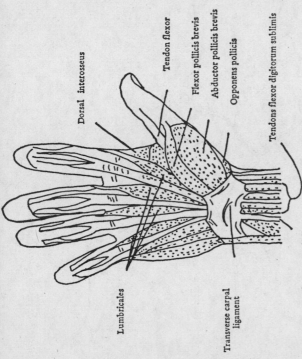

Dorsal interosseus

Tendon flexor

Flexor pollicis brevis

Abductor pollicis brevis

Opponens pollicis

Tendons flexor digitorum sublimis

Lumbricales

Transverse carpal ligament

Tendon carpi radialis

Muscles of the hand, palm view

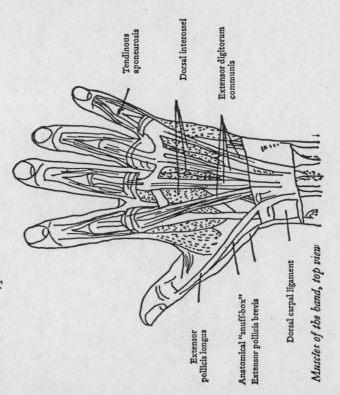

Tendinous aponeurosis

Dorsal interossei

Extensor digitorum communis

Extensor pollicis longus

Anatomical "snuff-box"
Extensor pollicis brevis

Dorsal carpal ligament

Muscles of the hand, top view

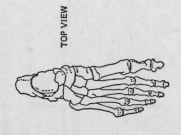

TOP VIEW

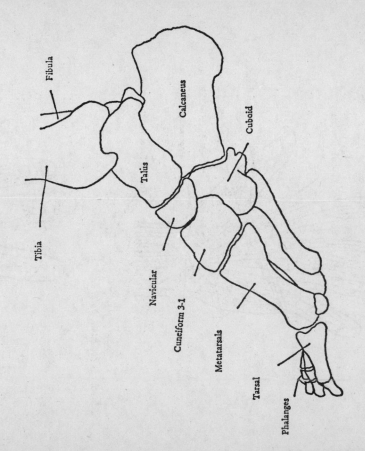

Fibula

Tibia

Talus

Calcaneus

Cuboid

Navicular

Cuneiform 3-1

Metatarsals

Tarsal

Phalanges

Bones of the foot, right inside view

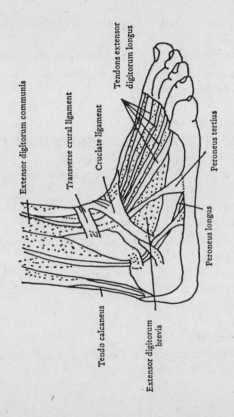

Extensor digitorum communis

Transverse crural ligament

Cruciate ligament

Tendons extensor digitorum longus

Peroneus tertius

Peroneus longus

Tendo calcaneus

Extensor digitorum brevis

Muscles of the foot, outer view

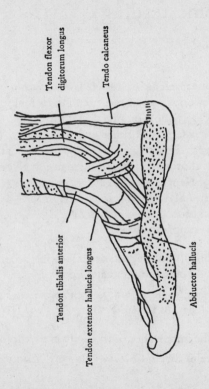

Tendon flexor digitorum longus

Tendo calcaneus

Tendon tibialis anterior

Tendon extensor hallucis longus

Abductor hallucis

Muscles of the foot, inner view

Some reading

About massage itself there is not much more to read. Older books on massage tend to be funky but extremely short on practical information. One good book is Gertrude Beard and Elizabeth C. Wood, *Massage: Principles and Techniques*, W. B. Saunders. The most thorough standard reference work on anatomy is Gray, Henry, *Anatomy of the Human Body* (edited by Charles Mayo Goss), 1973, Longmans. Clem W. Thompson, *Manual of Structural Kinesiology*, Kimpton, is interesting and cheap.

A difficult but important philosophic account of the relation between mind and body:
Maurice Merleau-Ponty, *The Phenomenology of Perception*. Routledge & Kegan Paul.

On the importance of the body in psychology:
Wilhelm Reich, *Character Analysis*. Vision Press.

Wilhelm Reich, *The Function of the Orgasm*. Panther.

Several overviews of the human potential movement:
Abraham Maslow, *The Farther Reaches of Human Nature*. Penguin Books.

On gestalt therapy:
Frederick Perls, Ralph F. Hefferline, Paul Goodman, *Gestalt Therapy*. Penguin Books.
Frederick Perls, *Gestalt Therapy Verbatim*. Bantam Books.

On techniques you can use at home to get more acquainted with yourself and your body:
Bernard Gunther, *Sense Relaxation Below Your Mind*. Macdonald.
Howard R. Lewis and Dr Harold S. Streitfeld, *Growth Games: How to Tune In Yourself, Your Family, Your Friends*. Souvenir Press.

On meditation:
Christmas Humphreys, *Concentration and Meditation*. Robinson & Watkins.

Philip Kapleau, ed., *Three Pillars of Zen*. Harper & Row.
Claudio Naranjo and Robert E. Ornstein, *On the Psychology of Meditation*. Allen & Unwin.

On yoga:

B. K. S. Iyengar, *Light on Yoga*. Allen & Unwin.
Ernest Wood, *Yoga*. Penguin Books.

More About Penguins and Pelicans

For further information about books available from Penguins please write to Dept EP, Penguin Books Ltd, Harmondsworth, Middlesex UB7 0DA.

In the U.S.A.: For a complete list of books available from Penguins in the United States write to Dept CS, Penguin Books, 625 Madison Avenue, New York, New York 10022.

In Canada: For a complete list of books available from Penguins in Canada write to Penguin Books Canada Ltd, 2801 John Street, Markham, Ontario L3R 1B4.

In Australia: For a complete list of books available from Penguins in Australia write to the Marketing Department, Penguin Books Australia Ltd, P.O. Box 257, Ringwood, Victoria 3134.

Physical Fitness

5B X 11-MINUTE-A-DAY PLAN FOR MEN
XB X 12-MINUTE-A-DAY PLAN FOR WOMEN

2 Series of Exercises developed by Royal Canadian Air Force

In an age when more and more people drive to their desks on wheels, physical fitness has become an almost universal problem. The need for exercise is felt, but we do not all have the time, the taste, or the facilities for organized games.

With this kind of situation in mind, the Royal Canadian Air Force developed its now famous Plans 5BX and XBX for men and women. The basic exercises, which are clearly detailed with diagrams in this book, can be performed without any special equipment in the most confined space. They can be completed daily in eleven or twelve minutes without any danger of exhaustion since the advance to fitness has been gently graded.

These exercise plans do appear to offer a practicable answer - with no Olympic standards of training in view -- to the modern problem of getting fit, feeling fit, and keeping fit, in a mechanized age.

The permission of the Royal Canadian Air Force for making the text of this training pamphlet available is gratefully acknowledged.

Slimnastics

Pamela Nottidge and Diana Lamplugh

Correct exercising is as important as correct eating in achieving a good figure – and losing weight in the right places.

In an effort to teach women how physical fitness, as well as weight control, is vital to healthy living, two slimnastics enthusiasts have produced a book about the kind of exercises to do while you slim.

They define their subject as a combination of slimming and gymnastics in a group: the group therapy is emphasised strongly, since better results can be achieved in the company of others who are having to cope with similar problems.

'They provide graded exercises, dieting and beautycare details, with courses catering for everyone from teenagers to grandmothers. They encourage women to get together in groups on a living-room floor for their keep-fit sessions' – *Yorkshire Post*

A Penguin Handbook

The Slimming Business
John Yudkin

John Yudkin was Professor of Physiology at Queen Elizabeth College, University of London, until 1954, when he became Professor of Nutrition and Dietetics. There are not many men, therefore, who are better qualified to give authoritative advice about slimming and draw the lines between fact, fashion, and fad.

Although a good deal of nonsense is printed in some women's magazines about slimming, Professor Yudkin shows in this readable and often entertaining handbook that the effort involved in carrying extra weight can be harmful and may lead to a number of ailments, some fatal. For other than merely fashionable reasons, therefore, it is wise to watch your weight – without being too impressed by the so-called average weight tables – and, if necessary, take sensible steps to reduce it.

This *Slimming Business* is not heavy reading. Light verses by Ogden Nash help the author's easy style to keep the weight well down. And in this fourth edition Professor Yudkin notes the intriguing results of recent research into individual control of weight, the effects of activity, and the distribution of meals during the day.

A Penguin Handbook

Skin and Hair Care
Edited by Linda Allen Schoen

What is the best treatment for acne?

How safe are eye cosmetics?

What causes dandruff?

Would plain lanolin make a good night cream?

Can oral contraceptives cause hair loss?

Is there a danger of skin cancer from using a sun lamp?

Do rejuvenating creams really eliminate wrinkles?

These and literally hundreds of questions of daily concern to everyone are answered in the three parts of this handbook along with questions about such special topics as birthmarks, excessive hair, and aesthetic surgery.

A Penguin Handbook

Praise for Deryn Lake's
previous John Rawlings Mysteries:

Death in the Dark Walk
and
Death at the Beggar's Opera

'John Rawlings and the Blind Beak are developing into
my favourite historical mystery heroes – tenacious in
their search for villains, daring as they outwit them, yet
always ready to pause for a moment of delightful
domestic life. I really enjoyed the first two in the series,
and I'm eager for the next!'
LINDSEY DAVIS

'An effervescent tale . . . the author organises her large
cast and colourful background with skill and gusto
through a racily readable drama'
FELICIA LAMB in the *Mail on Sunday's
Night & Day* Magazine

'A wealth of marvellous characters parade across the
pages, their dialogue is lively and John Rawlings is
proving to be a real charmer'
Eastbourne Herald

Death at the
Devil's Tavern

Deryn Lake

NEW ENGLISH LIBRARY
Hodder and Stoughton

Copyright © 1996 by Deryn Lake

First published in Great Britain in 1996 by
Hodder and Stoughton
a division of Hodder Headline PLC

A New English Library Paperback

The right of Deryn Lake to be identified as the author of
this work has been asserted by Deryn Lake in accordance with the
Copyright, Designs and Patents Act 1988.

10 9 8 7 6 5 4 3 2 1

A CIP catalogue record for this title is available from the
British Library.

ISBN 0 340 67427 X

Printed and bound in Great Britain by
Mackays of Chatham PLC, Chatham, Kent

Hodder and Stoughton
A division of Hodder Headline PLC
338 Euston Road
London NW1 3BH

In memory of
ZAK PACKHAM,
my dearest friend and companion,
a true gentleman,
who will live on for ever in the persona of
Joe Jago.

Acknowledgments

*M*y thanks are due to several people who have generously given their time to help me with this book. First, I would like to mention P.C. Keith Gotch of the Metropolitan Police Thames Division, Curator of the Thames Police Museum, Wapping. Keith not only discussed the state of bodies in the river with me, but also gave me the idea for the implement which killed Sir William Hartfield. Further, he advised me on tides, about the amount of shipping in the Thames in the 18th Century, and of the rewards given to watermen by the Coroner for bringing in a corpse. In short, his knowledge of the river during that period is excellent and I thank him for sharing it with me. I would also like to praise Christopher Reeves, landlord of The Prospect of Whitby, and his staff, Joseph Tchikou and Michael Chapman, who showed me all over that wonderful pub and were generally very kind and helpful, not only to me but to the artist Kenny McKendry, when he went to research the beautiful cover which he has painted for this book. Thanks too, as always, to that stoic researcher Beryl Cross, poet extraordinaire, who was with me as we sailed down the Thames to Greenwich and the idea for DEATH AT THE DEVIL'S TAVERN was born. Last but not least, I must express my gratitude to Philippa Pride, my editor, who handled the traumatic situation in which I found myself when Zak died just as I reached the deadline for this book, not only with genuine compassion but with love. Thanks to you all.

Chapter One

*I*t being a blustery March day, the wind booming down the
Thames with a jolly laugh, teasing the great ships at anchor
into fine humour as they bobbed a merry dance upon its surface,
John Rawlings, having cautiously emerged into the street from the
confines of Apothecaries' Hall, clutched at his hat as it rose swiftly
from his head and blew away in the direction of the river. In fact
so playful was this breeze that, in order to retrieve the wayward
garment, John was forced to break into a fast trot of pursuit, an
undignified gait for one who had just been granted his Freedom of
the Company and was, at long last, a Yeoman of the Worshipful
Society of Apothecaries, with all the gravitas that such a title
implied. Scurrying down Water Street in the direction of Black
Friars Stairs, he finally caught up with his hat at the entrance to
Glass House Yard, and rammed it back upon his head so hard
that his neat white wig, bought especially for the occasion, slipped
slightly, thus giving its owner a rakish air quite unsuitable for a
man of learning. Unaware of this, John Rawlings continued upon
his way with as much decorum as he could muster in view of his
bubbling good spirits.

His progress to Freedom had not been without difficulty and now
the relief of finally reaching his objective was like a bumper of
champagne. Originally, John had been released from his indentures
in the late spring of 1754 but had not made his first application to
be admitted to the Company until 22nd August. However, on that
occasion the court had broken up before his appeal could be heard
and on 5th December, the first date on which he had been able
to attend again, a similar fate had befallen him. But now it was
13th March, 1755, and he had just seen for himself the official
entry which had been made in the Court Book. Provided he paid
his fees and passed an examination, Mr John Rawlings, a Foreign
Apothecary, was made Free of the Company by Redemption.

Thinking about the day's events and grinning uncontrollably, the

1

new Yeoman let out a whooping sound far more suited to come from the lips of a savage, and tossed the offending hat aloft, barely retrieving his headgear as the high-spirited wind sported with it once more.

As was usual on the days when the Court of Assistants met in Apothecaries' Hall, a flotilla of wherries was waiting at the foot of Black Friars Stairs to row the men of medicine back to their various destinations. John, seizing the opportunity to engage the services of one of the smaller craft plying for hire, bounded down the stone steps, almost slipping in the wet as he did so. Then, with his cloak flapping round his ankles, he clambered aboard from the landing stage, hoping that the journey to the shipping basin of Wapping would not prove as rough as the saucy wind promised, for the wide river was wild with waves which slapped savagely against the shore.

Seeing John's somewhat anxious gaze, the waterman, part of a breed known for their coarse behaviour and foul language, laughed evilly. 'Do you want my hoars, Scholar? Or are you afraid of spewing up?'

The Apothecary, ignoring the waterman's deliberate mispronunciation of the word oars, attempted a dignified expression, no mean feat in view of the swaying craft and the desire of his rebellious hat to be airborne once more. 'I am an excellent traveller, thank you,' he answered, somewhat crisply.

'Then take a seat. Now, where would your scholarship be going?'

'Down river, to Wapping. Can you land me just below The Devil's Tavern?'

The wherryman adopted a look of mock concern. 'Are you sure, Scholar? I wouldn't go there if I was you, not a refined gentleman like yourself. There's lowlife gets in there, Sir. Not fit company for a man of learning. Who knows what bad habits you might clap in to.'

John gazed at him blandly. 'How subtly put. Now, are you going to take me or would you prefer that I hire another craft?'

The wherryman rolled his eyes. 'I was only trying to do me Christian duty, Scholar. If you wants to get your throat cut in a dark alley, or anything else cut for that matter, then don't say I didn't warn you.'

'If that fate befalls me I doubt I'll be in a fit state to blame anyone,' the Apothecary answered succinctly, and took to staring out across the wide stretch of waterway, thinking, as they cast off, that today it resembled the ocean more than a river with its plumed waves and churning blue reaches.

Yet there was a certain truth in what the waterman had said, for John had chosen for the rendezvous with his old friend Samuel Swann, one of the most extraordinary and notorious areas of London. Frequented by sailors and riverfolk, Wapping was full of taverns and brothels, halls where mariners danced with slatternly women, and dens in which opium, a powder produced from poppies and a substance which John used in the process of healing, was smoked. But like all localities of dubious reputation, Wapping held a certain fascination and it was considered *de rigueur* by the *beau monde* to visit the place at least once in order to see for oneself the unimaginable way in which the maritime fraternity lived. To say nothing of tasting some of its lowlife pleasures.

Pulling into mid-stream, the wherryman, who was undoubtedly foul but ferociously strong, strove against the unfavourable tide, rowing his passenger past Lime, Dung and Timber Wharves to where St Paul's dominated the landscape.

John gazed upwards. 'What a truly beautiful building it is, especially from this river view.'

The waterman shrugged. 'It means little to me, Scholar, seeing it every day.'

John nodded but did not reply, his attention now caught by the south bank of the river, these days consisting mostly of tenter grounds, flat spaces used for stretching cloth by means of securing the material to the earth with tenterhooks. However, this bank had once had a livelier reputation and some of the places of entertainment so popular in the previous century were still visible. The Apothecary, whose very profession was dedicated to the relief rather than the inflicting of pain, turned his eyes away with a shudder from the Old Bear Gardens, where wretched animals had once endured the agony of baiting.

Directly before him lay London Bridge, dating back to the twelfth century and one of the wonders of the realm. Standing on eighteen arches, its double row of shops and houses perched higgledy-piggledy upon its stone back, journeying under it was a known test of both nerve and skill. Timid passengers were inclined to land at Old Swan Stairs on the north bank and rejoin their boat below the bridge. But John, relishing the adventure, clung on hard as the wherry crashed through the roaring cataracts formed by the arches, and almost enjoyed being soundly washed as the foam drenched through to his skin.

Now the whole mood of the river changed, for between the Bridge and Greenwich lay one of the most important shipping basins in the world. Eight thousand vessels lay at anchor in this reach of the Thames, to say nothing of the lighters, bumboats and other craft which serviced them. To add to the confusion, colliers bearing coal and barges bringing produce to the capital competed for space on the crowded waterway. Indeed, at the Legal Quays, where all dutiable cargo was obliged to unload under regulations dating from Elizabethan times, shipping formed a queue that stretched for a mile. And it was into this extraordinary maritime mêlée that the Apothecary now plunged as the wherryman skilfully negotiated his way past the Quays and the Custom House where the mighty masted sailing ships clustered close together.

Passing beside the grim edifice of the Tower of London, John stared thoughtfully at Iron Gate Stairs, situated directly below the Iron Gate to the east of the fortress. It was here that immigrants fleeing from persecution or starvation landed, making their way into the ghettos around the Tower. The poor Jews, often the Ashkenaze, lived in Poor Jewry Lane, while the richer Sephardi had their own quarter around the Guildhall, further west. Hungry Irish also made their way into London through this same entrance. A sad reflection of the harshness of the times.

The Apothecary felt himself growing introspective even at the contemplation of so much poverty and despair, no mood for such a celebratory day as this one, and forced himself into conversation with the wherryman to lift his spirits.

'Do you live in Wapping, by any chance?'

'No, Scholar. I'm from Redriff, me. And what about you? Do you hail from the City?'

'No, from Soho. Nassau Street, to be precise. Do you know it?'

The waterman shook his head. 'No, too far inland for me. So what were you doing at Black Friars Stairs today?'

'I had attended the Court of Assistants. I'm an apothecary.'

'I guessed as much, Scholar. Though I can't say you look the part.'

'Oh? What should apothecaries look like?'

4

'Not like you,' answered the wherryman, and chortled that this scampish young man with his dark red curls peeping from beneath his crooked wig, his vivid blue eyes and irregular smile, should be a member of the profession usually associated with sombre dress and grey beards.

'I see,' said John, and did not know whether to be pleased or annoyed.

They were fast approaching the bend in the river and the wherryman pulled with all his might, striving against the wind and tide as they approached Execution Dock Stairs, the place where pirates were put to death, their corpses left to dangle in the breeze as a warning to others. Thirty years before John had been born, in 1701, Captain Kidd had been hanged on this very spot. Apparently the execution had been so mismanaged that Kidd could quite easily have escaped but was so full of liquor, presumably imbibed in order to keep his courage up, that he was unable to move when the opportunity presented itself.

'Is it much further?' the Apothecary asked.

'No, Scholar. I'll land you at the sixth set of stairs from here. They are built right by the tavern and will lead you straight to it.'

John consulted the fob watch which his father, Sir Gabriel Kent, had given him for his twenty-first birthday three years earlier. 'I see I'm somewhat early for my appointment.'

The wherryman gave an evil leer. 'Then stroll about, Scholar. You're sure to find many things that will interest you. Wapping High Street, now, there's a place that might tickle your fancy.'

'I've heard about it,' John answered, 'and I think I'll wait until my friend joins me.'

The wherryman grinned, busy with his oars as he pulled into a landing stage from which rose a flight of wooden steps. Beside these steps and jutting out over the water was the place John had come to visit. The Devil's Tavern, once a timber-framed country house but now an inn frequented by river people, thieves and smugglers, loomed above him. Standing up, John reached for his purse and gave the waterman a generous tip on top of his fare. What he lacked in charm, the fellow had more than made up for by his tremendous effort.

The waterman bit the coin John had given him, then rumbled a laugh. 'Take care, Scholar. There's much that's been lost within those walls. Purses, watches, jewels, virginity – even life.'

5

John smiled his crooked smile. 'I'll guard everything that I still posess, never fear.' Then he set off to climb the rickety steps.

He had been bobbing like a seagull on the surface for so long that his land legs had deserted him, and he could still feel the motion of the river as he made the somewhat treacherous ascent. In fact so strong was the sensation that he had to lean against the wall of the inn momentarily in order to regain his balance. The feel of its surface was cold and clammy to his touch, obviously where the spume thrown by the tide had hit it, and it was as much as John could do to conquer a sudden moment of irrational fear. Telling himself not to be foolish, he shook his head and looked around to get his bearings.

To his left ran Wapping High Street, that infamous thoroughfare of vice, while to the Apothecary's right was a seedy alley called Fox Lane. Directly in front of him, however, John could see some gardens and a church spire. Though very far indeed from being pious, the Apothecary decided that a house of religion might well be the safest place in which to while away an hour's waiting time, rather than risk wandering alone through Wapping's festering streets. Guessing that the church must be the famous St Paul's, Shadwell, known even as far away as Nassau Street as 'the Church of the Sea Captains' and therefore worth a visit, John felt in his pocket for his pistol, a necessary precaution in such a dubious locality, and strode out in the general direction of the spire.

Fox Lane widened out, turning from a mean alley to a sizeable walkway running beside both a cooper's and a timberyard. Then it grew positively pleasant and became a path between some gardens and the back of the churchyard. It was at this moment, as John walked on, enjoying the greenery, that the mighty wind, dormant for a while, gusted so heartily that the Apothecary found himself practically blown round the building and in through the pillared entrance. Rescuing his hat, attempting escape once more, John straightened his apparel and went inside.

Extremely interested in the church's maritime connections, the Apothecary stared about him, hoping to find evidence of the great mariners in their place of worship. He even took a few bold steps down the aisle, only to pull himself up short. For he was not alone in the church of St Paul's. Greatly to his embarrassment, the Apothecary saw that he had inadvertently interrupted a wedding. Somewhat flushed, he hastily took a place in a back pew on the left-hand side of the church, the side traditionally occupied by the family and friends of the bride, and attempted to become invisible, staring into his lap in an ostrich-like manner.

It was the sound of crying that first attracted his attention to the fact that all was not as it should be. Above the coughing and shuffling of the congregation, not very many to judge by the noise, rose the plaintive wail of a weeping woman. Raising his eyes, John allowed himself a good hard stare at the bridal party and was quite shocked to see that other than for the bride herself and an older woman, presumably her mother, he was the only person sitting on the left-hand side of the church. Of the bridegroom there was absolutely no sign, though a tall thin figure clearly dressed in his best suit, a fine affair in lavender silk, sat miserably crouched in the front right-hand pew, his head bowed and his hands clasped between his knees. This, John took it, must be the bridegroom's witness, also kept waiting.

The parson, meanwhile, very red in the face and obviously extremely flustered, was stationed before the altar, Bible in hand. In between frantic glances at the church door, he occasionally muttered soothing words to the hysterical young woman, fast disintegrating into an inconsolable heap of wretchedness quite incapable of going through a marriage service. With his expressive eyebrows dancing, John took a cautious glance round to see the effect of all this on the other guests.

Confirming his earlier impression, he observed that there was only a handful of people present, all sitting at the back, clustered together like an unkindness of ravens, clad in starkest black, looking as if they would be more suitable at a funeral than a marriage.

''Sblud!' he muttered beneath his breath, and would have studied these freakish visitors more closely, had not the sound of the priest clearing his throat attracted his attention once more to the front. The cleric, plainly much discomfited, had produced a fob watch from beneath his cassock and was staring at it with furrowed brow. He had obviously set himself some kind of time limit before he declared the ceremony null and void and sent everyone on their way. And now, it would seem, that time was up. Heaving a great sigh, the unhappy man shook his head in the direction of the bride and closed his Bible with a thump. Behind him, John heard the definite swell of a muted cry of triumph drown the pitiful sobs of the young woman as she rose to her feet and, leaning heavily on the arm of her attendant, made her way from the church, head bowed.

As she passed by where he sat, the Apothecary observed that despite the fact she was by now unattractively flushed and her eyes were both reddened and sore, the deserted bride was an extremely pretty girl of no more than twenty-five, her figure neat and pertly breasted, her hair a glorious colour, pale yet rich, the shade of wheat. Whoever had jilted her, John caught himself thinking, had to be mad.

The other guests, however, clearly did not share his opinion. No sooner was the unfortunate young creature outside the door than they burst into excited conversation, laughing heartily, one or two of them, whilst the others chattered away cheerfully. It would appear that they had won the day, that the non-appearance of the bridegroom – clearly a friend or relative of theirs – was exactly what they wanted. Still keeping his seat, the Apothecary watched them go out.

Leading the way and having much deference paid to her in the process, was an elderly woman leaning upon a stick, a middle-aged female, presumably a relative, fluttering at her elbow. Next came a monstrous beau, past his best as regards years, but for all that dressed within an inch of his life despite his sober black garb. As he went out he caught John's enquiring eye and flashed a sudden smile, adding a winsome wave of his fingers as if he had known the Apothecary for years.

A rugged young man, somewhat square of shoulder, followed, escorting a small bird-like woman, with darting brown eyes. Then came the last to leave, a redheaded beauty of striking good looks – or rather two of them! John stared in open admiration at a pair of twins, as alike as brother and sister could possibly be, and quite the most attractive couple of siblings he had ever set his eyes on. As soon as the last of this extraordinary black-clad party had gone, the gentleman in lavender scuttled out of the church, looking neither to the right nor left of him. John had one quick glimpse of a hawkish man with dark arresting features as the bridegroom's witness hurried past.

Outside, the wind was still gusting furiously, tugging at the garments of the poor little bride as she clambered into her carriage, lugged the older woman up after her, and set off at great speed towards the City. Meanwhile, the others were also getting into their conveyances, still laughing and joking as if they did not have a care in the world. The Apothecary, frankly amazed by the entire spectacle, stood and stared until the last of them had disappeared from his sight.

'Well, that's a sorry business,' said a voice at his ear.

John, who had a range of suitable expressions which he assumed according to the occasion, put on his honest, puzzled face and turned round. Standing beside him, shaking his head as the last of the carriages vanished into the distance, was an individual whom the Apothecary took by his dress to be the churchwarden.

'Indeed it is,' he answered in a sorrowful tone. 'In fact I've never seen anything quite like it. I am but a visitor to this parish, Sir, and entered the church for its fame as the sea captains' place of prayer. So do please tell me what is afoot.'

The churchwarden shook his head once more. 'It's a jilting, Sir, in plain language. The bride and her mother have been waiting this last hour but the groom did not appear. His witness knew nothing of his whereabouts, having arranged to meet him here. A sorry business for all concerned.'

'Who is the groom? Do you know?'

'A local ship owner I believe, born in the parish of Shadwell. I do not have his name. The wedding was arranged in something of a hurry and I was therefore not asked to assist.'

'Is that common?'

'When the ceremony is a quiet one, yes. There's many a runaway comes here before they sail for the Colonies.'

'The priest does not object?'

The churchwarden sighed. 'He must eke out his miserable stipend somehow or other.'

John nodded, thinking that St Paul's, Shadwell, no doubt provided its incumbent with a good living and that conducting runaway marriages would hardly be necessary to make ends meet. However, that was not the affair at issue.

'Who were all those extraordinary people in black?' he asked, his look bewildered.

The churchwarden lowered his voice, though there was not another soul in sight. 'The bridegroom's family, I believe. It seems they got wind of the match and came here to make unpleasantness.' He fingered his chin. 'Perhaps that is why the groom did not appear. Perhaps he wanted to avoid a scene.'

'In that case he would surely have informed his bride and witness.'

'Yes, you're right of course. It is quite inexplicable.' The churchwarden raised his hat. 'Well, I must be on my way. Good day to you, Sir.'

John returned his salute, clutching his headgear in a firm grasp. 'Good day, Sir. It has been most enjoyable speaking to you.'

Turning up his coat against the wind, the churchwarden headed off in the direction of the path, now dark with shadow, and John, glancing upwards, saw that the sun had sunk low in the heavens. Looking at his watch, he realised that there was no time left in which to explore St Paul's, in fact he had only fifteen minutes to spare before his appointment with Samuel. Intrigued by all that he had seen and wondering how the poor bride was faring in the face of such a catastrophe, the Apothecary retraced his steps and hurried back in the direction of The Devil's Tavern.

It was the noise that first struck John. Even as he left Fox Lane and crossed to where the door of the inn opened on to the street, a fierce discord of sound was already assaulting his ears. Several voices were raised in a song of some foreign tongue, distantly a woman was screaming, though whether with laughter or fear it was difficult to tell, while at the tops of their lungs two men were arguing ferociously. With a delicious mixture of trepidation and eagerness, John pushed the door open and went inside.

The downstairs area consisted of a long low room at the far end of which were two windows looking out over the Thames. The bar, or what the Apothecary could see of it for the press of bodies standing close by, appeared to be made of pewter and stood upon barrels. This highly unusual feature ran the length of the building and was attended by a rough looking fellow with a beard. Looking round for his old friend and simultaneously guarding his pocket, John took stock of his surroundings. The air he was breathing was thick with tobacco smoke, the smell of drink, of bodies, and above all the river. The light was dim, thrown by tallow candles. In a dark corner a sailor was making love to a slut. It was one of the most dangerous and exciting environments into which he had ever ventured, and the Apothecary relished the prospect of the wild evening ahead.

'Over here!' called a great voice, and peering through the gloom John saw that Samuel had arrived ahead of him and had already secured a place, his powerful frame squeezed onto a settle beside some sailors, who were regarding him with a great deal of suspicion.

'Coming,' John shouted in reply and made his way through the throng, still guarding his valuables, for beyond doubt thieves and pickpockets, eager for pickings, would be mingling amongst this crowd of riverside scum.

Samuel stood up, dislodging a mariner as he did so. 'There's very little room. Do you want to stay here?'

'Certainly I do.' The Apothecary stared round. 'Look, there are two places by that table.'

And he made a dive to where a wooden bench, very old and dishevelled but still standing, occupied a space beside a table in front of one of the windows and comfortably close to a cheerful fire. On the table a man lay sprawled, dead drunk.

Samuel looked doubtful. 'Do we really want him for company?'

'Of course.' his friend answered. 'He'll be far less trouble than anyone else in this unruly mob.'

'How very true,' Samuel answered, and eased his broad build onto the protesting bench.

He was a very powerful young person, tall and largely made, and extremely handy to have around in times of trouble. As yet he still carried no excess fat, though this would undoubtedly gather with the passing of the years, but none the less Samuel gave the impression of girth and size, and always reminded John of a tower or windmill. And now that impression was endorsed as Samuel Swann threw a vast arm round his friend's shoulders.

'Well, my dear chap, how did it go?'

'I've been made Free,' answered John, pumping Samuel's hand. 'I am a Yeoman of the Worshipful Society of Apothecaries. And not before time as you well know.'

Samuel responded by giving John a slap on the back that sent him reeling. 'What splendid news. I wonder if they serve champagne here.'

'Bound to. The place is always teeming with quality folk come to see how the other half lives. A clever landlord will cater for their tastes, sure as fate.'

'Besides, it's an inn as well as a tavern. People stay here, waiting to board ship. I'll go and order some.'

11

And Samuel rose to his feet, looming over the assembled company, and made his way through the throng towards the pewter bar.

The drunken man let out a terrible belch and a voice said in John's ear, 'Disgusting pig. Could we not roll him onto the floor?'

The Apothecary turned to see who addressed him and found himself staring into the prettiest pair of blue eyes he had seen for a long time, the colour of forget-me-nots and fringed by a pair of long jet lashes. Their owner, a neat comely little thing, simply dressed and smelling strongly of the sea, gave him a dimpling smile. John immediately guessed her to be one of the fraternity who haunted the banks of the Thames alongside the watermen and sailors, taking their craft down to the Estuary in order to fish.

'I think,' he said, rising and making her a small polite bow, 'that if we wake him up it could be dangerous, for who knows what state of anger he might be in. Might it not be best to let him rot?'

She flashed her eyes, and Samuel, returning with a bottle of champagne and two somewhat rough looking glasses, regarded her with open admiration. 'I don't think I've had the pleasure.'

She stared at him. 'What?'

'I haven't had the pleasure of being presented to you. John . . .'

The Apothecary's mouth curved. 'Miss . . . er . . .?'

'Kitty.' She held out her small workaday hand. 'I'm Kitty Perkins of Wapping. Oyster girl by trade. Evening to you both, gents.'

She descended to the floor where she sat cross-legged at John's feet, such an inelegant move and posture that any person of breeding should have been filled with horror at the sight. Yet, coming from her, there was so much charm about it that both John and Samuel found themselves gazing at her in fascination.

'Like me, do you?' she went on.

'Very much indeed,' the Apothecary answered enthusiastically. 'But are you comfortable down there? Are you sure you wouldn't like my seat?'

'Do have some champagne,' Samuel added, and passed her his glass.

She raised it in a toast. 'Here's long life to you, gents.' She drank deeply. 'Reckon you've never met a working woman before, other than for your servants.'

'On the contrary,' John answered, grinning crookedly. 'The ladies of my acquaintance nearly all have some occupation or other.'

Kitty looked at him mischievously over the rim of her glass. 'Indeed? And what work might that be, Sir?'

'My closest female friend was once a card sharp and gamester,' he answered, amused by the astonished expression on her face. 'And amongst my circle there are several actresses.'

Samuel chortled. 'I rather thought Miss Coralie Clive should be described as a friend rather than merely a member of your group.'

'As you are well aware,' John answered severely, 'I have seen little of that lady since Christmas. She has been appearing at Drury Lane a great deal and has had little time for socialising.'

'Ooh!' said Kitty knowingly, and Samuel chuckled once more. 'I'd give her a piece of my mind if I was you.'

The Apothecary instantly felt irritable and could not think why. 'Miss Clive and I do not have that kind of relationship,' he said pompously. 'We are merely people who meet from time to time. I have no right to tell her what to do, nor she me.'

'More's the pity, eh?'

Samuel tactfully changed the subject. 'Where do you get your oysters, Miss Perkins?'

'Kitty to you. I goes down the Estuary and brings 'em back from Essex. Sometimes I gets as far as Whitstable, but it's quite a distance.'

'And do you bring them back by the barrel-load?'

'Yes, and sells 'em all around. I brought a haul in here tonight. Would you like some?'

'I certainly would,' answered John keenly, and stepped up to the bar to put in the order. And it was then that he saw the bridegroom's witness, sitting in a dusky corner, consoling himself with a bottle of brandy. He had changed from his lavender suit and now wore plain grey worsted, but there could be no mistaking his long spare frame and hawkish features. Much intrigued, for it had not occured to him that the man could possibly be local, the Apothecary studied him surreptitiously.

He was about thirty-five years of age, and handsome in his dark saturnine way. He was also, in marked contrast to the rest of the customers, immaculately clean. Looking at his hands, John noticed how long and elegant they were and thought to himself that this man had never done a day's labouring work in his life. Fascinated, he returned to the table, bearing three great plateful of oysters.

'Kitty, you come from Wapping, do you not?' John asked as he sat down.

'Yes,' she answered, finishing her glass of champagne and pouring herself a refill.

'Do you see that man sitting alone over there? The dark one in grey.'

She craned her neck. 'You mean Mr Randolph?'

'I'm not sure who I mean. Is he drinking brandy?'

'Yes.'

'That's the one I want to know about. What can you tell me?'

'His name is Valentine Randolph,' she replied promptly. 'He works for one of the ship owners. I think he manages their office. He lives across the river at Redriff. He rows himself over every day.'

'Redriff?' repeated John, frowning. 'Where *is* that? The waterman referred to it earlier today.'

'It's also known as Rotherhithe,' said Samuel importantly. 'There's quite a pretty fishing village clustered round the church, and one or two expensive properties as well. One of my customers lives there. He had a very fine gold necklace made for his wife's birthday.'

'That's as may be,' Kitty answered spiritedly, 'but we locals call it Redriff. Redhra – sailor. Saxon, see.'

John shook his head. 'No, I don't.' He smiled encouraging. 'Tell me what else you know of Mr Randolph.'

'Nothing really. Like I said, he lives across the river and works in Wapping.'

'Is he a married man?'

She shrugged. 'He could be. Though come to think of it I've never seen him with anyone. In fact most of his family sailed for Virginia a long time ago, leaving him by himself. Reckon he's got no friends.'

'Well, he's got at least one,' John said thoughtfully.

'And who might that be?'

'The missing bridegroom,' the Apothecary answered, and laughed to himself at the perplexed expression on both Kitty and Samuel's faces.

Chapter Two

*I*t had been one of the most exhilarating and colourful nights of John Rawlings's life. As the evening had progressed, the bar of The Devil's Tavern had filled with a motley collection of characters, all quite terrifying in their different ways and therefore tremendously thrilling to watch. Sailors of every nationality, or so it seemed, had leant against the bar, flaxen-haired Scandinavians rubbing shoulders with those of a far more swarthy hue. Pocket divers and cutpurses, clearly on the look out for members of the *beau monde*, cast their eyes over John and Samuel but decided that in their sober garb – John had dressed quietly that day in order to attend the Court of Assistants – they were probably not worth robbing. In one corner a gypsy told fortunes, in another a slut plied her trade, lowlife abounded in plenty. Sitting at their table, feasting on oysters and champagne, the Apothecary and his friend watched it all and were intoxicated by the swashbuckling, insecure atmosphere. The tide had risen while they had been in The Devil's Tavern, so high that, with the driving wind behind it, the water now lashed against the window by which they sat. Staring out into the darkness, looking at the lights of the great ships which rode at anchor, John wondered where they had come from and what their next destination might be, and what great and mysterious cargoes they carried in their holds. Again and again, he felt his eyes drawn to the square rigger which bobbed mid stream directly opposite the hostelry, its lantern lit masts reflecting pale pools of gold on the black waters beneath, wondering who slumbered on board there in its cramped and coffin-like confines.

It was midnight, the hour of dark thoughts, candles were burning low and many of the patrons had gone to their lodging. Still at his feet, Kitty was singing quietly to herself, while Samuel slept, leaning forward on the table, his head a mere few inches away from that of the drunken man. In the thrall of a strange mood, the Apothecary felt as if his soul were flying out over the river enabling him to see the tide falling again, exposing the mud flats which banked the wild waterway on either side. Above him, the sky was a velvet cloak of deepest blue, scattered with sequinned stars. Below, the Thames looked like a tinker's ribbon woven with glittering threads. Then John's head fell forward and he realised that he had been on the point of dropping off to sleep.

Kitty looked up at him slyly. 'You've been dozing and I didn't like to wake you.' She stood up, yawning and stretching her arms over her head. 'Well, I must get to my bed. Do you want to come with me? I promise I'll wash.'

John smiled. 'I'm too tired for such pleasures, alas. Also I need to see my friend gets home safely. For all his size, he's a bit vague when it comes to practical matters.'

Kitty hitched her skirt up so that her ankles were uncluttered for walking. 'Well, I'll say goodbye then. Don't forget, you can usually find me here of an evening and I'd like to drink with you again.' She gave him rather a sad smile, then walked out into the dangerous darkness.

The bearded ruffian came towards them from behind the pewter bar. 'You'd best put up for the night, Sir. There's not many that would row you back on so black and windy a river. And those who might would charge you a pretty fortune.'

The Apothecary nodded. 'Do you have a good room?'

The landlord laughed, an oddly musical sound. 'Aye, good enough for a bride.'

John woke up fully. 'A bride you say?'

'One slept here last night, on her way to her wedding.'

'She was to be married locally?'

'At St Paul's, Sir. But then there's many that do. It's handy for embarkation, you see.'

'You did not know her?'

'No, I'd never seen her before in my life.' The landlord stared at John hard. 'Why do you ask? Was she something to do with you?'

'Nothing at all,' the Apothecary assured him. 'It's just that I have a lively curiosity.' He leant over Samuel and shook him by the shoulder. 'Wake up, old friend. It's time to go to bed.'

His companion leapt to his feet and flailed his arms. 'What's going on? Is there trouble?'

'Not at all,' John answered soothingly. 'It's simply that the hour is so late I have booked a room.'

Samuel returned to consciousness. 'A wise move. I feel fit to drop.'

'You already have,' the Apothecary commented wryly.

'Then that being settled, I'll escort you, gentlemen,' said the bearded landlord, and took up a candle stuck in a bottle from the many that rested on the bar.

It was precisely at that moment that the door leading onto the street swung open and John saw a waterman standing there, dripping wet, soaked through from head to toe.

'Daniel,' gasped the newcomer. 'We needs to borrow the cock fight place, urgent like.'

As if this were some secret code between them, John, suddenly extraordinarily alert, saw the landlord stiffen. 'Where?' he asked.

'Bottom of the stairs.'

'Well, I'll just see these gentlemen off to their room and then I'll join you. Have a brandy, you look drenched, man.'

'It's an evil night,' answered the waterman in a different tone, and the Apothecary had the distinct impression that he and Samuel had been surveyed, put down as town folk, and that nothing further would be said in front of them.

'Come on Mr Swann,' he ordered over-loudly. 'We must let this good man have some rest.'

'Yes indeed,' his friend answered heartily, clearly aware that something strange was taking place.

'You have one of the rooms overlooking the river, Sir. The best in the house,' and Daniel led the way upwards, his candle throwing dancing shadows on the wall.

The wooden staircase, well worn with generations of ascending feet, swung round on itself, then continued upward by means of a spindly narrow stairway leading to the top floor. When The Devil's Tavern had first been built in the reign of Henry VIII, it had served a turn as a timber-framed private riverside residence, and evidence of that was clearly revealed as John and Samuel made their way up to what would once have been the servants' quarters, now transformed to bedrooms. Yet the chamber into which the landlord showed them was unexpectedly well furnished and neat, albeit small. It occurred to John that many of the tavern's guests were members of the *beau monde* too drunk to return to their homes until morning, and this room had been specially set aside for that type of visitor. Those, and eager young brides of course.

John looked round him for any sign of the former occupant, but the room had obviously been cleaned since the woman had departed and there was nothing left that could give any indication as to her identity. Removing his coat, the Apothecary was just about to strip down to his small clothes when from outside the building came a faint but unusual sound, a sound which immediately caught his attention. Somebody, or perhaps even two persons, were dragging something heavy up an outside stairway which John had not even known existed. A staircase that was quite definitely not Pelican Stairs which lay to the right, whilst this noise came from the left.

Turning to Samuel who had instantly crashed down onto the bed, John motioned him to listen, but to no avail. His friend was already snoring, mouth wide. With a small click of annoyance, John went to the window and stood close behind it in order to overhear as much as he could.

There was the low murmur of voices and the muffled dragging continued to the top of the stairs. Then came the sound of the object, whatever it was, being deposited in the room exactly below the one in which John stood listening. Knowing that the tavern and the riverside were both a haunt of smugglers, he assumed that contraband had been brought ashore and was being secreted away within. Certain that he was spending this night within a nest of villains, the Apothecary lay back down on the bed, though sleep eluded him.

On two previous occasions he had worked with John Fielding, the phenomenal blind magistrate known to both the underworld and the *beau monde* as the Blind Beak, to help him bring a murderer to justice. And now the habits he had learned at the hands of such a great master were beginning to exert their influence. Supposing it was not contraband that had been carried so laboriously up the stairs. Supposing it was a human being, wounded and in need of his help. If that were so then he had no right to be lying on his bed considering the matter. He should be investigating the source of the disturbance. With a slight groan, John got up and padded to the door in his stockinged feet.

Like many of his fellow Englishmen, the Apothecary had no dislike of smugglers and had, indeed, purchased smuggled goods in his time, tea amongst them. Further, he had commissioned a sailor to bring in from those exotic lands across the sea, the bitter sweet nuts of the moringa tree, the oil obtained from which was so

18

useful in treating everything from ears to cramps caused by wounds. John had also ordered his contact to fetch him the zizyphus or Christ thorn which, when mixed with other ingredients, was an unbeatable remedy for cooling the anus. No duty had been paid on these imports and the whole matter had been treated as a private transaction. Therefore, it was no desire to peach or inform that led John to creep down the cramped stairs in search of what the watermen had brought in, merely a need to satisfy himself that there was nobody in distress.

By now the tavern was quiet, not a sound from the main room below, even Samuel's snores silenced. Aware of the floorboards creaking as he moved along, the Apothecary made his way cautiously downward, his only light the candle he was carrying. The attic steps petered out and swung round, joining the main staircase. Not quite sure in which direction to go, the Apothecary turned and saw a room leading off almost directly opposite, a long heavily panelled room with a large square window overlooking the river. Close to this was a door leading on to an open porch and a wooden balcony beyond. From outside the lights of the moored ships, coupled with some faint moonlight, threw a glow of luminescence and aided by this, John stepped within.

At first he could see little, just the vague outlines of a few crude benches, all pushed well back, whilst two trestles with something lying on them stood in a far corner. There was a pungent smell of sweat in the air and it suddenly occurred to John that this room was used not for fighting birds but fighting men. He remembered now that during the course of the evening there had been muffled shouts and cheers coming from upstairs, and had thought at the time that somewhere a bare knuckle contest between sailors was taking place. This, then, would appear to be its location. And it would also appear to be the hiding place of the contraband. Half smiling, John went towards the table to see what the watermen had brought in.

It was as he stepped closer, the flame of his candle wavering in a draught from the window, that the first frisson of fear crept the length of his spine. There was something odd about the shape of the cloth covered object that lay on the makeshift table, something that seemed all too alarmingly recognisable. Suddenly afraid of what he might be about to see, John Rawlings held his candle high and plucked the concealing sheet to one side.

How he did not cry out, even prepared for the worst as he was, he never afterwards knew. For a pair of open eyes looked up at him, eyes that appeared to stare straight into his with a dark secretive glare all their own. Catching his breath, the Apothecary put out his hand and touched the freezing cheek, also exposed by the removal of the cloth, then withdrew his fingers fast, aware that he was alone in the cockfighting room of The Devil's Tavern with a dead man. Controlling an urge to run away and fetch Samuel, John put the candle where it would throw most light and thought of the words of his Master, the apothecary to whom he had been apprenticed. He had taught his pupil that only the living can harm the living, the dead can never do so. Having proven the truth of this in the past, John now composed himself and set about seeking even the faintest signs of life.

There was no heartbeat, no pulse, no breath. The man had been dead for hours and, judging by his saturated garments, had drowned in the river Thames. Yet despite this, John continued with his examination, wondering if there was anything to be discovered about the man which might show how he came to be in the water in the first place. Finding another couple of candles and lighting them with the flame from his own, the Apothecary set to work.

He was looking at the body of a man aged about sixty, perhaps a little more. Yet a good looking fellow for all his advancing years. Delicately undoing the corpse's coat and waistcoat, John eased up the shirt and saw that the body bore many abrasions, presumably caused by knocking against things as it floated in the water. However, the man's flesh was firm and not as lined as he would have expected. Similarly, the legs, though grazed, showed little sign of veining and the genitals seemed healthy. So it was not an obvious illness that had driven this man to suicide, if, indeed, suicide it had been and not accident. Somewhat puzzled, the Apothecary was just about to draw the corpse's clothes back decently, when his attention was caught by a bulge in the coat's inside pocket. Feeling rather like a grave robber, John drew out a pocket book, dampened by the water but still intact for all its time in the river. Holding it up to the light, he turned out the contents.

There was a bag of money containing quite a considerable amount, this attached to the inside of the book. There were also several pieces of paper, none of them of any particular interest. But it was the final document to be unearthed, neatly folded and still legible despite its soggy condition, that made John's flesh creep. It was a licence to wed.

Once again in his mind's eye, the Apothecary saw that cruel black wedding party, sitting so stark and grim in the back of St Paul's, Shadwell. Could this be the missing bridegroom that he was presently examining? Bringing the licence close to the candle, John read the words on the damp paper, protected as it had been by being tucked within the pocket book. Sir William Hartfield, Kt of St James's Square and Kirby Hall, Bethnal Green, and Miss Amelia Lambourn of Queens Square. Thinking about that evil group of guests cast a cruel suspicion in the Apothecary's mind, and he rapidly searched the body for signs of robbery, as if to give the lie to his own unpleasant thoughts. The dead man's rings and watch, presuming he wore them, were missing. But his jewelled snuff and pill boxes, concealed in an inside pocket, were still in place. Sir William Hartfield, if this indeed was the identity of the body, had not met his end at the hands of cutpurses and footpadders, for they would have removed everything. Feeling deathly cold, the Apothecary turned his attention to the corpse's head to see if any clues as to why he had drowned lay there.

There was no damage on the handsome old face but the victim had sustained a blow to the brow, probably striking something in the river, possibly as he fell in. Closing the eyes, still staring in that unnerving fashion, John brought one of the candles nearer and examined the mark. Though he had a thick growth of white hair at the back, the man was balding, and had shaved what hair he had left on top to facilitate the wearing of his wig. And it was on this bald area, just above the temple, that the clout had been sustained. The Apothecary peered closely, wishing he had his quizzing glass with him.

All the blood that such a blow would have caused had been washed away by the water and it was impossible to tell from the wound what had produced it. Very gently, John touched the place with his long and sensitive fingers. It had been a hard knock for there was a marked indentation, he could feel it distinctly. Drawing so close that the dead man was only an inch away from him, John shone the candle directly onto the injury.

There was a pattern in it, of that much he was certain. Whatever had crushed the dead man's skull had borne a design of some sort and the shape of it had marked the balding head, a phenomenon that John knew of but had never actually witnessed before.

'God's mercy!' the Apothecary whispered aloud as he strove to see what it was.

And then everything became clear as, just for a moment, the vague outline took shape and he knew, for certain, that this man had been struck by a human agency. For there on his head, imprinted on the flesh, was the faint contour of an ornamental fox's head. The dead man had been smashed by a stick bearing such an object as its handle and had probably, if the force required to leave such a mark were anything to go by, been dead when he entered the water. With a sense almost of resignation, the Apothecary came to terms with the fact that he was looking at a case of murder.

Questions formed in his mind. Could the watermen themselves be guilty of such a crime? But, if so, why leave the body lying here so openly, not even bothering to close the door of the room? Surely, John thought, they had simply found the corpse floating and had brought it to the shore. In fact they probably had an arrangement with the landlord to leave anyone discovered in the river in this very spot once the hours of darkness had fallen. Certain that he was going to be called upon to remember every detail, John made one final careful study of the dead man, painting a picture of the scene in his mind. Then, having carefully placed the marriage licence in his own pocket, the Apothecary blew out the candles and went back to his room.

As was to be expected, John slept fitfully and woke as soon as the first slivers of daylight shone through the gaps in the closed curtains. Just for one blissful moment he lay quite still, listening to the sounds of the mighty river and the bustling people who inhabited its banks, then he was up, splashing his face with cold water and calling to Samuel to wake. The Goldsmith groaned blearily.

'What is it? What's going on?'

'Oh God's dear life,' John answered impatiently. 'Do you spend all your time sleeping? If you go on like that you'll be unconscious for more years than you spend awake.'

His friend looked at him quizzically.

'Now mark this,' the Apothecary continued. 'While you were couched supine, snoring like a grampus and resembling nothing so much as a bumboat becalmed, I was examining a body.'

Samuel sat bolt upright. 'A body?'

'Yes,' said John, and told him all that had taken place.

They struggled into their clothes in a mad kind of race which the Apothecary won. 'I'm off for a second look,' he announced, heading for the door. 'Are you coming with me?'

'I hope I'm up to such a sight before breakfast,' Samuel answered, fastening his cravat.

'Of course you are. Now come along,' John ordered firmly, and taking his friend by the elbow propelled him down the spindly staircase to the room in which cockfighting had once been the order of the day.

Beyond the window the mighty waterway leapt and danced in the early morning wind, and the Apothecary saw that the square rigger which had been moored mid-stream was preparing to sail with the tide. Matelots swarmed in the rigging and the canvas was swelling in the freshening breeze. The sight was one of such exuberance that momentarily he went to the window and forgot all about the fact that he was in the presence of death.

'I love this river,' he said, almost to himself, and then Samuel brought him back to grim reality.

'Where's the corpse?'

John turned. 'Over there, on that table.' But even as he spoke his voice was dying away.

'What's the matter?' asked his friend, reading the Apothecary's expression.

In consternation, John seized him by the arm. 'It's gone, Samuel. By God's holy wounds, the body has gone.'

They stared at one another in amazement, though there could be no doubt about it. The dead man and even the cloth that had covered him, were no longer there. The table was empty.

Chapter Three

*D*espite the horrors of the night, neither John Rawlings nor Samuel Swann found themselves to be impaired in any way as regards appetite, indeed both consumed a great deal of pickled meat and fresh oysters, to say nothing of quite a lot of beer, at the breakfast served to them before they departed the mysterious confines of The Devil's Tavern. Then, having settled their account with the pot boy, the landlord being mysteriously unavailable, they stepped out into the colourful world of Wapping by day. But instead of heading for the river, John turned back in the direction of St Paul's, Shadwell.

'Where are we going?' asked Samuel, surprised.

'I want to show this soggy but legible certificate to the incumbent of St Paul's. Sam, I have the strangest feeling that that sinister wedding I told you of and the disappearing body are somehow connected. Because if they are not it is the most extraordinary coincidence that the corpse should be carrying a licence to marry.'

Samuel nodded. 'Too great a coincidence for my liking. I reckon that the bridegroom did not appear because he was already dead.'

'I agree. Now, let it be hoped that the priest knew the groom by sight and can describe him for us.'

As luck would have it, the vicar of St Paul's was already present when they arrived, appearing to be engaged in the humble task of dusting, a fact which John found more than a little endearing. He straightened as he heard the sound of approaching feet and dropped the duster into a pew, tugging at his cassock and snatching up a Bible which he hastily opened as if he had been studying it all along.

'Blessed are the meek,' he intoned.

'Blessed indeed,' responded John, and advanced on the cleric, his expression that of an earnest good citizen.

'Good morning, my friend,' said the vicar heartily. 'Are you new to the parish? I do not seem to know your face.'

The Apothecary decided on the expediency of a minor lie. 'Sir, I am actually present on the business of Mr John Fielding of the Public Office, Bow Street, and in that respect I *am* new to the parish. So may I just say how very much I admire your beautiful church, known as that of the sea captains I believe. In fact so much do I admire it that I will not hurry away when Mr Fielding's affairs are concluded.'

The priest cleared his throat. 'And what business could Mr Fielding possibly have with me?'

John looked grave and Samuel bowed his head. 'I wonder if you would mind looking at this, Sir.' And from his pocket he produced the wedding licence that he had found on the corpse.

The vicar took it with hands that trembled slightly. He was balding, pink and inclined to be porky but for all that obviously nurtured a sensitive soul. 'God bless us all!' he exclaimed as he read it. 'Where did this come from?'

The Apothecary's countenance was that of a professional mourner. 'I am sorry to be the bearer of ill tidings, Sir, but it was found on the body of a man pulled from the Thames last night.'

The priest blanched and sat down rapidly, dropping the bible onto the floor. 'Surely it could not have been that of Sir William himself?'

John shook his head. 'I don't know. Would you care to describe him for me?'

'I'll try,' answered the poor man, with such a sad note in his voice that the Apothecary found himself producing his smelling salts from an inside pocket. 'Here, inhale these,' he said gently. 'They will make you feel better.'

'I simply cannot believe any harm could have befallen him,' the distressed cleric went on, sniffing the salts dejectedly. 'He was a benefactor of the church and a good citizen. But when he did not attend his own wedding I began to have a sense that all might not be well.'

John felt a thrill of cold seize his spine as he realised that his guess had been correct.

'He did not attend his own wedding?' repeated Samuel, speaking for the first time.

'No, Sir. It was to have been here, late yesterday afternoon. But Sir William did not come.'

'Is he of this parish then?' Samuel continued, impressing John with his alertness.

'Not exactly, though he does have an office here. Sir William owns a fleet of ships, all of which sail from Wapping. But he was born in Shadwell, you know, and baptised by one of my predecessors. Therefore, I consider him to be one of my parishoners even though he does not reside amongst us.'

'And why did he choose to be wed here rather than nearer his home?' the Apothecary asked, administering the salts once more.

'Because he wanted his marriage kept secret,' answered the priest, his voice a whisper. 'There was family disapproval, or so he informed me. But they found out about it, you know. The church was full of them yesterday. In fact Mr Challon – he is Sir William's secretary and therefore known to me – told me on the very eve of the wedding that he thought Sir William's elderly mother might make a scene.'

'How ghastly!'

'Indeed so.'

'But they did not have that satisfaction,' put in Samuel.

'No,' said the priest, and wiped away a tear.

Genuinely sorry for him, John said, 'Sir, I do not wish to cause you further pain but I must ascertain whether the dead man and Sir William are one and the same. The body I saw, in my official capacity, was that of a handsome man in his sixties. He had a bald head, though with some white hair at the back. He was about five feet and eight inches in height and of a medium build. I believe that his eyes were blue. He carried a silver snuff box, very finely made and richly decorated with an emerald which, to judge by its clarity, probably originated in the Indies. Is . . . was . . . that Sir William?'

The priest straightened his shoulders and got a grip on his emotions. 'Yes, it was.'

'Then I am afraid your benefactor is dead, Sir.'

The vicar nodded his head and said very simply, 'Then I shall pray for his immortal soul.'

It had often been the habit of Sir Gabriel Kent, retired merchant of the City of London and man of elegance, to sally forth on a fine spring day and take the air for the sake of his health. And today being so capricious a March morning, with a merry breeze teasing the budding trees and pale sunshine splashing the walls of the houses in Nassau Street, Sir Gabriel called for his valet shortly

27

after breakfast in order to help him prepare for the occasion of progressing abroad.

As ever, Sir Gabriel wore clothes fashioned in black and white, never displaying colour upon his person as he did not consider it good taste to do so. On festive occasions or great fêtes, Sir Gabriel permitted silver to replace the paler shade, but this was as far as he was prepared to go in the interests of celebration. However, to his son John's addiction to high fashion and rainbow hues he was prepared to turn an indulgent blind eye, as he also was to the foolish escapades of youth into which his adopted offspring was prone to blunder from time to time.

Standing now before the mirror in his dressing room, Sir Gabriel fastened the cornelian clasp of his cloak – he conceded to colour in his jewellery – then asked his servant to affix to his head his second best tricorne. This was no easy matter for Sir Gabriel had a somewhat old-fashioned taste in wigs and still wore a towering three-storey affair, often seen in the reign of the Stuart kings but not so much in that of the Hanoverians. However, as Sir Gabriel was not the sort of man who would ever allow his hat to fly off in public, a masterpiece of pinning was a necessity, and this the valet undertook, muttering silently as he did so. Eventually, though, all was ready and Sir Gabriel, having been handed his great stick by a footman, stepped from his house and proceeded down Nassau Street in the direction of Leicester Fields and, ultimately, the far boundaries of St James's Park.

He was a formidable sight, standing tall and straight despite the fact that he was only a few weeks away from his seventy-first birthday. And though he may have leant a little more heavily on his stick than he had twenty years earlier, Sir Gabriel did not quibble with this and accepted it as part of life's natural progression.

At the far end of Leicester Fields stood Leicester House, usually occupied by the Princes of Wales, from which they set up a rival camp to the court of their fathers, whom they customarily detested. Now, however, there was a far more compliant prince. George II's grandson, another George, a pleasant but vulnerable young man, had on the death of his father, Frederick, Prince of Wales, become the heir. Staring up at the imposing building, Sir Gabriel hoped that George would continue to lodge there, if only in order to escape the attentions of his domineering mother and her lover, the Earl of Bute.

Striding briskly, Sir Gabriel passed William Hogarth's house, which stood at number thirty, and was just thinking how pleasant the walk was and how well the valet had secured his tricorne against the wind, when a hoydenish figure, hatless and with its stockings not neatly connected to the knee of its breeches, turned into the Fields from St Martin's Street, and began to run in a manner that Sir Gabriel could only think of as uncontrolled.

'Really,' he muttered beneath his breath, 'what are things coming to? Has no one ever explained to these people the meaning of the word deportment.'

And then he stopped in his tracks, a look of astonishment on his face, as the figure drew closer and revealed itself to be that of his son, out of breath, dishevelled and in need of a shave.

'Merciful heavens!' exclaimed Sir Gabriel. 'My dear child, what has happened to you?'

'I've been made Free,' answered John Rawlings, with a crooked smile. 'And I am also in search of a dead man.'

Sir Gabriel took him firmly by the elbow. 'I think we had better go straight home and then you can explain yourself further. There is no question of your opening the shop in that state.'

John nodded. 'This morning I had what could only be described as an extremely primitive wash. What with freezing water, no razor, and the thought of a body I had come across on the previous evening, a body, I might add, after which I am now in hot pursuit, it is surprising that I look as good as I do. So my dear and elegant Papa, please bear with me and take that disapproving expression from your face.'

As always, Sir Gabriel weakened, finding it impossible to be annoyed when his son cajoled him. 'I'll say nothing further,' he answered, 'merely that when you have completed your toilette I would like to be told all that took place on such a momentous day as you seem to have experienced.'

'I can think of nothing I would like to do more,' John answered cheerfully. 'Now why don't you take a further turn round the Fields and let me run on so that I can make a start? It will save valuable talking time, for later, I'm afraid, I must go to Bow Street.'

'You really *are* looking for a body?'

'Yes, Father. I regret to say I really am.'

*   *   *

An hour later, his attire and visage completely restored, the Apothecary sat with Sir Gabriel in the library of their home in Nassau Street and explained to him all that had taken place on the previous day, describing with much relish the Court of Assistants and the characters who had been present.

'There was one old goat who bleated on and on about my paying the increased fine for admitting Foreign Apothecaries. I explained to him I had first applied to be made Free last August so it was on those terms I should be let in, but he was such a know-all he couldn't listen to anything except his own voice.'

'But you won the day?'

'Yes. I paid the lesser fine. I have to go back to sit an examination but that is a mere formality. So, after all this time, I can really call myself an apothecary.'

'I am very proud,' said Sir Gabriel. 'And I apologise that I looked askance at your tatterdemalion appearance. You obviously have enjoyed an extremely exciting time.'

'It was all quite extraordinary,' John answered, and told his father everything that had happened once he had arrived in Wapping, including the wedding that did not take place, the finding of the body, and the reasons why he believed the dead man not only to be Sir William Hartfield but also to have been murdered.

'And now you want him found?'

'Yes. Bodies do not walk out by themselves. He must have been removed at first light.'

'And by this time might well be lying in a freshly dug grave.'

'Indeed he might. But whatever the case, it is my duty to inform Mr Fielding of all that I saw.'

'You know, it is my belief,' stated Sir Gabriel thoughtfully, 'that the watermen may have been acting under instructions.'

'What do you mean?'

'Perhaps it is their bounden duty to drag corpses from the river. Maybe it is they and no other who are responsible for keeping the Thames clear of carrion.'

'I think you're right,' John exclaimed. 'I'm sure I have heard that fact now you come to say it.'

'Then the sooner you get to the Public Office and sort this business out, the better it will be.'

John glanced at his watch. 'If I go now I might well be home in time to dine with you.'

'And what about the shop?'

'Just for today, it being rather an especial one, I shall let it stay closed.'

Sir Gabriel got to his feet. 'I've a mind to drive out with you. I can make a few calls while you are closeted with Mr Fielding. I shall send a footman forthwith to get the carriage brought round.' He turned at the doorway, the suggestion of a smile lighting his eyes. 'Would you like me to lend you a hat, my dear? You seem to have mislaid yours.'

The Apothecary gave an amused grin. 'I have my own second best, thank you. As to my other, the one bought especially for yesterday's ceremony, after a day of attempting to escape me it finally plunged into the Thames this morning. The last I saw of it, it was heading determinedly for the sea. Samuel offered to dive in and capture it but I declined his proposal. I did not relish the prospect of two dead men in the river.'

Sir Gabriel inclined his head. 'Just so. A wise decision.'

'I am glad you agree,' said his son, attempting to look serious.

The third house on the left-hand side of Bow Street, that is if one had made one's entrance from Russell Street, looked very much like the others, in fact there seemed nothing remarkable about it at all. Tall, four storeys indeed, and thin, it was built in similar style to the rest of the property in this mainly residential area. But here resemblance ceased. For it was this house which, some seventeen years earlier, had been the dwelling place of Sir Thomas de Veil, Colonel of the Westminster Militia and Justice of the Peace. And it was from here, his own home, that he had administered equity to the city of London. Thus the Public Office in Bow Street had been born. After Sir Thomas's death, the house had been occupied by the author and magistrate, Henry Fielding, but his declining health had led to his half-brother, John, taking his place. And it was to see this man, already becoming something of a legend because of his blindness, an affliction which seemed to handicap him not in the least, that John Rawlings was presently making his way.

As Sir Gabriel's coach, a dark affair drawn by snow white horses, pulled up before the door, the Apothecary got out swiftly, remembering the stark terror he had felt when he had first laid eyes on the place, suspected as he had been at the time of committing a murder. Now, though, he was glad to see the house's graceful lines rise before him, knowing that he could share the burden of his belief that a man had been done to death, with one of the sharpest brains in London. It was a disappointment, therefore, to be told that not only was the court not in session but that Mr Fielding was away from home, having driven out with Mrs Fielding for the purpose of visiting friends.

'Would you like to see Mr Jago, Sir?' asked the fellow in charge of the Public Office.

John nodded gladly. 'Indeed I would.' For if the formidable Magistrate was not available, the next best thing was to talk to his clerk, the foxy faced, sandy haired Joe Jago, a man whose origins were something of a mystery to John, for he spoke with the accent of one who had started life amongst the criminal fraternity yet worked on the side of law and order.

'Then take a seat, Sir, and I'll go and fetch him.'

But already a voice was saying, 'Why, bless me, if it ain't Mr Rawlings,' and Joe himself was coming into the room, some papers in his hand. 'Well now, Sir, and what can I do for you?' he went on.

The Apothecary stood up and made him a polite bow. 'There is a certain matter I have to report to this office. May I talk to you?'

'By all means. Step into Mr Fielding's study. He's gone abroad with Mrs Fielding and Mary Ann. But if you tell me what you want to say, I shall report back to him faithfully.'

The clerk sat down on the other side of a paper-covered desk, pushing back his wig and scratching his head with his quill pen. 'Now then, Mr Rawlings, I'm all attention.'

'I'll come straight to the point, then. Last night I stayed at The Devil's Tavern in Wapping. I was there with Samuel Swann, my friend the goldsmith, whom you know of old, celebrating the fact that yesterday I was made Free of the Company.'

'And about time too. Well done, Sir.'

'Thank you. Anyway, just as we were going to bed a waterman came in, soaking wet, and told the landlord that he needed the cock fighting area. This seemed to be some secret code between them because Samuel and I were rapidly shown to our room. After that I heard the sound of footsteps and something being carried up an outside flight of stairs. Later, when all was quiet, I went to investigate and found a dead man lying on a table in one of the first floor rooms.'

He paused for effect and Joe Jago said, 'And in the morning he was gone, I suppose.'

John gaped at him. 'How did you know?'

The clerk scratched his head so hard that his wig fell over one ear. 'Because the watermen would have moved him on to the mortuary by then. Bless you, Sir, for every body they bring in they are entitled to a reward from the Coroner of anything between four shillings and sixpence and five shillings. Obviously, late at night they cannot deliver the goods, so to speak, so they would leave it somewhere until morning. No doubt they have an arrangement with the landlords of various hostelries to lodge the corpses with them till daylight comes. There's nothing illegal about that.'

The Apothecary nodded. 'My father suggested as much. But there is one thing, Mr Jago, that I feel you ought to know.'

'And what might that be?'

'I examined the body, albeit in very poor light, and came to the conclusion that this particular man had not drowned, either by accident or his own hand. There was a mark to his head which had left a pattern of the object that made it. And can you guess what that mark was?'

Mr Fielding's clerk sat up straight. 'No, Sir, I cannot.'

'It was an ornamental fox's head. Unless I am much mistaken, the victim was given a blow to the skull by a great stick bearing a handle of that design, then was thrown into the river, either dying or dead, in order to make it appear that he had drowned.'

'Or hopefully to vanish for ever more,' Joe said thoughtfully.

'Or that too.'

The clerk drew a piece of paper towards him and began to write on it, then looked up as a thought struck him.

'Were there any identifying effects on the body, Mr Rawlings? What was in the dead man's pockets?'

John smiled grimly. 'The victim's rings and watch were missing . . .'

'Anything that might *fall off* in the river does so, if you take my meaning, Sir,' interrupted the clerk, smiling cynically.

'Quite, but concealed in his pockets were valuable snuff and pill boxes.'

'Did you remove them?'

'I did not like to do so. Such an act smacks of grave robbing.'

Joe Jago gave another wry grin. 'Whether they are still on him when we go to look depends on the honesty of the mortuary keeper. You should have taken them, Mr Rawlings. They might have helped with the matter of identification.'

John ignored the mild rebuke and produced his trump card. 'I did, however, remove this.' He took the paper from his pocket. 'It is a marriage licence in the name of Sir William Hartfield. Acting upon it, I went to see the priest at St Paul's Church, Shadwell, earlier today. From his description it is safe to assume that Sir William and the victim are one and the same man.'

A look of admiration stole over Joe Jago's features as he examined the licence to wed, then he gave a loud, appreciative guffaw. 'Well, bless my cods, if that don't beat all. We don't need the Runners with rum dukes like you around, that's for certain.'

The Apothecary winked an eye. 'To be honest, I had a sniff of it before I found the document upon him.' And he explained to the clerk, who wrote it all down carefully, exactly what he had seen in the church on the previous day.

'So it looks as if one of his family might have done away with the poor wretch in order to stop him marrying his pretty young bride,' Joe said thoughtfully.

'It is certainly possible.'

The clerk scratched his head violently then readjusted his wig. 'Tell you what, Mr Rawlings, I shall relay all this to the Beak as soon as he returns. No doubt he will be in touch with you straight away. Tomorrow, we shall send a Runner to the mortuary for the Wapping area to try to find the remains of Sir William.'

'Will he be there?'

'I am sure of it, Sir. Remember that the watermen do not get their reward until the body is delivered.'

'And what will happen after that, do you think?'

Joe Jago screwed up his ragged face. 'I reckon someone or other will have to go to Sir William's home and find out what's what amongst that family of his.'

'I see,' said John, an ominous feeling coming over him.

The clerk's bright eyes glinted. 'Course, who that someone is depends entirely on the wishes of the Principal Magistrate. It is he and he alone who will decide precisely how to deal with this particular case of murder.' His grin broadened. 'Well, Mr Rawlings,

I reckon you're going to be kept very busy. In fact it would be my guess that you're probably going to be very busy indeed.'

'What exactly do you mean?' asked John cautiously.

'Now that you've been made Free, of course,' answered the clerk innocently. 'What else could I possibly be talking about?'

Chapter Four

Relieved that Sir Gabriel Kent was not entertaining friends to cards and supper, John Rawlings had gone to bed early that night, mixing himself a draught before he did so to ensure that he got a good ten hours' rest. Then, feeling somewhat hypocritical in view of his recent remarks regarding Samuel and his sleeping habits, the Apothecary had retired at nine o'clock, the hour when the *beau monde* was customarily setting forth to seek its nightly entertainment.

He woke the next morning in rather a fine mood, certain that Mr Fielding was going to ask him to assist in the investigation of Sir William Hartfield's death, and pleased about the challenge. He was also pleased, though he would not admit it even to himself, that this would probably mean meeting the beautiful female twin and getting to know her better. In high humour, John tied his cravat with a large bow atop, and whistled his way down the stairs.

'I see that you are quite restored from yesterday's excitments,' said Sir Gabriel as John arrived at the breakfast table.

'Indeed I am,' answered his son, 'but will you forgive me if I do not have more than a cup of coffee with you? I am most anxious to get to my shop before the rumour goes round the neighbourhood that it has closed down permanently.'

'A wise precaution,' answered his father, and smiled to himself as John took a seat, decided to spread a piece of toast with a large helping of fruit conserve, murmured something about eating lightly but none the less took a second slice, then gulped down his coffee and departed.

As was always his habit when the weather was fine, John walked the short distance between Nassau Street, Soho, and Shug Lane, Piccadilly, passing down Gerrard Street, then turning left towards The Hay Market, hurrying the last quarter of a mile in order to get to his shop. For whenever he stepped through its door, into his magic world of exotic bottles and jars, of alembics and crucibles, of pewter pans which shone brightly, and row upon row of herbs hung aloft to dry, then he was truly happy. And today was no exception. As the Apothecary put on his long apron and started to remove the dust covers from the counters of pills and perfumes, he felt the contentedness of familiarity come upon him. In fact he was so far away in thought, enjoying his routine and thinking of a brew he wanted to make for the cure of loose teeth, that he did not hear the tramping feet of two chairmen, nor notice that they had set their burden down outside his shop. It was not until the door opened and the bell rang, that John finally looked up, only to have his day made complete. Serafina de Vignolles stood radiantly in the entrance, holding out her hands to him.

'My dear friend,' she said, 'how very nice to see you.'

'Madam,' John answered, and bowed, before taking her fingers between his and kissing them. 'May I say that your beauty grows daily,' he added, meaning it.

Serafina grimaced slightly and put her hand to her body. 'Something down here is growing daily. Why John, I resemble a grape. But it is kind of you to be so flattering. Indeed that is why I came. To hear soothing words from my favourite young apothecary – and to buy a remedy for heartburn.'

They knew each other so well, John having met her during the dangerous summer of 1754 and fallen madly in love with the challenge of her, that now he took the liberty of surveying his visitor from head to foot, his expression professional. 'On the contrary, Comtesse, you are carrying your child gracefully. And you are still one of the loveliest women in London, and always will be for that matter.'

She smiled up at him. 'Why did I not take you for a lover when I had the opportunity?'

The Apothecary smiled back. 'We could never be the kind of friends we are now if you had.'

'And talking of lovers,' said the Comtesse with a glint in her eye, 'how is Miss Coralie Clive these days?'

John shook his head so that a curl of dark cinnamon-coloured hair appeared from beneath his wig. 'I haven't seen her since Christmas. Not since that time when we were all together at Sarah Delaney's home, in fact.'

Serafina raised her exquisite eyebrows. 'Why is that?'

The Apothecary turned away, busying himself looking for a bottle. 'She is very occupied with pursuing her career as an actress. I believe it is her intention to become as famous as her sister, Kitty. Furthermore, I hear tittle-tattle that the Duke of Richmond is set to make her his Duchess.'

Serafina allowed herself an undignified snort. 'Oh, what stuff! For a start Richmond will marry another title, you can be sure of that. For a second, I do not see Coralie as the kind of girl who would sit around, incarcerated in his estates, doing nothing but stare at the wall. When she marries it will be to someone of enormous interest, not to a lecherous little Duke.'

John chuckled. 'How colourfully put. Let it be hoped that you are right.'

'Of course I am. My dear, why don't you write to her, invite her to meet you? She does not work in the theatre every night of her life surely.'

The Apothecary found the bottle that he was looking for and took it down from the shelf. 'Here you are, Comtesse. Drink this after each meal, warm and with a little sugar. Your digestive problems will vanish.'

Serafina took the physic and stared into its depths. 'What is in it?'

'Star anise, camomile flowers, gentian roots, lemon balm, to name a few of the ingredients. All perfectly harmless, I assure you.'

'There is no need. I trust you and your compounds more than I do those of any other apothecary alive.'

'And you may call me that at long last. I was made Free the day before yesterday.'

The Comtesse let out a cry of delight. 'John, this is wonderful news. You must come and dine with us in order to celebrate. Louis will be so pleased.'

'And how is your gallant husband?'

Serafina rolled her eyes. 'Preparing for fatherhood as if the condition were unique to him alone. No woman has ever been *enceinte* before, no man has ever sired a child. Why, if he had his way I would be lying at home on my *duchesse en bateau* and would not shift until the babe was born. It is all tremendously endearing and enormously trying.'

'It sounds very like him.'

'Yes. I have come to the conclusion that the greater the philanderer, the better the father. I'll swear it is because they know the perils their child might fall in to.'

John looked slightly startled. 'Philanderer? But surely, Louis . . .'

The Comtesse shook her head. 'Don't worry. He is completely cured of all that. It is as much as I can do these days to get him to leave my side, which is a pity.'

'Why?'

'Because occasionally, just very occasionally, I have this overwhelming urge to don a disguise and make for Marybone or some other gaming house, and there to gamble as once I used. Oh John, it was a dangerous life – but it was so exciting!'

The Apothecary smiled. 'The mysterious Masked Lady, the most enigmatical figure in the *beau monde*.'

'And who was it who unmasked me?'

John spread his hands and bowed. 'I apologise.'

Serafina kissed him lightly on the cheek. 'It was worth it in order to find the happiness I now enjoy.'

'You're sure? Promise me you aren't bored.'

'No, it is only a small wicked streak in me that wants to go back to the old life.'

John nodded. 'Talking of that life, did you ever come across a man called Sir William Hartfield during your travels?'

Serafina frowned. 'The name seems vaguely familiar.'

'He was in his sixties, not bad looking for a man of his years. He owned a fleet of ships.'

'Hartfield? Hartfield?' Serafina repeated. 'Did he have a son called Julian by any chance?'

'I don't know. Why?'

'Because I took a tidy sum from that young man, a pretty fellow with flaming corkscrews of hair upon which his wig did not sit easy. He believed himself a regular gamester but did not have the flair to make his belief reality. He was in debt to many, the foolish creature.'

'And were those debts honoured?'

'Oh yes. And by his family I imagine. If this Sir William was his father, I pity him.'

'How interesting,' said the Apothecary reflectively.

'Why do you ask? Has something happened? John, you have a

certain look upon your face. Are you working with Mr Fielding again?'

The Apothecary grinned, just a fraction sheepishly. 'You know me too well, Madam. But the answer is no, not as yet. Though I expect the summons at any moment.'

'And can I assume that this Sir William Hartfield is involved somehow?'

'Indeed you may. The poor wretch was thrown into a watery grave, the river Thames to be precise. But he was dragged out and is now lying in the mortuary. The Blind Beak has just cause to believe that his death was in suspicious circumstances, I can assure you.'

Serafina gazed at him, her face suddenly pale. 'Be careful, John. If the Julian Hartfield I knew is part of the family, then there is a great deal of money involved. And a fortune makes people grow vicious, particularly when they want to get their hands on it.'

Just for a moment John enjoyed the luxury of holding her close to him. 'Don't worry, I shall be a mere outside observer.'

'I don't think so,' the Comtesse answered slowly. 'If I know anything about you, my fine young friend, you will find it practically impossible to remain out of harm's way for long.'

The letter from the Principal Magistrate arrived during the course of the afternoon, written in the strangely neat hand of Joe Jago though the signature was John Fielding's own, his pen guided for him. It read simply:

'Mr John Fielding presents his compliments to Mr John Rawlings and has the pleasure to acquaint him of his desire that he should dine with the above at Bow Street this night at five. He remains Mr Rawlings's most obedient servant,

J Fielding.'

It was somewhat quaintly worded and John smiled to himself, as he hastily wrote a reply and gave it to the waiting Runner.

'Can you tell Mr Fielding that I may be a little late. I have to see to the closing of my shop.'

'He will understand that perfectly, Sir. It is the Beak's expressed wish that he should never interfere with your working life.'

But he does, John thought, and just for a moment had a doubt about whether he should become involved in yet another of John

Fielding's investigations into violent death. Yet there was a fascination to it, a honing of the wit against that of the perpetrator, which no other pastime could satisfy. The Apothecary supposed that as Serafina was addicted in some degree to gaming, so was he to the art of catching murderers.

So it was with mounting excitement that he closed his shop punctually at half past four and hired a sedan chair to take him to Bow Street. And it was with pleasure that John climbed the staircase to the private dwelling above the Public Office and allowed a servant to usher him to the doorway of the large airy room used by the Fieldings as their salon. It being a typical March evening with a sharp wind that had a hint of snow in it, the curtains had been drawn across the three large windows, while a log fire sent forth a comforting radiance. Seated in a chair beside this glow, the colour of it reflecting warmly on his face, was the man whom the population of London either greatly feared or greatly respected, according to the degree of honesty which they practised. John stood for a moment in silence, realising that John Fielding was not yet aware of his presence, and studied the Blind Beak.

He was already something of a legend, yet the Apothecary knew for a fact that the Magistrate was very far from old, only thirty-four in fact, having been born in the winter of 1721. Tragically blinded in an accident at the age of nineteen, his desire for a career at sea had thus been brought to an untimely end but, with almost superhuman power, John had followed in his half-brother Henry's footsteps and become a magistrate. Not only that! He had ably improved Henry's scheme to employ the court's officers as a law enforcement brigade, a body nicknamed the Beak Runners by the population at large. The policing of the lawless capital had sprung into life at the hands of an author and a blind man.

Hearing a movement in the doorway, the Principal Magistrate turned his head. 'Is that you, Mr Rawlings?'

'It certainly is, Sir.'

'Then pray step inside and take the seat opposite mine. There is some punch keeping warm by the fire. If you would be good enough to help yourself.'

John did so, bowing before he sat and wondering what it was about the Blind Beak that made everyone treat him as if he were sighted. But there was no time to dwell on it for the Magistrate was speaking again.

'Joe Jago tells me that you were made Free of the Company on the day before yesterday. Many congratulations, my young friend.'

'Thank you. I must confess it is a very satisfying feeling after all this time. I had half convinced myself that it would never happen.'

'You certainly suffered from several set backs as far as that matter was concerned, some of which I fear may be my fault.'

'What do you mean, Sir?'

'That the pursuit of certain facts on behalf of the Public Office may have stopped you attending the Court of Assistants.'

'I can truthfully assure you that is not so. It came near to it last December but I did get to the Court despite the difficulties.'

'Then all is well.' Mr Fielding held out his glass and John refilled it, then he drank and paused before he said, 'And now it would seem that we are on the trail of a killer once more.'

'Joe Jago told you the tale?'

'Yes, all of it. Further, two of my men went by water this morning to the mortuary where the bodies found at Wapping are lodged. They returned with these.' The Magistrate produced from his pocket a velvet bag and handed it across the space to John. 'Are these the snuff and pill boxes you found upon the corpse?'

John turned the contents onto his lap, the brocade waistcoat that he kept in his shop lest he should be invited out unexpectedly, reflecting in the silver snuff box decorated with its emerald from the Indies.

'They are, Sir. So the mortuary attendant proved to be an honest man.'

'Either that or frightened by the sight of the Runners.'

'But he released the articles in question without demur?'

'Not until my men had been to and fro the Coroner till they were giddy. Anyway, the situation stands that the Coroner is now convinced that the deceased was Sir William Hartfield, having been shown the wedding licence and told where it was found. Not withstanding that, he will release the body to no one but the dead man's family as he is not at all convinced of foul play.'

'The mark on the body presumably vanished as it bloated.'

'Yes, you were lucky to see it so soon, my friend. Had you not, this case of unlawful killing might well have gone undetected.'

John refilled his glass and topped up that of Mr Fielding. 'Joe Jago told you of the extraordinary wedding party, Sir?'

'Yes, very clearly. He said that you described the guests as more suitably clad for a funeral than a festivity.'

'The first of which they will very soon have to attend! Yes, they were a most baleful bunch, there to make trouble according to the churchwarden.'

'Yet one of them may well have known that the bridegroom would not be present.'

'You think a member of the family is responsible?'

Mr Fielding sipped his punch thoughtfully. 'I believe a great deal of money is involved in this case. If Sir William were about to remarry and to make a new will in favour of his beautiful young bride, then that may very well be so.' He paused, then said, 'Tell me of the bridegroom's witness. Jago said he was one of Sir William's employees.'

'Yes. He was obviously much embarrassed by the whole affair and scuttled away as soon as the vicar announced that the ceremony would not be taking place. I saw him later in The Devil's Tavern, drowning his sorrows. A local girl told me that his name is Valentine Randolph and that he lives across the river in Redriff. Apparently, he works for one of the ship owners so I am surmising that it must have been Sir William.'

'I think you are moderately safe in doing so. With an antagonistic family who else would one choose to act as witness but a trusted employee?'

'Yes,' agreed John thoughtfully.

There was a brief knock on the door which then flew open to reveal the prettiest of little girls. 'Mary Ann!' exclaimed the Apothecary, with pleasure.

'Mr Rawlings, how very nice to see you again,' she answered, and dropped a demure curtsey. She turned to John Fielding. 'Uncle, Aunt Elizabeth has asked me to say that dinner will be served in five minutes.'

'Then tell her we shall join her shortly. Now, I have a few more matters to discuss with Mr Rawlings.'

'Very well.' And bobbing another curtsey, the charming little thing went out.

'How well you have taught her,' John commented, expressing his thoughts aloud.

'As you know, she has been with us since she was six. My wife brought her to the marriage as a dowry.' The Blind Beak laughed gently. 'She is Elizabeth's niece, of course, but to us she is the child we never had.'

His manner changed suddenly and entirely and he leant towards the Apothecary, his black bandaged eyes, prominent nose and strong features giving an almost frightening impression. John Rawlings found himself thinking, yet again, that John Fielding was one of the most powerful men he had ever met and he pitied any poor miscreant dragged before him.

'My friend,' said the Magistrate softly, 'you will be well aware by now that I would very much like you to help me find Sir William Hartfield's murderer – and yet I hesitate to ask you.'

'Because you believe you might be taking me away from my livelihood.' John did not pose this as a question being so sure of the answer.

'Indeed. We compromised in the past by agreeing you should work for the Public Office on alternate days, but I do not consider that arrangement to be satisfactory if it means that you must close your shop.'

'But if I do not do so, how can I serve you?'

'Have you thought of getting an assistant?' Mr Fielding answered one question with another.

'An apprentice certainly.'

'What age need this person be?'

'About fifteen or sixteen.'

'Would someone a little older be unsuitable?'

'It depends. Why do you ask?'

'Aha,' said the Blind Beak mysteriously, 'I will come to that matter when we have eaten our repast.'

Chapter Five

*T*he cold March night had deepened and beyond the walls of the house in Bow Street, the wind which had played such havoc with the Apothecary's hat during the last two days could be heard howling like a caged beast, apparently having lost its sense of humour. Occasionally it blew gusts down the chimney of the salon, sending smoke into the room and causing the candles to flicker wildly. But generally the place remained cosy and John, stretching his legs out to the flames and drinking Mr Fielding's finest port, felt his mood grow expansive, so much so that he began to dread the idea of turning out into the cold. Aware that he must gather his dulling wits, the Apothecary asked a question.

'Do you want me to call at Sir William Hartfield's town house tomorrow?'

Mr Fielding nodded. 'Pray do so. Say that you have come to inform the family of some grievous news and take the snuff and pill boxes with you as a means of identifying the dead man. I shall give you a letter of authorisation in which I shall request them to cooperate fully with my representative. Then I suggest that you get one of them to accompany you to the mortuary to arrange for the release of the body. Observe them as closely as you can, Mr Rawlings. Something will be revealed, sure as fate.'

John downed his port and sat up in his chair. 'I have become so comfortable that I don't want to leave. But leave I must. There is a great deal to be done and I think an early start is indicated in the morning.'

The Blind Beak laid a restraining hand upon his arm. 'Wait one moment before you depart. There is someone I very much want you to meet. It will only take five minutes.' And getting to his feet, he felt his way to the door and called down the stairs, 'Nicholas, some more wood for the fire if you please.'

'Yes, Mr Fielding,' a distant voice responded, and a few moments later the Apothecary heard the sound of a servant humping a heavy basket up the staircase. Somewhat surprised, he turned to look as the salon door reopened.

A youth stood framed in the doorway, a young man of about seventeen or eighteen years old, clutching a basket of logs to him, both arms at full stretch round it. Normally, John would have taken little notice of a kitchen lad come to tend the fire but there was something so arresting about this boy that he gave him a second glance. It was the newcomer's hair which first caught his attention, so black it had almost a blue tinge about it, its vibrance in tremendous contrast to the pale face beneath, clearly etched with the lines of enormous suffering. The Apothecary instantly put the boy down as a charity child, one who had been abandoned by its mother, probably left to die by the roadside, but who had survived to be brought up by the parish.

'Is that you Nicholas?' asked Mr Fielding, hearing the young man enter the room.

'Yes, Sir.'

'This is Mr Rawlings. I want you to tell him about yourself. Speak up and use a clear voice.'

It was pathetic, and the Apothecary hardly knew how to sit emotionless, as the pallid creature turned to him and recited a speech he had obviously learned by heart.

'My name is Nicholas Dawkins. I was born in Deptford and lived in my grandmother's house until I was three years old, when she died. My mother died at my birth and there was no one to care for me so I was brought up by the parish. I was apprenticed to a sailmaker when I was twelve years old but he beat me so cruelly that I ran away to sea. However, an injury to my leg resulted in my being unfit for service. I came to London looking for work and became involved in petty crime. I appeared before the Principal Magistrate who took an interest in my case and has given me a job as a servant. Thank you.'

John did not know whether to laugh or cry. 'How very interesting,' was all he could think of saying.

Nicholas fixed his clear russet eyes, an almost identical shade to the sails of a Thames barge, onto the Apothecary. 'Very good, Sir,' he answered, just as if he were still at sea.

'Thank you, Nicholas,' said John Fielding, and there was silence as the young man carefully placed some more logs on the fire, piled the remaining few in the basket by the grate, then quietly limped from the room.

The Blind Beak turned his unseeing gaze in John's direction. 'Well? What did you think of him?'

Very puzzled, the Apothecary answered, 'His is a sad tale but not all that an unusual one. It was kind of you to give him a home here. Will he continue to be honest, do you consider?'

'Oh yes, I believe so. He only took up thieving in order to feed himself. But the fact is, Mr Rawlings, there is something about him that interests me.'

'And what is that?'

'When he was apprehended by the Runners he was searched and found to be carrying two items, one a document written in a foreign tongue with a post script in English, the other a ring, not tremendously valuable in itself, though made of gold. It bore a crest upon it.'

The Apothecary, who had been wondering why he had been detained just to look at the log boy, suddenly became interested.

'Yes?'

'I had the document translated. It was written in the Muscovy language and dated June, 1698. In it the writer, though he does not state exactly who he is, acknowledges that he has sired a bastard by one Nell Dawkins and asks that the reader should do all he can to protect the child with the money provided. Though as to whom that reader actually was is not made clear. Then there was the post script, added in 1737. This states that the child of the union, a certain Katrina Dawkins, gave birth to yet another bastard, one Elisabeth, who died giving birth to a son, Nicholas, and that he is now in the care of Katrina. An unusual name for an English woman, don't you think? Furthermore, the ring, when examined by an expert, appeared to emanate from a noble Muscovite house.'

'But how in heaven's name,' asked John practically, 'did the boy manage to protect such items from discovery all those years?'

'He wore them in a bag which he stitched to the garment nearest his skin. He appears to have continued this practice as he grew and his clothes wore out.'

'Is it possible that a Muscovy bastard could get itself to Deptford?'

'Indeed it is, Mr Rawlings. Many years ago, in 1698, Tsar Peter lodged in Sayes Court in that very place in order to see the Deptford shipbuilding yards and study their work practices. He had members of his court with him. No doubt, the eager young beauties of the neighbourhood were kept busy attending to their amorous requirements. They probably left behind them a goodly brood of babes. At least this one's father gave something to support his love child.'

'What a curious tale,' said John intrigued, then suddenly and quite clearly saw the purpose of his being asked to stay late. 'You want him to work as my assistant, don't you? Am I right, Mr Fielding?'

The Magistrate, feeling carefully, poured out two generous measures of his excellent port. 'Yes, that was my intention,' he answered, and laughed his tuneful chuckle.

'I see.'

'Perhaps you don't quite. The lad can read and write, taught by the captain of his ship so he told me. He is also highly intelligent and has some trace about him of his exotic heritage, a certain indefinable air which cannot be learned. I also believe that from now on, having been cherished in this house, he will continue on the path of honesty. Mr Rawlings, I am not asking you to take him as an apprentice, that would be too much. What I am suggesting is that while you act as my eyes, hunting down the killer of Sir William Hartfield, he works in your shop on the days when you are about the business of the Public Office.'

John hesitated. 'Can you guarantee that he can be trusted with money?'

'As much as one can about any human being, yes.'

The Apothecary grinned, considering that once more he had been manipulated by the sharpest brain in London, and decided to compromise just to prove his independence.

'Then, Sir, send him to my house at seven o'clock tomorrow morning, sharp. If my father considers him suitable I shall take him on until this particular quest is completed.'

'My dear Mr Rawlings,' the Blind Beak replied solemnly, 'I had hoped all along that you might say that.'

Whatever other bad characteristics Nicholas Dawkins might prove to have, unpunctuality was not one of them. At half past six on the following morning, while Sir Gabriel lay in a darkened room, a small mask protecting his eyes from the cold light of dawn, and

John whistled while he shaved, a habit which demanded certain facial contortions, there came a tentative knock at the front door. The footman who answered it was astonished to see standing on the step an extremely pale, very thin, dark-haired young man, scrubbed scrupulously clean and wearing a threadbare but servicable worsted coat and breeches, stating that he had come on the business of Mr John Fielding. And when he produced the documentation to prove it, he was allowed admittance and told to wait in the smallest receiving room of all until Master John came downstairs.

Half an hour later, as the Apothecary entered the breakfast room, he was given the message that a certain young man desired to see him.

'Then show him in here,' John told the astonished servant, 'he may as well have something to eat before he starts work.'

A few minutes later Nicholas came in, treading diffidently, his limp even more pronounced than it had been on the previous evening. Studying him, it seemed to the Apothecary that the young man had difficulty in smiling, so hard had been the blows that life had delivered him.

'Well now . . .' he began, but Nicholas interrupted him with one of his rehearsed speeches.

'If you decide to employ me, I promise to be an industrious and honest assistant, Sir. You will not find me lacking when it comes to the call of duty. I am deeply grateful for the trust that you have put in me in giving me this opportunity. Thank you.'

John's eyes twinkled. 'Noble sentiments, nobly expressed. Have you had breakfast?'

Nicholas's dark eyebrows shot up in surprise. 'Some bread and cheese, Sir. That is all.'

'Then sit down and have some more. You have a long day's work ahead of you and a lot of learning to do. I want you nourished and strong for such an enterprise.'

So saying, he tucked in heartily himself, motioning Nicholas to sit opposite him and ordering that another cover be laid for Sir Gabriel. Somewhat hesitantly, indeed as if he thought that the chair might break beneath him, Nicholas sat down and took a small piece of bread which he spread thinly with marmalade. He was just about to bite into this when the door opened and John's father appeared, a black velvet turban upon his head, a quilted nightrail flowing from his shoulders in a cascade which rippled about his ankles. It was an awe inspiring sight and Nicholas promptly leapt to his feet and stood at attention, just as he must have done before the captain of his ship.

Sir Gabriel looked at him, an expression of much amusement on his face, then addressed himself to the Apothecary. 'And whom do we have here?'

'Nicholas Dawkins, Father, a protégé of Mr Fielding. It is the plan that, if you approve of him, he will help out in my shop while I go in pursuit of Sir William Hartfield's slayer.'

Sir Gabriel's attention temporarily shifted from the newcomer and he stared at John with interest. 'I presume from that remark that the Beak has now tracked down the missing body?'

'He has, Sir. It is in the mortuary and the Coroner is satisfied that the dead man is indeed Sir William. So it is my duty, this very day, to go to St James's Square and inform the family of the tragedy.'

'He lived at number thirty-two,' put in John's father, 'I looked him up last night in Pigot's street directory.' He turned back to Nicholas. 'And so this young fellow might be in charge of your shop. Tell me, lad, how old are you?'

'Eighteen this year, Sir.'

'And where do you hail from?'

'From Muscovy, Sir.'

'Muscovy!' exclaimed Sir Gabriel in astonished tones.

'Via Deptford,' the Apothecary added quickly. 'It's a long and interesting story. I'll tell it to you later.'

Sir Gabriel took a seat at table, his robe swirling as he moved. 'Well then, John, I should take the lad on if I were you. It is not every day that one is offered a Muscovite as an assistant.'

His topaz eyes were sparkling but his expression was severe. John, catching his mood, looked equally stern. 'Umm. Do you really think so?' But he could continue the teasing no longer as Nicholas's mouth, delicately moulded in his pallid face, began to tremble with anxiety. 'Be of stout heart, Nick,' the Apothecary added quickly, 'the appointment is yours if you would like to have it.'

The waxen features transformed into a smile, like spring in frost. 'You won't regret it, Mr Rawlings, nor you Sir. I'm a quick learner, so the captain used to say, and I swear to do my best.'

'Then that's settled,' said John, winked his eye at his father, and continued with his breakfast.

*　　*　　*

An hour later he and Nicholas had opened the shop in Shug Lane and the boy had started to write a list of what potions, pills and physicks were suitable for which particular complaints. He had also made a tour of inspection, noted what each cupboard and drawer contained, and sniffed several bottles of perfume. The exertion of mastering this in so short a space of time had brought a slight tinge of colour to his face and his russet eyes looked livelier than John had seen them. All in all, he seemed to be a useful enough lad to have around the place.

'Tonight you are to put all the money in a bag and deliver it to my father. That is after you have carefully locked up the shop,' John ordered, wondering if he was making the greatest mistake of his life.

'You can rely on me, Mr Rawlings.'

'I sincerely hope I can,' the Apothecary said under his breath, as he went out into Piccadilly to hail himself a hackney coach to take him the short journey to St James's Square.

He was now entering one of the most fashionable parts of London for the entire area of St James's was considered excessively smart and *bon ton*. Not only had the Prince of Wales been born there but the street directory listed several Dukes and Earls amongst the residents of the Square. Furthermore, the inhabitants of this stylish quadrate had their own church, namely St James's, Piccadilly, and their own club, White's, which stood on the east side of St James's Street. John considered, as the hansom dropped him outside number thirty-two, an imposing building if ever there was one, that Sir William Hartfield must have been rich indeed to have owned a house in so élite a quarter.

He had dressed sprucely but not ostentatiously for this occasion, a dark green cloth suit with gold decoration seeming to fit the bill perfectly. His waistcoat of matching material had perhaps just a fraction more embroidery on it than should have befitted one of Mr Fielding's representatives, but the Apothecary considered this to be a personal statement of his love of fashion and did not let the matter concern him. And he had never been more grateful that he had turned himself out well than when the door was opened by a footman with a face as long and pompous as a viola da gamba, attempting to look down his nose at the visitor.

Forestalling any effort to turn him away, John said, 'I am calling here on behalf of Mr John Fielding, Principal Magistrate, of the

Public Office, Bow Street. I do not have an appointment but it is imperative that I see the head of the household immediately. I have some grave news to impart.'

Momentarily startled, the footman instantly regained his usual sang-froid. 'Sir William Hartfield is not at home, Sir.'

'I am aware of that,' John answered quickly, covering his bad choice of words. 'I have come to see his next of kin.'

There was no mistaking the meaning of that and the front door opened immediately, allowing John into a magnificent hallway, part of a spacious mansion built, so he guessed, in the 1660s.

'If you will take a seat in the antechamber, I will fetch Mr Roger Hartfield. Who shall I say has called?'

'John Rawlings.'

'Very good, Sir.'

The servant departed, his expression bemused, leaving John to study the room into which he had been shown. Though small, it shouted aloud of Sir William's wealth. Tall jars imported from India glinted azure and argent in the cold clear sunshine, rich brocades hung at the window, while a Chinese cabinet inlaid with gold stood beneath a decorated porcelain looking glass. Sitting carefully, the Apothecary took a seat in a velvet-covered chair which, by its graceful shape, denoted that it had been made in the reign of Queen Anne.

The noises of the house bore in on his consciousness. The ticking of the great clock in the hall, footsteps descending the stairs, the distant sound of a harpsichord, a girl laughing. Wondering whether it was the female twin, John got to his feet and was just about to cross to the door to have a look outside, when it opened.

'Mr Roger will see you in the salon,' the servant intoned expressionlessly. 'Would you follow me, Sir.'

They crossed the vast area of the hall and turned down a passage leading off to the right. At the end of it lay two large doors which the footman threw open, announcing as he did so, 'Mr John Rawlings, Sir.'

'Come in,' said a voice, and John stepped beyond the bowing servant into a room of unbelievable grandeur. Yet before he could take in his opulent surroundings, his eye was drawn to the figure that stood before the fireplace, one elbow resting nonchalantly on the mantelpiece.

'Did he say Rawlings?' it asked, and raised a quizzing glance to get a better look at the newcomer.

John stood thunderstruck, staring, mouth agape, at the fantastic creature who was regarding him, recognising him at once as the monstrous beau who had waved bejewelled fingers at him in St Paul's Church, Shadwell.

A vast periwig sat on top of the man's head, covered with the very finest powder, it being the current fashion to powder one's headpiece, particularly in the winter months. But if the wig was overpowering, the beau's clothes were even more so. A coat of pink silk lined with white, revealed beneath it a white satin waistcoat embroidered with silver, unbuttoned at the top to display a shirt of fine cambric with Valenciennes lace ruffles at the neck, these held in place by a glittering ruby brooch. The breeches, when John's astonished gaze finally worked down to them, were of crimson velvet and encompassed the wearer's knees without a wrinkle to be seen anywhere. On the legs themselves, which were rather fleshy in the calves, the Apothecary noted, were white silk stockings, these rising from shoes of blue Meroquin bearing stamping red heels and diamond buckles, which winked and glinted and rivalled the shafts of sunlight that fell on them through the many windows.

'Yes, I am Rawlings,' said John, his voice hoarse with wonderment.

The man smiled, displaying a fine set of large white teeth. 'Roger Hartfield,' he said, holding out his hand. 'How may I help you?'

And with that he made a little *moue* with his mouth, gave a silvery laugh, and pulled the bell rope.

'Champagne, champagne,' he shouted carelessly to the bowing footman who came almost immediately. ''Tis not every day that a pretty fellow such as this crosses my path. Now, my dear chap, tell me why have you called?'

'Sir,' said John gravely, 'I fear that I may be the bearer of ill tidings. Be good enough to prepare yourself.' He fished in his pocket and drew out the bag containing the snuff and pill boxes. 'Mr Hartfield, do you recognise these?' he asked.

Roger threw them a disinterested glance. 'Can't say that I do, no.'

The Apothecary was dumbfounded. 'They are not the property of your father?'

The beau shrugged. 'Could be, I suppose. Damme, man, one snuff box is very like another.'

'Even bearing an emerald such as this?'

Roger was about to reply when the door opened to admit the footman bearing a silver tray with glasses and champagne upon it.

'Gibson,' ordered the beau, 'come over here.' The servant did so, having first set down his burden on a side table. 'Does this belong to my revered Papa?' Roger went on.

The footman took the snuff box in a white gloved hand. 'Indeed it does, Sir.'

'There you are,' said Roger triumphantly, as if he had just solved the riddle of the universe. 'Why d'ye want to know?'

'Because,' John answered solemnly, 'it was found on a body dragged out of the river Thames. A body that the Public Office has every reason to believe is that of Sir William Hartfield.'

'Damme!' exclaimed Roger violently. Then he rolled his eyes up in his head, turned white as chalk beneath his enamelled face paint, and crashed noisily to the floor, sending an exquisite clock flying as he did so.

'He's fainted!' screeched the startled servant, taking a step backward.

'So,' answered John, reaching for his salts, 'it would appear.'

Chapter Six

*R*oger Hartfield was far more heavily built than his elegant clothes would suggest. Bending over to pull the unconscious man into a sitting position, John found his arms straining in their sockets and was obliged to call the terrified footman, not an ideal companion in a crisis, to heave alongside him. But finally, as a result of their combined efforts, they managed to roll the beau into a ball and John thrust the head of the patient between his silk stockinged knees, simultaneously administering the salts to his flaring nostrils.

'What, what, what?' screeched Roger, sniffing, and cast a bleary eye in the Apothecary's direction before once more lapsing into oblivion.

Fighting off a terrible suspicion that the beau was playing the scene to the full, John controlled himself and looked professional. 'I need cold compresses for his head. I think that's the only way I'm going to bring him round. Can you get me some ice and cloths?'

'Certainly, Sir,' the footman replied with alacrity, and left the room with considerable speed.

The door had barely closed behind him when it opened again. Turning from where he knelt beside Roger's body, John found himself the subject of a very cold stare emanating from an extremely arresting woman. 'And who might you be?' she asked the Apothecary coolly, making it quite clear that she did not enjoy entering her own salon to find a member of the family lying on the floor with an entire stranger leaning over him.

John adminstered more salts. 'John Rawlings, Ma'am. An apothecary. Presently calling on you on behalf of Mr Fielding, the Magistrate.'

The cold look did not falter. 'And what possible business could that man have with us?'

'The business of identifying a dead body,' John answered, somewhat irritated by her attitude. He stood up and brushed at his knees.

The woman came into the room and closed the door behind her. She had grown paler but had lost none of her chilling attitude. In fact she seemed to glare even more as she said, 'What body is this? Explain yourself more clearly.'

'It was that of a man found floating in the Thames. Certain articles upon the victim's person have led the Coroner to the conclusion that the remains are those of Sir William Hartfield.'

She drew in breath sharply. 'Are you sure?'

'Perhaps you would like to see for yourself.' And John passed the snuff and pill boxes into her reluctant hands.

She looked at them for a moment, then said quietly, 'Yes, those belonged to my father-in-law.'

From the floor Roger began to make sounds of recovery, groaning noisily as he struggled to sit up. Seeing the newcomer, he exclaimed, 'Lydia! I thought you were out.'

'I returned and walked into the room to find you splayed upon the ground,' she answered tartly. 'This man, here, told me you had fainted.'

Helped by John, Roger struggled to his feet. 'It was the shock. Apparently, a body has been found in the river which they believe to be Papa's. God's life but the strength went clean out of me when I heard the news.'

'Well, it may not be so. It might be that of a common cutpurse who had stolen the goods and died with them on him.'

'There was also a marriage certificate in the name of Sir William Hartfield and Miss Amelia Lambourn found in the dead man's pocket book. I doubt very much that a thief would have bothered to keep that.'

Roger clutched his throat. 'It all makes a terrible sense. That would explain why he did not appear at the wed . . .'

Lydia cut across him. 'There's no need to go into all that now. I'm sure our visitor would not be interested in family gossip.'

'On the contrary,' John answered evenly. 'I might be very interested indeed. You see, we have very good reason to believe that Sir William was murdered.'

Two pairs of eyes regarded him in consternation, and John was alarmed to observe that Roger's were rolling once more, the whites much on display.

'Mr Hartfield, do sit down,' he ordered firmly. 'I would not like you to fall over again.'

But Roger ignored him, instead rushing from the room with his hand clapped over his mouth, making the most unpleasant retching sounds.

'He's a sensitive soul,' Lydia said dismissively, then turned the full beam of her attention on John. 'Now, tell me everything.'

The Apothecary paused, looking at her in silence, doing his best to sum her up before he spoke.

The creature he was regarding was a tall woman in an age of small people, almost as tall as John himself, a fact that she used much to her advantage, staring him straight in the eye without hesitation. Lydia was also well set up about the body, creating an overall impression of being both strong and muscular and not particularly feminine. However, giving the lie to this, there rose from her mannish shoulders a lovely neck, long and swan-like, black hair, waves and waves of it and unpowdered, looping down in curls around its whiteness. Lydia's brows, as dark and defined as ravens' feathers, rose in two curves above enormous eyes, deep blue and secretive. Yet despite the beauty of these, her main feature was a long strong nose which dominated her face above a full red mouth.

Wondering how he could possibly have missed so striking an individual at the wedding, and thinking that only sober black dress could have hidden such a smouldering loveliness, John gave a polite bow. 'Madam, you have the advantage of me. You are aware of my name but I do not know yours. Nor, indeed, your position in Sir William's household. Would you be so kind?'

'I am Lydia Hartfield, widow of Sir William's second son, Thomas, who was drowned at sea on one of his father's ships,' she answered promptly. 'As I had no children, my father-in-law invited me to live in his house. I have been here for the last six years. I think it was generally considered that I would meet another husband and before too long leave the Hartfields in peace, but alas that has not happened.'

'By fate or design?' John asked.

The lips of the red mouth, until now harshly compressed together, relaxed, and Lydia smiled for the first time. 'What do you mean?'

'Did you meet nobody suitable or was your heart still set on the man you had lost?'

The smile vanished. 'You are a very impertinent young person, has nobody ever told you that?'

'Oh they have,' John replied, walking a tight rope in his assessment of her. 'But as an apothecary I am interested in how people think. You see, my old Master believed that the mind and the body are closely related and that the one could bring about ailments in the other. That is why I ask questions.'

She thawed a little, but not as much as he had hoped. 'Well, the answer is that I met nobody who could come up to Thomas's standard.' She motioned him towards a chair. 'Now pray sit down, Mr Rawlings, and tell me about the body found in the Thames. I find myself hard put to believe it was Sir William's.'

'Then I am afraid you must be prepared to change your mind. The corpse was that of a man in his sixties, of average height and build and well preserved for his years. He had white hair but was balding, his head shaved for his wig . . .'

Lydia caught her breath and put both hands to her mouth. 'You are describing my father-in-law exactly.'

John nodded. 'I feared as much. You see, the vicar of St Paul's, Shadwell, has also given me a similar description.'

The deep blue eyes flashed then narrowed. 'The vicar? How did you come to see him?'

The Apothecary leant forward, his clasped hands between his knees. 'I am not going to waste your time, Mrs Hartfield, by indulging in minor deceits. I know about the wedding ceremony that did not take place. I am aware that most members of the family attended the church, all dressed in black, though I am not certain that you were one of them. I am also sensible of the fact that the bride left in a storm of tears because Sir William did not appear. Now, I think, we all know the reason why, though maybe she does not. Perhaps, therefore, you could tell me where I may locate Miss Amelia Lambourn, for that is her name, isn't it?'

The widow's ferociously beautiful features contorted. 'In answer to your first question, no I was not present. I am not the type that dances on the grave of another. And a grave it would have been if he had married her, for the weeping bride is no one to be pitied, you can believe me. She is a wretched little schemer and an unprincipled slut. As to her whereabouts, I have absolutely no idea where she can be found. I believe Sir William had set her up somewhere, no doubt in the lap of luxury. But if you want her exact address, you'll have to ask Luke Challon.'

'Luke Challon?' the Apothecary repeated.

'My father-in-law's private secretary. He is privy to all his affairs.' Lydia laughed bitterly at the double entendre.

John assumed his most sympathetic expression. 'I take it that Miss Lambourn was a thorn in the family's side?'

'Then you take it correctly. She is a common strumpet after every penny she can get hold of. While my father-in-law is that archetypally foolish figure, the old man clinging desperately to his youth by means of an association with a female considerably younger than he is.'

'The seasoned campaigner struggling to win his last battle. Alas, I have many such patients.'

For no particular reason that John could see, this struck Lydia as extremely funny and her forbidding face lit as the red lips turned up at the corners and she burst out laughing. 'Oh la la!' she gasped. 'And what a battle it is, no doubt.' Then she sobered. 'But he lost his, didn't he, poor old fellow? Oh Mr Rawlings, how did Sir William die?'

'He was struck over the head with a great stick, or at least by something that bore an ornamental fox's head for handle. Then he was thrown into the river.'

Lydia swung to the other extreme and became immensely still. 'God's life,' she murmured. 'Who could have done such a thing?'

'Someone who wanted to prevent his marriage at all costs, perhaps.'

She regarded him solemnly. 'But only his family desired that, and none of us would have harmed him.'

John looked at her very seriously. 'For all that I will have to ask your relatives questions. Do you have a few moments to tell me about them?'

Lydia stood up. 'No, I don't think I have. I believe it best that you request Luke Challon to help you. He can give you an impartial view whereas I cannot.'

The Apothecary nodded. 'And where may I find this Luke?'

'He's at the country house in Bethnal Green at the moment. He was very concerned when Sir William did not turn up for the wedding and I believe has gone there to initiate enquiries.'

'I see. But you were not?'

Lydia frowned, the black brows sweeping downwards into a line. 'Not what?'

'Not concerned when your father-in-law didn't appear?'

'It was the general belief that he had seen sense at last, had decided not to proceed with the marriage, and consequently was lying low for a few days.'

'And what would you have done if he hadn't returned?'

Mrs Hartfield looked marginally irritable. 'I don't know. Someone would have gone in search of him, I suppose.'

John got to his feet and bowed. 'Thank you so much for giving me your valuable time. Tomorrow I shall call at Bethnal Green. But meanwhile I am going to have to ask Mr Roger Hartfield to accompany me to the mortuary to claim the body. The Coroner will only release it to a member of the family.'

'Oh dear, why him?' Lydia exclaimed. 'Can't Luke do it?'

'I am afraid not. It has to be kin.'

'Then why not ask horrible Hugh. He would be far more suitable.'

'And who is he?'

'My brother-in-law, the third of the four brothers. As he displays all the emotion of a swabbing bucket on every occasion, I think he would perform the task best.'

'Is this particular Mr Hartfield readily available?'

'No, Sir, he is not. He has gone on a short journey.'

'Then Roger it must be. That body must go for decent burial without undue delay.'

Lydia whitened. 'Please say no more. I will try and find out where he is and the current state of his nerves.'

And with that she left the room, her extraordinary face drawn and tense. Thinking that she was rather a splendid woman despite her inclination to be agressive, John crossed to the window and looked out, only to hear the door open behind him once more. He turned to see who had come in and felt his eyes widen at the sight of the newcomers. For there stood the twins, just as fascinating and brilliant as he remembered them. Well aware of the fact that he was staring in open admiration, John made them a formal bow.

They were as similar as any two people can be who are not of the same sex. Burnished red hair, tight in natural corkscrew curls, whirled round the girl's head, and though the boy had shaved his short in order to accomodate his wig, today he wore none and it was clear that had he allowed his curling locks to grow they would have been identical to his sister's. Their eyes were of the same light blue, a disconcertingly unusual shade like a certain variety of meadow butterfly, while their features had been cast in a precise mould, the only difference a certain hardness of the boy's skin caused by shaving. In physique, too, they were of equal build, both inclined to be small, though there all similarity ceased, for the girl had pretty feminine curves which the Apothecary considered alluring.

He bowed again. 'My name is Rawlings, John Rawlings. Whom am I addressing, please?'

They responded together, bowing and curtseying simultaneously. In any other situation it would have been amusing, but knowing that a close relative, presumably their father, had been done to death, John found himself unable to smile.

The girl spoke first. 'I am Juliette Hartfield, Sir, and this is my brother Julian.'

The two men bowed to one another.

'Do please tell us what is afoot,' Juliette went on. 'We glimpsed your arrival and were much intrigued that whatever you said caused Roger to take to his bed declaring billiousness. Also that Lydia swept from the room looking more like a fury than ever. Do you know something about them? Something scandalous, that is?'

The Apothecary shook his head. 'No, it isn't that. I had some news to impart to them, news that they were not happy to hear. And before you ask me what it is, let me say that I do not feel it my place to tell you.'

Identical eyes exchanged a glance and the twins's entire aspect changed.

'It's Father, isn't it?' asked Julian tightly. 'I felt certain when he didn't appear at his wedding that all was not well.'

Juliette clung to her brother's arm. 'Is he dead? Is that why he hasn't been seen?'

John, knowing that they would have to hear the ill tidings sooner or later, decided to tell the truth. 'Yes, I'm afraid he is. Please accept my sincere condolences.'

Both of them fought back tears, a sad and touching sight. 'How did he die?' asked Juliette in a whisper.

The Apothecary cringed, not wanting such a terrible duty. 'I fear he fell victim to a murderer's hand, and that is why I am here,' he said quietly. 'I represent Mr Fielding of the Public Office, Bow Street, and it is my task to try and find the perpetrator of this evil crime.'

Juliette gave a snort. 'If financial gain was the motive then I doubt you need look further than my father's mistress.'

'That's not fair,' Julian responded roundly. 'Papa was entitled to his happiness. Just because Amelia comes from a lower walk of life there is no need to lay all ills at her door.'

'Huh,' his sister answered in a most unladylike fashion, 'to hear you talk anyone would think you had a fancy for her yourself.'

'How dare you!' Julian replied furiously, and then he pulled himself up short. 'Juliette,' he said in a completely different tone, 'here we are arguing while Father lies dead. We should be ashamed.'

'Don't, don't,' she answered, and fell sobbing into a chair, while he made fists of his hands and gulped furiously in order to stop himself doing likewise.

'Take deep breaths,' the Apothecary advised gently.

Julian turned a stricken glance in his direction. 'But what a terrible thing. Our own father victim of an assassin's blow. Surely robbery must have been the reason for his death.'

'If so, not a great deal was taken,' John answered grimly. 'His rings and watch were missing, that is presuming he wore them . . .'

Julian nodded. 'He did.'

'. . . but it seems that those are considered honest pickings by the watermen whose duty it is to land bodies.'

'God's life, are you telling me that he drowned?'

The Apothecary shook his head. 'I think not. It seems more likely that he was thrown into the river after he was killed.'

Once he had spoken, John wished he hadn't said a thing, for this grim picture finally reduced Julian to tears. But with the extraordinary communication that exists between twins, Juliette stopped crying at that moment and rising from her chair went to comfort her brother. Thinking that he had handled it all very badly, the Apothecary produced his smelling salts and passed them to her.

She gave him a perceptive glance. 'What's this? Have the Beak Runners taken to carrying medicines?'

John smiled sheepishly. 'No, the truth is I am an apothecary. I only work with Mr Fielding from time to time.'

'I see.' Juliette administered the salts to her brother. 'Come Julian, we must rally. Let us give Mr Rawlings what help we

can. We shall have plenty of time for grief after he has gone.'
She turned her lovely streaked face back in John's direction. 'Do
you really mean to find the person who killed our father?'

'I'll do my best, though a cunning criminal could well elude
me.'

Juliette looked at him pleadingly, her expression hard to resist.
'I beg you not to let that happen. Now, Sir, what can we tell
you? Would a description of the events leading up to Papa's
disappearance be of any use?'

John motioned her to sit down, tactfully turning the two chairs
away from Julian, who was struggling hard to control himself.
'Could you go back a little further, Miss Hartfield? Perhaps you
could tell me how Sir William came to be involved with Miss
Lambourn in the first place. I mean, how long has he known her?'

She crinkled her delightful nose. 'I am not certain about that. I
believe some time. Probably before our mother died.'

'How long ago was that?'

'Only seven months. It is all quite, quite shameful.'

Julian interrupted from behind them. 'It was a natural thing,
Mr Rawlings. Ten years ago, when Juliette and I were nine, our
mother suffered a stroke which led her to be paralysed. My father
was quite hale and strong at the time, in the early part of his fifties,
and I believe sought the comforts of marriage elsewhere. My twin
and I were too young to know about such things but we overheard
family gossip and had the long ears of childhood. Then he met
Amelia and she became his mistress. My grandmother found out and
took great exception to this, as did other members of the family who
considered her a money-seeking flap. However, my father obviously
cared for the girl because he planned to wed her.'

'I know about that,' John put in.

'The marriage was to have been secret but Grandmama got wind
of it . . .'

'How?'

'By terrorising Luke Challon into telling her. Then she ordered
us all to go, dressed in black, to try and put a stop to it.'

'But how could you have done that?'

'Had the marriage proceeded she intended to shout out yes when
the preacher asked if anyone knew any just cause or impediment.'

'But she had no right. Your father was a widower after all.'

'She considered that Mother – who was her daughter by the way

65

– was not yet cold in her grave. Why, she swore that she would go to any lengths to see that her son-in-law did not remarry. Did she not, Juliette?'

'Yes,' said his sister, going pale as the full import of the words dawned on her.

John glided over the akward moment. 'And what was your opinion of Miss Lambourn, Mr Hartfield? I presume from your general tone that you take a man of the world's view of your father's transgression. Am I right?'

Julian blossomed and the Apothecary, remembering that the young man considered himself something of a gamester and blood, smiled inwardly.

'I certainly did not disapprove. She is a very pretty delicate soul, albeit something of a dell.'

'Really, Julian,' said Juliette crossly, 'she is a lowlife little harlot and well you know it.'

'Men and women see these things differently,' he answered carelessly.

Sensing that they were about to bicker again, the Apothecary determinedly changed the subject. 'Tell me of the other members of your family apart from your grandmother. Describe them to me.'

'Well, there's Aunt Hesther, Grandmama's daughter and our late mother's sister. She never married and now acts as the old lady's companion, poor creature.'

John nodded as into his pictorial memory flashed a picture of a fluttering female and a nasty old woman sitting together in church.

Juliette took up the tale. 'Father had five children, Roger, Thomas – who drowned at sea – Hugh, then us. Roger never married . . .' She exchanged a sudden mischievous look with her brother which spoke volumes. '. . . so he brought no wife to the house, though Thomas did. You've met her, Lydia the dark lily. She's odd, a bit maddish, in total contrast to our brother Hugh, who is such a prim it is hard to believe he is a Hartfield. And the same can be said about his wife Maud. Needless to say they have no children. Julian reckons that they don't know how to set about getting one.'

She giggled naughtily, her radiance restored, and John considered how ephemeral were the emotions of youth. Then, as if she had picked up his thought wave, Juliette's face grew stricken again. 'We shouldn't be laughing, should we, with poor Father dead?'

'On the contrary, you are grieving for him in your heart so smiles are not forbidden. Now, is that the picture of your family complete?'

'All but for Luke, though he is not actually related. My father took him on as secretary some years ago. I believe he is a younger son of some noble house with no hope of an inheritance. Anyway, despite the fact that he is not tied to us by blood, he lives with the family and seems one of us. He is as devoted to Papa as a dog. *Was* as devoted . . .'

Her voice trailed away sadly and Julian put his arm round her shoulders. 'Shall we go now? Controlling emotions can be very difficult and the strain is beginning to tell on you, I think.'

Intensely sorry that two such burnished and beautiful individuals were having to carry so cruel a burden of sorrow, John got to his feet.

'I regret that I have been the bearer of such grievous news.'

'Someone had to tell us,' Julian answered sensibly.

'But a family member might have been better.'

'Not at all,' Juliette continued. 'They are all so strange, in their different ways, that I preferred to hear the facts from you.' She curtsied and held out her hand. 'Goodbye Mr Rawlings. I hope that we can meet again soon.'

'So do I,' said John, and bowed.

A voice spoke from the doorway and all three of them turned to see that Roger, very white in the face and clad from top to toe in black, in fact in the very same clothes he had worn to Sir William's wedding, had come silently into the room.

'Lydia has informed me that you wish me to accompany you to the mortuary, there to lay claim to my father's remains,' he said theatrically.

'And to make formal identification of the body to the Coroner.'

'I thought that had been done.'

'No, Sir. Identification has been surmised from the effects. It is the duty of a close friend or relative to do the rest.'

Roger staggered slightly. 'I hope I am up to this.'

'Of course you are,' said Julian shortly, as he led his twin from the room.

'It's all very well for him,' remarked Roger pettishly as the door closed behind his younger siblings. 'He hasn't got to do the ghastly task.'

'I'll be there,' said John. 'And I can give you some physic before you go in which will help to keep you strong.'

Roger looked at him moist-eyed. 'How very charming of you, my dear fellow. I shall hold you to that.'

'Do,' said the Apothecary and held the door politely as his companion went out.

In order to avoid putting any extra strain on Roger's fragile nerves, it was decided that the first part of the journey, beyond London Bridge as far as Billingsgate Stairs, should be undertaken by coach. Consequently, John found himself bobbing down the length of The Strand and Fleet Street in one of the most luxurious and expensive equipages in which it had ever been his good fortune to travel. Wealth and opulence breathed from the highly polished wood of the bodywork, the large and finely balanced springs ensuring as comfortable a ride as possible to the passengers, while the four generous windows allowed a good view of the passing parade. Outside, the carriage was decorated by panels depicting roses and fat naked cupids with bouncing buttocks. Within, luxurious padded red velvet covered the seats and there was a hand-painted chamber pot discreetly hidden beneath one of them lest there should be an urgent call from nature.

Seeing John's admiring glances, Roger said carelessly, 'Do you like it?'

'Very much.'

'It's mine. Father would never have allowed such ornamentation on his carriage. He was somewhat staid, you know.'

'Not as regards keeping a mistress, though.'

Roger frowned. 'Oh you've heard about that, have you? It's true, alas. He fell in with a grasping chit who insisted upon marriage once my poor mother had gone to her rest.'

'But Sir William never attended the ceremony. Presumably because he was already dead.'

The beau blanched even paler. 'Oh don't talk about it! The very thought turns my stomach.'

'Will you be all right to travel by water?' the Apothecary enquired anxiously.

'Probably not.'

John's heart sank and he fished in his bag. 'Do take this,

Mr Hartfield. It is pleasant to the taste and really should help to settle any queasiness.'

'What does it contain?'

'A little secret of my own,' the Apothecary answered swiftly, covering the fact that he had filled his holdall in such a hurry he could scarcely remember what he had put in it.

Roger uncorked the phial and downed the contents in a single swallow. 'Excellent,' he said, his eyes lighting up. He lowered his lids. 'By the way, do call me Roger.'

John gulped noisily. 'Er . . . yes . . . of course.'

Climbing Ludgate Hill and Ludgate Street, the carriage skirted round the back of St Paul's Church Yard and into Cheapside, where the daily market was in full swing and the conveyance reduced to walking pace in order to avoid the various stalls. Passing St Mary-le-Bow, whose famous Bow Bells had rung out the curfew in the Middle Ages, they made their way along Poultry, then into Cornhill, where they turned right as if going down to London Bridge itself. However, after a sharp turn into Thames Street, the coachman came to a halt, the way no longer being wide enough to permit entry. Cautiously, John alighted, realising that they were right by Billingsgate Fish Market, as famous for its foul oaths as it was for its fish. Guessing that one sight of Roger, albeit in black, would set the fishmongers off, John walked with eyes down, his ears assailed by obscenities, most of them casting doubt on Roger's masculinity, until he and his companion had reached the relative safety of Billingsgate Stairs where, clustered amongst the many tall masted ships riding at anchor, some wherrymen waited for custom. It was a profound relief to take to the water and finally escape the catcalls.

Contrary to the Apothecary's worst fears, the beau endured the journey well and showed no further signs of faintness until they reached the morgue itself. But once there the sickly scent of death that pervaded the place, despite the herbs and other aromatic substances used to combat the odour of decay, proved too much for him. Dragging a lace trimmed handkerchief to his nostrils, Roger let out a high pitched shriek and leant heavily upon his companion.

'God's mercy, John, what's that terrible stink?' he gasped.

'These corpses await burial, Sir,' the Apothecary answered honestly.

'Oh lud, can *you* not identify my father? One further step and I swear I shall vomit.'

'You won't,' John stated firmly. 'The physick I gave you will hold your stomach firm.'

'But it's heaving now.'

'Oh come along. It won't take a moment.' And John propelled the miserable man forward, his hand resolutely beneath Roger's elbow.

The mortuary attendant approached, striding between the cold slabs and their sheet covered occupants with the nonchalance of one who lived amongst the dead and never gave the fact a second thought.

'We've come to see the body believed to be that of Sir William Hartfield,' the Apothecary informed him.

'Very good. This way, gentlemen.'

Roger made a loud retching sound which John ignored as they followed the assistant through the maze of slabs and finally drew to a halt before one particular corpse. Without ceremony, the attendant twitched back the concealing sheet and Sir William's face appeared.

John turned to the beau, who had gone a glorious shade of pea green. 'Yes?' he said.

'Yes,' gasped Roger, and bolted for the door.

'That's a pretty fellow!' commented the attendant with a laugh.

'Rather delicate I fear,' John answered, grinning. He motioned to the body. 'Do you mind if I have a closer look? I am an apothecary and interested in advancing my knowledge.'

'By all means, Sir. As long as you leave him tidy.'

John nodded, pulling the sheet right back so that only Sir William's feet were covered.

Under the shroud, the corpse had been stripped naked and John could see at a glance that it had undergone a considerable change since he had last examined it. The hours in the river had bloated the body up so that now the skin was stretched tautly over the flesh and had a blueish shade about it. In fact so marked was this inflation that John, bending towards the balding head, found that the pattern made by the fox's head handle was no longer visible. He thought then that whoever had killed Sir William might well have known the effect water would have on his victim, and had chosen the river as a place to dispose of him with much care. But then again, John considered, the murderer might have been in a panic and pushed the body into the Thames as the most expedient way of getting it out of sight. With a sigh, he gave one last long look before drawing the sheet back over all that was left of Sir William Hartfield.

Outside, Roger was leaning against the wall, drawing deeply from a silver hip flask. 'Can we go now?' he puffed, applying the handkerchief to his eyes.

'Not until we've visited the Coroner and asked him to release your late father's remains.'

'Oh pox it!' said the beau, stamping his foot like a petulant child. 'I've had enough of death for one day.'

John put on a sympathetic expression and nodded, despite a growing certainty that Roger was very far from being as distressed as he wanted the world to think.

Chapter Seven

*T*he journey back from the mortuary to St James's Square, two ill-matched points of destination if ever there were any, was not without incident. Twice Roger called for the coach to be stopped, on the first occasion that he might vomit behind a bush, on the second in order to take air and consequently avoid faintness. All in all, John, who had most reluctantly attended the beau as he heaved and gasped, had never been more glad to see civilisation return, and would have jumped straight into a hackney and gone home had not Roger insisted that he borrow his carriage. So it was that the Apothecary returned to Nassau Street in the beau's equipage, a sight which much amused Sir Gabriel, who stared long and hard through his quizzing glass at the abundantly buttocked cupids.

'My dear, how could you allow yourself to be seen in such a thing?' he asked eventually.

'I rather like it,' answered his son, supressing a smile. 'It is amusing, exuberant.'

'Ah,' said Sir Gabriel, putting away the lorgnette, 'is that what it is?'

'Don't tease me,' John replied, undaunted. 'It belongs to a man of style, a beau of cutting fashion, who happens to be the eldest son of the deceased.'

'And a fiend of poor taste if his conveyance is anything to go by.'

'Father, you are getting very intolerant. I am sure Mr Roger Hartfield would consider you staid in your outlook.'

'That,' answered Sir Gabriel crisply, 'would be entirely up to him.'

John looked at his watch. 'Is there time for us to have sherry before supper?'

'Of course there is. Let us go to the library. I am sure you have a great deal to tell me.'

'And I want to hear all about Nicholas. Has he behaved himself?'

'Impeccably. I made it my business to take a stroll to Shug Lane, partly for my health you understand, partly to see how the Muscovite was faring.'

'And . . .?'

'There he was, firmly ensconsed, selling a bottle of your most expensive perfume to an eager young widow. To say nothing of a cure for foul breath to a rotten-toothed barrister's clerk.'

'Did he bring you the day's takings?'

'Most certainly, and I gave the boy a shilling out of it as an advance against his wages.'

'I presume from this that you approve of him?'

'Indeed I definitely do.' Sir Gabriel opened the library door. 'I consider that Mr Fielding served you well with that introduction. Nicholas seems an industrious worker and, besides, the young man has something of an exotic air about him which is obviously favoured by females.'

'How can you be so cynical?'

'With ease,' answered Sir Gabriel, and poured two generous measures of sherry into crystal glasses. He took a seat and smiled at his son blandly. 'A youth of Nicholas's stamp is very good for trade and there's no denying it.'

John took his glass. 'Has he told you his story by any chance?'

'Oh yes. We chatted in the shop while he made me tea.'

'Do you think Tsar Peter was his great grandfather?'

'It's possible I suppose.'

'What an interesting thought.'

'Isn't it.' Sir Gabriel paused, then went on, 'You have an abstracted air, my child. Is the murder of Sir William Hartfield presenting you with a fascinating puzzle?'

'The entire affair is fascinating. First the wedding that never took place, then the bridegroom's witness who ran from the church, then the body being held fast by the ship moored close by the very place where I was celebrating.'

His father shook his head, his daunting wig towering. 'I don't know about that. Tell me.'

'There was a square rigger, a beautiful, powerful vessel, moored in mid stream, just beyond The Devil's Tavern. I could see her through the window until it grew dark, when the lamps on her masts shone on the river like suns. Anyway, according to the Coroner, Sir William's body was found by the watermen, caught up in her mooring ropes. So all the time that I was staring at her, the victim was probably there, lying beneath the water.'

Sir Gabriel refilled both glasses. 'But that means he could have been thrown in anywhere and drifted with the tide until something finally ensnared him.'

'It certainly does. So what I have got to discover is where Sir William spent the night before his marriage. For that is the place where he most likely met his end.'

'He was not at his St James's Square address then?'

'No. Roger Hartfield told me on the journey to Wapping, between bouts of sickness and swooning, that though he was not at home himself, he was informed by the servants that his father left the house on the night prior to the ceremony and did not return.'

'What about his country residence? Was Sir William there?'

'That I shall find out tomorrow when I visit Kirby Hall. By the way, did you ask Nicholas to come here in the morning?'

'He offered to call every day to see if you needed him.'

'What a stout heart he is!'

Sir Gabriel smiled a sagacious smile. 'I think that young man will very soon make himself indispensable to you.'

'To say nothing of rapidly worming his way into your affections.'

John's father gave a cry of laughter. 'No, to say nothing of that at all.'

As dawn shivered the sky on the following morning, John rose and performed his ablutions by candlelight, before dressing in sensible riding clothes. Then the Apothecary made his way through the quiet streets to the livery stables in Dolphin Yard where, in response to a note sent round the previous evening, a grey mare of impeccable character answering to the most unlikely name of Godiva, stood already saddled up, awaiting him. With a leg up from the hostler, John secured a bag containing a change of clothes to the back of the saddle, and trotted off, heading down towards The Strand, before the clocks had so much as struck six.

Even at this hour of the morning, the City of London, which horse and rider entered by way of Temple Bar, was full of people, street traders and hawkers clashing with carts and wagons as they made their way along the thoroughfare, all attempting to avoid the miry ditches on either side, awash with pestilential filth from which indescribable odours came forth to poison the air. It was not easy to make progress, for the middle of the street was equally treacherous, full of cavities which harboured dirty puddles packed with garbage. It was considered great sport by carters and coachmen to charge their horses through these morasses when they had reached full tide and drench from head to toe any poor unfortunate pedestrian who happened to be passing at the time.

Above John's head as he carefully picked his way through, swung the elaborately carved signs of the shopkeepers, each giving the name and profession of its owner, one of the most fanciful belonging to a hosier who had erected a pole hung with stockings. As if taking up the challenge, a shoeblack working on the street corner beneath, was flying a shoe on the end of a stout stick, below which he squatted on his three-legged stool, his pipkin of oil and soot, his brushes, and a cast-off periwig for removing mud, spread out before him. Walking at a snail's pace, the Apothecary proceeded through the stalls of Cheapside market, then on into Poultry, its very name indicating the kind of produce on sale there, before turning left into Threadneedle Street where the shadow of two great buildings, the Bank of England and the Royal Exchange, cast a gloom over both horse and rider.

The path became clearer as John cut across into Bishopsgate Street, leaving the markets behind him. Now he was heading for the Bishops' Gate itself, one of the principal entrances into the City, the others being the Cripple Gate and the Moor Gate. Passing through the ancient portal, there since medieval times when London had consisted of a walled citadel and little else, and so named because it had been the route into the City used by the Bishops of London, the Apothecary found himself in Bishopsgate Street Without, meaning beyond the city walls.

The open ground of the Moor Fields, where the medieval population had played football and practised archery, even skating on the marshy land when it froze over, stretched out to John's left, beyond them the Artillery Ground, where the Fraternity of Longbows, Crossbows and Handguns had trained in the time of Henry VIII. As a harsh reminder of the suffering of the present day, the London Workhouse could be glimpsed nearby and, further away, Bethlem Hospital, better known as Bedlam, where for an entrance fee of 2d. the *beau monde* could go and gaze at the antics of the insane. Not wanting to dwell on such a grim prospect, John coaxed his grey mare across the rough terrain of Shoreditch, emerging by the brewhouse off York Lane. From here it was but a quarter of a mile to Cock Lane, which led away from all signs of habitation and into the open countryside, ultimately going to the pretty rural paradise of Bethnal Green. Well aware that these fields were much frequented by highwaymen, the Apothecary checked that his pistol was in his pocket and took Godiva at a hard canter along the farm track which Cock Lane quickly became.

The March sun now being high in the heavens and John seeing an extremely welcoming hostelry named The George standing beside the thoroughfare, he dismounted, leading his horse round to the stables. Catering as it presumably did for many travellers, the Apothecary was directed by the hostler to a Bog House in the field nearby, a rare luxury not offered by all. However, the odour emanating from the grim looking building was enough to send him in search of a tree. After which relief he went into the bar to order ale, hoping to get into conversation with the landlord so that he might seek information.

As luck would have it, a young woman was serving, presumably the host's daughter, for she tossed her head pertly as John approached and said, with a saucy spark in her eye, 'And what may I do for you, Sir?'

'Oh several things I expect,' he answered, catching her mood and winking, 'but first I would like a flagon of ale, and then directions as to how I can find Kirby Hall.'

There was a sudden stillness in the flagstoned room and the few people who had been sitting on the rough hewn benches, consuming their daily beverage, stopped speaking and stared at him. John instantly came to the conclusion that news of Sir William Hartfield's death had already reached the village and that curiosity was running rife. He decided to play the total innocent and adjusted his features accordingly.

The serving girl looked at him closely. 'Well, it's not far, Sir. About another mile down the road. It's the sizeable house built near to the watch tower. The lane leading to it is called Drift Way.'

She was longing to ask him why he wanted to know, that was obvious, but clearly could not summon up the gall. The Apothecary decided to give her a helping hand.

'I believe there's an elderly lady living there. I have been asked to call on her to discuss her aches and pains. You see,

I am a man of medicine and her family think I might be able to help her.'

'Oh, that would be old Lady Hodkin,' the girl said knowingly. 'It's true she's always complaining. But I'm not sure you'd be welcome there today, Sir.'

John's eyes shone earnestly. 'Oh? Why is that?'

'There's been a bereavement, a tragic death. It's said that Sir William Hartfield, he was the owner, has drowned in the river.'

The Apothecary looked horrified. 'Good gracious! When?'

'I don't know, Sir. One of the gardeners rushed in here this morning to say that during the night a messenger had come from Sir William's London house to inform the family of his death.'

'What a shock. And for you, too. May I buy you a nip of gin?'

The girl dimpled an impudent smile. 'I always enjoy a drink with a gentleman. And my name is Suky, Sir, if you'd like to call me that.'

The Apothecary bowed. 'Rawlings. John Rawlings.'

His companion lowered her voice. 'What's worse, Mr Rawlings, is that Sir William was about to get married. Secretly though, nobody was supposed to know.'

'How very interesting.'

Suky warmed to her tale. 'One of the under footmen who thinks he's sweet on me, overheard Sir William and Luke Challon talking about it. That's how I found out. Just to think of it! Off to get married and then he dies.'

Wondering to how many other people the servant had passed on this choice piece of gossip, John said, 'It's beyond belief! But why was Sir William being so furtive about getting wed?'

'Because he had been misbehaving with the bride for years. She was his kept woman, his fancy piece.'

'Are you telling me that was during the time of his first marriage?'

'Of course I am.'

John held out his tankard for some more ale. 'How very shocking! Surely Sir William's family could not have approved. I have heard they are very respectable people.'

Suky gave a delectable smile. 'They'd like you to think they are. But it wouldn't do to dig too deep. I reckon all of 'em's got something to hide, even poor Miss Hesther.'

'Is she the old lady's companion?'

'Yes, her eldest unmarried daughter. Sir William's late wife's sister. I've heard it said . . .' Suky giggled. '. . . that she's nursed a passion for her brother-in-law all these years, ever since she and her sister met him as young women.'

'Then she must have been very hurt by the fact he was about to marry his mistress. That is, if she knew of it.'

'Oh, she knew all right. Job, that's the under footman, says they had all found out and were determined to stop it.'

'And now the bridegroom is dead,' said John without emphasis, watching her expression.

Suky looked extremely thoughtful. 'Yes, strange, isn't it. I wonder how Sir William came to fall in the river. Or was he given a helping hand, do you think?'

'That's naughty,' the Apothecary answered reprovingly, 'for surely no member of a loving family would harm another.'

'In a *loving* family, no,' she replied. 'But I'm not so certain that the Hartfields know too much about love. In fact I'd say that, between 'em, they know a great deal more about hatred.'

The whisper of spring was everywhere, in the wild flowers burgeoning beneath the hedgerows, in the swiftly important flight of birds, in the disturbing, primitive song of thrushes, in the sharp sunshine which lit the landscape with such crystal clarity. So it was in a mood of sparkling excitement, quite unsuited to the task in hand, that the Apothecary rode towards Kirby Hall on that mad March noontime. An excitement engendered by the fact that the world was coming back to life again after the winter and that he was young and alive and part of it.

Before he had gone to bed on the previous evening, John had searched through Sir Gabriel's library for a guide book and had found one dated 1754, the previous year. Looking up Bethnal Green, he had read, 'this Parish hath the Face of a Country, affording every Thing to render it pleasant, Fields, Pasturage-grounds for Cattle, and formerly Woods and Marshes.' And staring about him as he crossed over the Green, its few gracious houses nestling amongst the trees, the Apothecary thought how very accurate the description was, for he could not remember being in a prettier place for an age.

Immediately opposite him stretched a tree-lined track from which John caught a distant glimpse of a Watch House. This, then, must be where his destination lay. Trotting on, the Apothecary turned his eyes to the right and drew in breath in wonderment at the unashamed ebullience of the red-bricked Stuart mansion which met his gaze.

Surrounded by carefully tended gardens and lying back from the path, Kirby Hall consisted of a major central block, very grand and imposing, connected by several intervening ranges of elegant pavilions, a majestic gate tower with a clock and weathervane above, dominating all. Before the house stood a smooth arrangement of flower beds, known as a parterre, at its side, a bowling green. There could be no doubt, even at this distance, that great wealth had built this magnificent edifice and that considerable sums continued to maintain it. Wishing he were wearing something smarter, John walked Godiva up the drive then, having handed her to an hostler who seemed to have appeared from nowhere, went on foot up the path through the parterre and pulled the bell which hung outside the front door.

Already there were signs that this was a house of mourning. The curtains on the many windows had been drawn fast and the door knocker was carefully encased in dark flannel. The footman who answered wore a black ribbon over his livery and a long face to match it. Clearly expecting John to be a neighbour come to offer his condolences, his eyes widened in surprise at the travel-stained spectacle which the Apothecary presented.

'Yes, Sir?' the servant enquired, his voice solemn as the knell of doom.

'I have come to see Lady Hodkin,' John answered cautiously.

'I am afraid she cannot be disturbed, Sir. There has been a bereavement in the family and they are not receiving,' came the mournful reply.

'But I fear I *must* disturb her,' the Apothecary answered firmly. 'You see, I am here on the business of the Public Office, Bow Street, making an investigation into the mysterious death of Sir William Hartfield.'

The footman looked thoroughly startled, his eyebrows shooting upwards towards his white wig. News of foul play had obviously not reached the servants' hall. John wondered if it had even been relayed to the family by the rider who had come through the darkness to tell them of the loss of its head.

'I regret having to shock you,' he continued, very aware of how brutal and uncaring he must sound, 'but it is essential that I speak to someone. Are any of Sir William's sons available?'

'No, Sir. Mr Roger and Mr Julian are in London, and Mr Hugh is on a voyage to France.'

'Then what about Mr Challon, the secretary?'

'Mr Challon has gone to Wapping, Sir, to inform those who work in Sir William's office of the tragedy.'

'Then if Lady Hodkin is unavailable I will have to speak to one of the other ladies.' John softened his tone even further. 'I would not inflict this on them were the matter not so urgent.'

'Then I will try to find Mrs Hartfield or Miss Hesther. Please take a seat and I will make enquiries.'

With those words the front door opened wide and John found himself ushered into a stately grand hall, not typically Stuart in design, having something of an earlier style about it. From there he was shown into a small panelled room, somewhat dark and oppressive in atmosphere. Thinking how greatly all this contrasted with Sir William's London home, the Apothecary sat down, wondering what was going to happen next. If the ladies of the house stood firm against interruption to their mourning, there was little he could do. Even Mr Fielding's letter of authorisation would not get him past a determined set of weeping women. Hoping that one of them would decide to be cooperative, John sat listening to the ticking of the clock, pondering whether he would be able to get home that night or whether it would be too dark to leave Bethnal Green. A factor of great significance in view of the highwaymen who haunted the surrounding countryside.

The door opened and John saw that the footman had returned. 'Lady Hodkin will receive you now, Sir,' he intoned, his face expressionless though his eyes were beady with curiosity. 'Would you care to use our facilities first?'

And before John could say a word he was propelled back into the hall and into a niche containing an enormous mahogany projection, complete with holes, brass handles and cocks, the whole frightening edifice being known as a plunger closet. This monstrosity filled the space so closely that it was impossible to shut the door while the thing was in use. Holding his breath, the Apothecary availed himself of its noisesome services, then rushed out to wash off the dust of his journey in the sturdy tripod with basin and jug that thankfully stood outside the horrid little cabinet. A few moments later, in stark contrast, he was ascending the grandest of grand staircases, heavy with richly carved oak banisters, heading towards a landing with a very fine moulded plaster ceiling.

The footman glanced over his shoulder. 'Who should I say is calling, Sir?'

'John Rawlings.'

'Very good.' The man halted before a door and gave a deferential cough, then he knocked.

'Come in,' called a quavering voice.

'Mr John Rawlings, m'Lady,' he announced and made a rapid retreat, leaving the Apothecary to enter the room alone.

Here, too, both curtains and shutters were drawn, betokening a place of death, and John had to peer through the gloom to make out his surroundings. Staring round, he saw that he was in some kind of parlour which, in normal circumstances, must have been quite pleasant and cosy. Now, however, with its tapestry-hung walls and opulently ornate ceiling, the place appeared dismal and dark and just a little sinister. To add to the menacing atmosphere, the Apothecary was certain he could hear the faint sound of wheezing, as if some creature were struggling for breath in the blackness.

A voice spoke out of the shadows behind him. 'And who the devil might you be, young man?'

John started violently then whirled round, narrowing his eyes. Sitting in a chair, looking almost like a large bolster, was a dumpy shape that appeared to be human. Staring even more closely, the Apothecary was able to recognise the features of the odious old woman he had seen in the church. As best he could in the darkness, he made a bow.

'The name is Rawlings, Ma'am. Here about the business of Mr John Fielding, the Principal Magistrate.'

There was a snort of contempt. 'Common upstart, he and his brother both. Came from nowhere, no good breeding, and now they think they can lord it over us all. Well, he ain't got no jurisdiction here, Sir, so you'd best be off.'

John stared at her, utterly amazed and totally lost for words. Then a low growl echoed through the shadows, apparently her last say on the subject. The Apothecary felt the sweat break out on his brow, certain that he was in the clutch of lunatics. Then he became aware of something moving on Lady Hodkin's lap. Taking a step forward, John saw that it was an ancient and ugly pug, the source of the asthmatic sounds he had heard earlier. Disliking both the dog and its owner, he drew in breath and decided to ignore the speaker's great and venerable age.

'I'm afraid that that is where you are wrong, Madam. Mr Fielding's men have authority to go anywhere in the kingdom in search of villains. Which is precisely what I am doing now. I am seeking out the scoundrel who cruelly did Sir William Hartfield to death.'

There was a pause before she answered, 'Bah! What rubbish is this? My son-in-law drowned accidentally.'

The Apothecary advanced another step and turned on her a terrible gaze. 'Sir William Hartfield was beaten over the head with a stick and was then thrown into the river. I know because I examined his body shortly after it was retrieved. There can be no disputing the facts. And it is those facts which give me, acting on the Magistrate's behalf, the absolute right to question all those connected with the dead man. In fact, Madam, I'll go one better. Refusal by any person to cooperate can only be taken by those in authority as a possible sign of guilt.'

Lady Hodkin let out a feeble cry and it occurred to John that the old wretch was a past mistress at play acting.

'Hesther, Hesther, come to me at once,' she screeched. 'There is a man in here, threatening me.'

The far door, presumably leading to a bedroom, flew open in rapid response to this and a plump woman of mature years and completely nondescript appearance, rushed in breathlessly.

'Now, now, Mother. What's happening? Who are you, Sir?'

'An officer of the law,' John answered dramatically, and watched with a certain satisfaction as the poor creature gasped and sat down hastily.

'He's terrorising me, he's terrorising me,' the old woman bleated meanwhile. 'Oh, my heart. I'm going to have a seizure. I can feel one coming on.'

'Give her this,' said the Apothecary, passing Hesther his salts.

She stared at the bottle suspiciously. 'What is it?'

'A reviving spirit. Please trust me, Ma'am. It will do Lady Hodkin no harm, I assure you.'

She shot him such a grateful and pathetic look that John's heart went out to her. The impression he had received in St Paul's had been utterly right. Hesther Hodkin had devoted her life to caring for a selfish old tyrant who had ruined it for her in return.

'You didn't threaten her, did you?' Hesther whispered pleadingly.

'No, of course not,' John lied. 'I came to see her about the death of her son-in-law, that is all.'

Hesther's already pasty complexion turned even greyer. 'I cannot believe that William is dead.' She pressed her knuckles to her mouth. 'Roger's letter . . .'

'Yes?'

'It seemed to me that it hinted at foul play, though he did not come out and directly say so. Tell me . . .'

But she got no further. The old woman, beating the air with her stick, managed to land a glancing blow on her daughter's shoulders. Near to tears, Hesther administered the salts.

John could not resist it. 'I see you are very handy with your cane, Madam. Perhaps you should watch where you are aiming.'

Tossing the pug to one side, Lady Hodkin rose from her chair like a fury. 'Get out, get out I say. Common little beast. Don't you ever show your face round here again, do you hear me!'

'I shall show my face as often as Mr Fielding requires me to do so,' John answered with dignity, then looked in Hester's direction. 'I shall await you downstairs, Miss Hodkin. I am afraid there are certain questions I have to ask you.'

'You're not to speak to him,' yelled the old tyrant. 'He's a tradesman.'

'Oh Mother, really!' Hesther answered miserably as the door closed behind the Apothecary's retreating back.

Yet despite this very minor stand against her parent's domination, it still took the poor woman an age to extricate herself from Lady Hodkin's clutches. In fact John, waiting below in the same small chamber, was on the point of taking his leave when Hesther finally threw open the door.

'I am so very sorry,' she gasped. 'I'm afraid my poor Mama does suffer with her nerves.'

'Yet obviously still maintains her strength,' John answered drily.

'Oh yes, yes indeed.' Hesther glanced over her shoulder nervously. 'She has forbidden me to speak to you. She says that she is going to write a letter of complaint to Mr Fielding. In fact she is threatening all kinds of terrible things.' The unhappy woman paused for breath. 'Oh, Mr Rawlings, what shall I do?'

John gave her a reassuring smile. 'Could we not speak somewhere private, somewhere where your mother does not go?'

Hesther frowned. 'But where could that possibly be?'

'Out of this house, perhaps.'

She stared at him in horror. 'Oh, but that would not be seemly. I mean . . .'

The Apothecary looked at her intently. 'Miss Hodkin, I believe you were very fond of your late brother-in-law.'

She flushed unalluringly. 'Yes.'

'Well, then, I shall pay you the courtesy of telling you the truth about him. What you feared is, alas, a fact. Sir William was murdered and thrown into the river, his assailant, at the moment, unknown.'

Hesther clutched her throat and let out a terrible sob, but said nothing.

'That is where I enter the picture,' John continued. 'Mr Fielding has entrusted me with the task of finding his killer and bringing him to justice. The only way I can do this is by talking to everyone involved and sifting through their evidence. Therefore, I would ask that you meet me later tonight in The George, the inn by the roadside, little more than a mile from here. I am sure that you will be able to assist me enormously.'

Hesther looked at him, her eyes awash with tears. 'Do you really mean that?'

'Of course I do.'

'Then I'll come,' she said determinedly. 'I'll do all I can to help you cause that wicked being to answer for his crime.'

Impetuously, John kissed her fingers. 'I admire your courage, Miss Hodkin. Shall we say eight o'clock?'

She started to weep and turned her head away. 'Yes, eight o'clock,' she replied in a choked voice. Then she withdrew her hand and hurried from the room.

Chapter Eight

*F*or an hostelry set in so out of the way a place, The George appeared to do remarkably good trade. So much so, the Apothecary considered himself lucky to get the last room in the house, packed as the inn was with wayfarers and travellers. But once having dealt with the problem of securing himself a bed, John took the redoubtable Godiva round to the stables, unhitched his bag from the saddle and went briefly to the small chamber beneath the eaves which had been allocated to him. Then, having washed and changed into clean clothes, he hurried to the parlour, the smell of cooking reminding him all too clearly that he hadn't eaten a thing since an extremely early breakfast.

In common with most coaching inns, the dining arrangements at The George were divided into two, the humbler travellers eating in the kitchen, the people of quality in the parlour. And though the Apothecary would have much preferred to dine amongst the locals, for the kitchen was always the place in which the best gossip could be overheard, one glance told him that it was already full and he had little alternative but to make his way to the other location.

Taking his seat at an unoccupied table laid for four, John took a swift look round at the other guests already assembled. An over-painted lady of uncertain years, together with her maid, both sitting nearby, smiled as she caught his eye. A red-faced parson, studying a book, muttered a surly greeting. A London family, obviously setting off on a visit, ignored him entirely. Whilst a man with a loud voice, whom John took from his flamboyant appearance to be a member of the acting fraternity, shouted a loud 'Good evening'. Having bowed and smiled at them all, the Apothecary turned his attention to the bill of fare, determined to fill his stomach before Hesther arrived. Listed under the word 'Eating' was a choice of several dishes, all advertised at the price of One Shilling. Marvelling at the cheapness of it all, John ordered beef broth served with meat and vegetables, to be followed by pie, bread and cheese. All of this to be washed down with several tankards of ale. Then in happy anticipation of the meal to come, he sat contentedly, covertly studying the pecularities of the human race.

It was at this moment that two men walked in and took a seat at a table almost directly behind his; two men at whom, in normal circumstances, he wouldn't have given a second glance. But there had been something about one of them that had brought the Apothecary back to a state of full alertness. For though he had been unable to get a really good look, John could have sworn that Valentine Randolph, the man he had seen both at the wedding and later in The Devil's Tavern and whom he believed to be Sir William Hartfield's office manager, had just come into the room, an extraordinary coincidence to say the least of it. Wondering how he could turn round without obviously gaping, John hit on the scheme of knocking his salt cellar to the floor and, in retrieving it, making a close inspection.

The plan worked even better than he could have wished. The man at the table behind politely leaned down from his chair to be of assistance and thus came face to face with the Apothecary who, by this time, was scrabbling about on his hands and knees. It was Randolph all right, John was certain of it. Indeed, there was just the merest hint of recognition in the man's eyes, though of the kind that cannot recall where or when the meeting has taken place.

'Much obliged, Sir,' said the Apothecary gratefully, as the salt cellar changed hands.

'A pleasure, Sir,' answered the other, and turned back to his companion.

John strained his ears. '. . . was killed?' Randolph was whispering. 'I simply can't believe it.'

'Apparently it's true. Roger wrote a private note to me. It seems a man from Bow Street took him to the mortuary . . .'

Randolph gave a low but distinct chuckle. 'I'm sure he appreciated that!'

'. . . and there is talk of Sir William being struck before he went into the river.'

The voice died away again but the Apothecary clearly heard Valentine Randolph snatch in his breath. However, it was at this moment that his meal arrived, steaming in its generous bowl, together with Suky bearing more ale and a wink about the eye.

'Well, well,' she said. 'They told me you'd come back.'

John smiled. 'It was too dark to return to London so I decided to extend my stay.' He lowered his voice. 'Tell me, do you have a snug, or any other small room in which I could have a private conversation?'

Suky looked at him sharply. 'Why? Expecting company?'

'Yes, as a matter of fact.'

'A lady is it?'

'Yes. Miss Hesther from the big house. She wants to discuss her mother's health.'

Suky grinned, a cheeky expression on her face. 'Oh Miss Hesther!' she exclaimed noisily. 'I thought you meant somebody young.'

Acutely aware that Valentine Randolph and his companion had stopped speaking and that it was now their turn to eavesdrop on him, John motioned her to be quiet.

'Oh I'm sorry to be indiscreet, Sir,' Suky continued, reading his expression and changing her tone to a loud stage whisper. 'Yes, we do have a nice little snug leading off the bar you were in earlier. I'll see to it that the boy attends to the fire.'

Giving up, John held out his tankard for refilling, almost feeling the two pairs of eyes that were boring into his back. Certain now that Mr Randolph had indeed worked for Sir William, for how else could he have recognised poor Hesther's name, John conjectured as to the identity of his companion. And it would seem that he was equally the subject of speculation, for the conversation coming from the next table was now of so general a nature as to be ridiculous. Half amused by the entire situation, the Apothecary proceeded to demolish his meal with relish, sending for a second helping of tart with custard when the first was gone. Then, having secured a bottle of port, the finest the house could sell, he proceeded to the snug to await Miss Hesther's arrival.

Punctually at eight o'clock, John heard the sound of a chaise draw up in the inn yard and a coachman jump down from his box to open the door. Certain that it was his visitor, the Apothecary was just about to leave the snug and escort her inside when raised voices caught his attention.

'Miss Hodkin!' said one of them. 'What are you doing here?'

A more redoubtable dame might have told the speaker to mind his business but Hesther, victim of so many years of subservience, muttered something inaudible, the very tone of which told John that she was thoroughly nonplussed. Distressed that the poor woman should be browbeaten yet again, the Apothecary went to her rescue at speed.

Much as he had expected, she had been accosted by Valentine Randolph and his associate, both of whom stood talking to her beneath the light of a lamp which swung from the stable wall. Crossing the cobbles, John went to join them, making the trio an elegant bow.

'Ah, Miss Hodkin,' he said, bestowing a courteous smile on the two gentlemen, 'I am so glad you could keep our appointment. Pray step inside. A good fire awaits you.'

Mr Randolph's companion gave John a steely glance. 'I don't think I've had the pleasure . . .' he began.

'The name's Rawlings,' the Apothecary answered, his smile even more pleasant, 'come to call on Sir William Hartfield's family on behalf of Mr Fielding, the Principal Magistrate.'

The other's jaw sagged violently. 'What did you say?'

'I'm here on Mr Fielding's business. Now, Miss Hodkin, pray step within. We have much to discuss I believe.'

'I insist on accompanying the lady,' said the speaker.

'You may insist until the moon turns green,' John answered, and offered Hesther his arm.

'Oh please, Luke,' she murmured, red with embarrassment, 'don't make a fuss. I have met this gentleman before.'

'But you have no chaperone.'

'Mr Challon,' said John icily, taking Sir William's secretary completely by surprise at the use of his surname, 'if you do not let this lady pass you will leave me no alternative but to presume that you are deliberately trying to impede the course of justice.'

'Before you get so damned high-handed,' Luke answered, jutting out his chin, 'let's see your authorisation. You don't look like a Runner to me.'

'Certainly,' the Apothecary answered promptly, and drew John Fielding's letter from an inside pocket.

Luke Challon raised it to the light and scanned the contents, then passed it to Valentine Randolph, who read the document in silence. They looked at one another, then the secretary cleared his throat.

'So Roger wasn't exaggerating. Sir William really was murdered.'

'I fear so.'

'But who could have done such a thing? He was a highly respected man.'

Valentine interrupted, his words coming a shade too rapidly. 'He was obviously set upon by a cutpurse. He fell victim to a common thief, that's the truth of it.'

'Convenient though that answer would be,' John stated harshly, 'I'm afraid it is not the case. Valuables were found on Sir William's body, valuables that no footpad worth the name would have left behind him.'

'Then it must have been because of Amelia,' Luke said, almost to himself, then obviously regretted the words and looked horribly uncomfortable.

Hesther came to the rescue. 'I'm getting somewhat chilled,' she remarked in an apologetic voice. 'May we go inside?'

'Certainly,' said John. He turned to the two men. 'Gentlemen, I shall call on you both at Kirby Hall tomorrow morning. Much as I dislike having to pry into the private lives of others, I fear it is a necessary evil if a killer is to be brought to book. I trust I will have your cooperation.'

'I know very little,' Valentine Randolph answered, again in the same over-quick manner, 'but naturally I will be of what assistance I can. As to seeing me tomorrow, I am staying here, at the inn, so we may as well get the wretched business over tonight, after Miss Hodkin has gone.'

Luke sighed deeply. 'As Sir William's secretary I was privy to his affairs but have a natural abhorence about discussing them. Yet I suppose in the circumstances I must do so. I shall see you in the morning, Mr Rawlings.' He turned to the office manager. 'I shall tell Lady Hodkin that you will visit her tomorrow to express your sympathy.'

'She may not see you,' put in Hesther unexpectedly. 'She's not had a good word for Mr Randolph since the wedding.'

'The wedding!' Valentine repeated bitterly. 'I wonder how different things might have been if it had actually taken place.'

Luke gave him a warning look. 'Useless conjecture will get us no further.' He addressed Miss Hodkin. 'I shall await your safe return.'

John grinned to himself in the darkness. 'I promise that no harm will come to Miss Hesther in my charge.'

'Oh tush,' she said with an unanticipated show of spirit, and without addressing any of the gentlemen further, led the way indoors.

She was not, John thought, regarding his guest in the mellow glow of candlelight, altogether ugly. In fact, with the skilful use of cosmetic preparations, she could be reasonably comely. It was merely the fact that poor, pathetic Hesther had allowed herself to become so horribly drab, and all in the service of an odious old lady who did not deserve her daughter's unfailing devotion. Only wishing that he could do something to help her, John spoke gently but directly.

'I know it may not be easy for you to talk of the past, Miss Hodkin, but, believe me, it will be more than helpful if you do. As you know, I am not a Beak Runner by profession but an apothecary, yet on the occasions when I have been called upon to assist Mr Fielding, it has been my experience that the key to present circumstances nearly always lies in what has gone before.'

She gave a small cough but did not reply.

'Therefore, I would like to ask you some questions about things that happened many years ago. Do I have your permission?'

Hesther looked at him meekly. 'Yes, I suppose so.'

'But first let me offer you a glass of port. I really can recommend it as very soothing to the throat and chest. It will ease that cough of yours.'

'I hardly ever drink.'

'Not even for medicinal purposes?'

'Oh, very well then.'

Pouring her a generous measure, John replenished his own glass. 'Now, Miss Hodkin, I wonder if you would tell me in what circumstances you first met Sir William Hartfield. Is it true that you and your sister were little more than girls at the time?'

Hesther looked slightly discomfited. 'How did you know that?'

John tapped the side of his nose in the style of Joe Jago, Mr Fielding's clerk. 'The Public Office has its methods,' he answered mysteriously.

'Oh! Well, yes, it is a fact that I was twenty and Harriet eighteen, when we first encountered him.'

'And how did you meet?'

'William came to work in our father's office. The Hodkins are a Bristol family and have always been in shipping. As my father was only a middle son, he went to London to strike out on his own, and did very well for himself. In fact he became an alderman and was knighted.'

'How commendable. And William?'

'He had been at sea but decided that he would have a brighter future on dry land. My father took him on as an assistant. That is how my sister got to know him.'

'And so they were happily married.'

'Ye–es,' said Hesther, with the slightest note of hesitation.

'You sound a little doubtful. Why?'

'My mother opposed the match. She did not care for William, you see.'

'Indeed?'

Hesther downed her port in a noisy gulp. 'She said he had no breeding. When she enquired who his people were, she discovered that he was merely the son of a Shadwell rope-maker. He was also without money, owning only what he earned himself. In the end, he and Harriet ran away and were married secretly. I helped them and she never forgave me for it.'

John quietly refilled Miss Hodkin's glass. 'You obviously approved of him then?'

Hesther looked at him, her eyes brimming with unshed tears. 'I was very fond of him, yes,' she said softly.

'Were you, perhaps, a little in love with him?' the Apothecary asked.

She glared at him, hovering between anger and the desperate need to confide. John smiled at her encouragingly.

'If I read your glance correctly, Miss Hodkin, you despise me for my forward manner. But please believe that my only concern is to find Sir William's killer. However, there is no need for you to reply to any of my questions if you find them too personal.'

Hesther nodded. 'Then let us leave my feelings out of the matter.'

'Very well. I will pass on to something else. From information I have received already, I believe that some years ago your sister suffered a stroke which left her an invalid. Shortly after this, so I am told, your brother-in-law took a mistress, a certain Miss Lambourn, whom he recently intended to marry. Is this correct?'

Miss Hodkin nodded, this time quite fiercely, but said nothing.

'I see. Ah well, passion plays odd tricks with people I suppose.'

She snorted. 'Lust, you mean. He craved that avaricious strumpet, strained after her like some ghastly old goat.'

'I take it you did not like Miss Lambourn,' John commented trimly.

'I loathed her,' Hesther answered, tears pouring down her unrouged cheeks.

'A very strong reaction for a sister-in-law.'

She threw her head back with rare defiance. 'All the family felt the same.'

'I think perhaps you more than any of them,' John said very gently.

'I told you I was fond of William.'

'Very fond, I believe. Come, Miss Hodkin, you have nothing to fear from me. Did your fondness grow into love?'

'Yes,' she hissed, suddenly losing control, 'yes, you inquisitive and wretched creature, of course it did. Now are you satisfied?'

'Sir William hurt you very much, didn't he?' John answered soothingly.

Hesther burst into violent sobs. 'He wounded me beyond belief. When my poor sister died I honestly thought he might come to me at last. Only to discover that he had been keeping that whore, that slattern, that foul little bitch all along.'

'So your love turned to hatred,' said John softly.

She shook with emotion, but must have realised down what a dangerous path her words were leading her.

'No, no, never that. However badly William treated me, I had to accept the fact that he did not realise how cruel he was being. To him I was just Harriet's sister, the relative he had always known and been fond of. Believe me, I could never hate him. I cared for him too deeply.'

'Yet Sir William was obviously capable of stirring strong emotions in others. Did he have many enemies that you know of?'

Hesther pulled the strangest face. 'He fell out with his children from time to time, as all fathers do. He considered some of them too frivolous, others too grasping. But these were mere family tiffs. No, if you are seeking his killer, I suggest that you look no further than Miss Amelia Lambourn herself.'

'But why should she wish to murder her future husband?'

'Because he has left her all his money.'

'Do you know this for a fact?'

Hesther tossed her head, the first truly feminine gesture that John had ever seen her make. 'No, of course I don't. But it stands to reason.'

'Not necessarily.'

Aware that she was making something of a fool of herself, Hesther rapidly became stiff and formal. 'Is there anything else that you wish to know?' she asked in a clipped voice.

'Yes, just one small point. When did you last see Sir William alive?'

'About five days before he was due to be married. The ceremony was supposed to be secret but my mother suspected it was imminent and frightened Luke Challon into telling her the time and place. Anyway, a few days previously William came to Kirby Hall to supervise the redecoration of some of the rooms. Obviously it was being done for *her*. I suppose he intended to bring his bride home after they were wed. Can you imagine a more terrible situation?'

John attempted to picture Lady Hodkin dwelling beneath the same roof as her son-in-law's pretty young wife, and failed miserably. He shook his head.

'No, I can't. But that aside, how was Sir William on that occasion? Did he seem worried at all?'

'Not in the least. On the contrary, he was cheerful to a degree.'

'I see.' The Apothecary changed tack. 'How are you feeling now, Miss Hodkin? Is there anything I can get you? I have one or two medicaments up in my room.'

She shook her head. 'I am quite recovered, thank you, though somewhat ashamed that I broke down as I did. However, if you have no further questions I would prefer to take my leave. Events have become somewhat overwhelming and I would welcome a night's sleep.'

John got to his feet. 'Of course. Allow me to escort you to your carriage. If I think of anything else I can always ask you tomorrow.'

Hesther finished her third glass of port and stood up. 'What I said tonight will remain confidential, will it not?'

'If you mean am I going to tell your family, the answer is definitely no.'

She smiled at him tearfully and just for a second a look of

enormous charm peeped out. 'Thank you for that. My mother was quite wrong about you, you know.'

'I would imagine,' said John, with feeling, 'that your mother can be wrong about a great many things.'

It was cold outside the inn, the moon almost full, riding high in a sable sky brimful with galaxies of glittering stars. Looking upwards, John momentarily lost track of his surroundings and leapt with fright when a voice spoke to him out of the shadows.

'Mr Rawlings?'

'Yes.'

'Are you ready to speak to me now?'

'Is that you, Mr Randolph?'

'It is.'

'Then let us go inside and make the most of what is left of the fire. To say nothing of the remains of a fine bottle of port.'

'You don't seem like the usual type of Beak Runner,' Valentine commented as they stepped within.

'I only work for Mr Fielding on an ad hoc basis. I am an apothecary by profession.'

'How strange,' came the reply. But John did not elucidate further until they were comfortably settled in the snug, listening to the noise of the inn as both the building and its occupants settled down for the night. Then he spoke.

'Believe me, as I've already told you, I don't enjoy asking people intimate questions about their private lives.'

'Then why do it?'

'Because I love the search for the truth, the pitting of wits against those of a cunning killer. Further, Mr Fielding has asked me to help him with this case because I was the one who discovered Sir William's body.'

'And you consider that in the answers you are given lie the shreds of the solution to his murder.'

'Most certainly.'

'Then ask away. I was fond of my employer, in fact I owe him a debt of gratitude. I won't shirk from anything that will help track down his slayer.'

Valentine Randolph stretched his legs to the fire and John did likewise. 'Tell me, how long have you known him?'

'Fifteen years, since I was twenty, in fact. He rescued me from my own determined efforts to turn myself into a drunken sot by offering me employment in his office.' Valentine laughed softly. 'I considered myself dying of a broken heart, you see.'

'Why was that?'

'I was very much in love with a cousin of mine, a Jane Randolph. She was born and baptised in the same year as myself, 1720, but her father, a sea captain educated in the colony of Virginia, returned there before I was able to declare my passion.'

'What was he doing in London?'

'He had come over here to find a second wife after the death of his first. He was active in the slave trade and very prosperous.'

'What happened?'

'Jane married another colonist, Peter Jefferson, when she was nineteen. As a result, I decided on a life of debauchery until Sir William got hold of me, that is. Jane is now a mother, by the way – her son is called Thomas. I have remained a bachelor.'

John nodded. 'I see. Now, Mr Randolph, tell me what you know of Sir William's early life.'

It was strange to hear the same story that Hesther had told, this time from a different focus. The facts were identical, only the interpretation of them different. It seemed that Valentine had a similar view to Julian Hartfield. Sir William, with an invalid wife and no one to love him, had been perfectly justified in finding himself a mistress.

'And exactly where *did* he find her?' John asked curiously.

'At New Tunbridge Wells, I believe.'

'Do you mean Islington Spa?'

'Yes, the same.'

'All the London pleasure gardens are well known as meeting places, of course.'

'Yes, but she wasn't there as a visitor, Amelia Lambourn actually worked at the Spa.'

'Doing what?'

'Serving water from the Well.'

'Good God! So she had no pretensions at all to being *bon ton*.'

'None whatsoever.'

'Then small wonder Lady Hodkin objected so violently to the match.'

'She considered the whole situation a slur on the family honour.

I think she would have gone to any lengths to stop Sir William marrying the wretched girl.'

'So where did you stand in all this? You were going to act as bridegroom's witness, were you not?'

Valentine Randolph looked thoroughly startled. 'How do you know that?'

John smiled enigmatically. 'The Public Office prides itself on being well informed.'

'Incredibly so. No, as I have already told you, I believed that my employer was entitled to some happiness at last. Lady Hartfield's illness had been a long and painful one, in fact it had affected every member of the family in different ways. I felt as none of them dare oppose Lady Hodkin and stand up for Sir William at the ceremony, then I would do so.'

'But the marriage never took place.'

'No, he did not come. Somebody made sure of that.'

'Yes,' said John thoughtfully. 'You know, it will be interesting to see exactly how Sir William's estate has been disposed.'

Valentine nodded. 'I presume the will will be read after the funeral.'

'Do you know the name of your employer's lawyer by any chance?'

'He used two, one for business, the other for personal matters. I only dealt with the commercial man. Luke will be able to furnish the details of the second.'

'I shall ask him tomorrow morning when I return to Kirby Hall. You know, Mr Randolph, I feel that the contents of Sir William's last testament will tell us a great deal about why he had to die.'

'You mean that following his marriage the bulk of his fortune was going to be left to Amelia and that somebody was desperate to prevent that happening?'

'That is one possibility. The other, of course, is that she is already his heiress.'

'Then that would mean . . .'

'Yes. I think it is essential that I speak to Miss Lambourn without any further delay.'

'Only Luke knows where she lives, officially that is.'

'What do you mean?'

'That I am fairly certain others knew of her whereabouts.'

'What others?' John asked curiously.

But Valentine Randolph refused to be drawn further and took to staring into the dying embers of the fire without saying another word.

Chapter Nine

*I*t was still very early in the morning, but despite that the servants were up, preparing the mansion for the day. Granted admittance by a yawning footman, not the man he had seen previously, John was once more shown into the small anteroom to await the arrival of Luke Challon, who was presently at his breakfast. In this way, with not even a newspaper to amuse him, the Apothecary found himself listening to every sound and was intrigued when the muffled knocker was banged and the front door opened once more. There was a murmured conversation, followed by the sound of a man's footsteps echoing on the floor of the great hall. Then came the noise of running feet as somebody hurried down the grand staircase to greet the newcomer. John strained his ears.

The couple were speaking very softly but it was still possible to make out that they were a man and a woman. Convinced that they were Julian and Juliette, the Apothecary moved stealthily to the door.

'. . . anybody see you?' asked the female.

'No one of any . . .' The male voice dropped infuriatingly.

'Then you're safe,' the woman said clearly.

'On the contrary . . .' The speaker started to whisper. '. . . gone terribly wrong.'

The female let out a little shriek. 'You don't mean . . .?'

'Yes,' he answered, quite forcibly yet with a break in his voice. 'I'm afraid I do.'

Longing to peer out but terrified of revealing himself, John slid his eye to the crack, but the couple were already climbing the stairs and had gone out of sight. Positive that it had been the twins who conversed, the Apothecary sat down again, puzzling over what they could possibly have been talking about. It was then, with John lost in thought, that the door opened and Luke Challon, still chewing, came furtively into the room, his whole manner uneasy, his short squarish body restless.

John stood up. 'Mr Challon, how nice . . .'

The secretary's finger flew to his lips, while his uncomplicated and rather boringly handsome face creased in a grimace. 'Shush, keep your voice down for the love of God.'

The tense atmosphere was catching and the Apothecary felt a clutch of fear. 'Why? What's the matter?'

'Lady Hodkin has forbidden you the house. There will be hell to pay if she discovers you are here.'

'Forbidden me the house?' John repeated incredulously.

'Yes. She swears that you menaced her yesterday. She has sent a letter of complaint about you to John Fielding, complete with a rider to transport it. Furthermore, she says that she refuses to cooperate in this investigation unless someone is sent to see her who is of her own social standing.'

'The evil old beast!'

Luke looked fraught. 'Mr Rawlings, please take my advice and go. Now!'

'But there is certain information I simply have to have.'

'I am aware of that. Look, I am journeying to London, to the St James's Square house, later today. Could I not call on you somewhere?'

John fished in an inner pocket. 'Here's my card. It has the address of my shop on it. My home is at number two, Nassau Street, Soho. Can you remember that?'

'I'll go and write it down straight away. Now, I beg of you, take your leave in good order.'

'One question before I do. When is Sir William's funeral to be held?'

'The body is coming here today to lie in state during tonight and tomorrow. He will be buried the day afterwards.'

'Where?'

'St Matthew's, Bethnal Green.'

'I shall be there.'

'But what about Lady Hodkin?'

'Even she cannot stop me taking my place in a church open to all.'

'That's true.'

'And Amelia Lambourn, do you know where she lives?'

'Twelve, Queens Square, just across the park from St James's Square.'

'How very convenient.'

Luke Challon smiled wryly, his grey eyes suddenly unreadable. 'Oh yes it was. Very!' he said.

John rode hard, stopping for nothing, and within an hour had passed through the gate leading into the City. Then having gone down Fleet Street to The Strand, John turned up The Hay Market and thence into Shug Lane, wondering whether he would surprise a riot of customers upset by his absence. But from the outside, at least, all was calm, and noticing how very clean the windows looked, the Apothecary pushed open the door, setting the bell in motion, and stepped within.

It was not only the windows which were sparkling. Shelves had been scrubbed, bottles washed, pestles polished and mortars cleaned out. The entire shop had been spring cleaned in the Apothecary's absence and now gleamed like a prism. Very much impressed, he took a step forward, only to hear a stirring in the back room. Then with a grand gesture a figure stepped forth, a figure wearing a towering wig and enclosed in John's long apron, a figure which solemnly took its place behind the counter. The Apothecary's eyes widened, as did his smile. He was staring straight at Sir Gabriel Kent.

'So,' said John, erupting into laughter, 'this is what you get up to when my back is turned, is it?'

'You're not to be angry, Sir,' put in Nicholas, appearing from behind his mentor. 'It was only right and proper that someone should supervise me.'

'Actually,' Sir Gabriel answered loftily, 'I found that I rather enjoyed being here. There is no question of anyone watching over you, my lad. I came to the shop because it amused me to do so.'

'Well, you seem to have made a very good job of it between you,' said John, looking round.

'That's my training at sea, Sir,' Nicholas explained. 'We had to keep things neat in such a confined space.'

John caught Sir Gabriel's eye. 'And has trade been good?'

'Excellent. What Nicholas lost in being unable to prescribe physicks, he gained in the sale of perfumes.'

'Which of course,' John put in, turning to look at the young man, 'is not part of an apothecary's trade at all.' Nicholas frowned, and John went on, 'The selling of scents is really the job of the perfumers and nothing whatever to do with the calling I follow.'

'Then why do you blend them, Sir?'

'Because, ever since I was an apprentice, I have been fascinated by the perfumer's art, the mixing of exotic ingredients to make rare and beautiful smells. Years ago and in secret, because I knew my Master would not have approved, I started to experiment with perfumes, and the creation of scents soon became my hobby. I have always enjoyed trying things out and inventing. One day I might do more of it.'

'So your shop is unique in stocking such things?'

'Yes, I fear it is.'

'But surely there is nothing to say that you cannot make and sell perfumes if you so desire?'

'I am certain the more pedantic of my colleagues would frown upon such a frivolous thing.'

'Then let them,' answered Nicholas with spirit. 'Let the old miseries criticise and speak by the card. Think what pleasure you give, Sir. To hell with those moaning old mumble crusts.'

'Now there's a show of dash,' said Sir Gabriel. 'Well said, boy. That must be your Muscovy blood talking.'

John smiled, pleased with this display of loyalty. 'Have you paid Nicholas for the last two days?' he asked.

'So far he has received only one shilling.'

'Then he shall have two more.' And reaching inside the drawer where the cash was kept, he paid the young man his well-earned dues. 'And now,' he said, still smiling, 'I would like you to run an errand for me.'

'Certainly,' said Nicholas, removing his apron.

'I want you to take the rest of the day off and go home to Bow Street, where I presume you are still living.' The boy nodded. 'In that case would you seek out Mr Fielding and tell him I will call on him tonight, after dinner. There is a great deal I have to discuss.'

'I have a better plan,' interrupted Sir Gabriel. 'Why don't you ask Mr and Mrs Fielding to dine with us at five o'clock. Then we can deliberate over a good meal.'

Nicholas looked as pleased as if he were going to eat the food himself and John, regarding him closely, thought that the boy was starting to lose the terrible paleness which had so singled him out.

'I think you're in better condition,' he said.

'That's because I'm enjoying myself,' the lad answered cheerfully and, struggling into his sensible worsted coat, whistled his way from the shop, leaving the two others to wink at one another behind his retreating back.

Punctually at five, just as the March evening started to darken, a carriage drew up outside number two, Nassau Street and, contrary to custom, Elizabeth Fielding stepped out first in order to assist her husband down the steps and into the house. Glimpsing the sight from one of the upper front windows, John as ever felt a moment's sadness that such a great and powerful man as the Magistrate should be reduced to such dependency upon another. But once inside and seated in the library, the Blind Beak having tapped his way across the hall with his cane, the Apothecary felt himself yet again totally in the thrall of John Fielding's potent personality.

Sipping his sherry, the Magistrate rumbled a laugh as he described his interview with Roger Hartfield, who had been requested to attend the Public Office in order to state formally that the body he had seen in the mortuary had been that of his father.

'What a pretty fellow he sounded, and what a pretty stinkard into the bargain. Why, the downstairs rooms were redolent with his perfume for an entire day after his departure. What does he look like, Mr Rawlings?'

'A trifle fleshy but a piercing beau for all that, dressed in the very latest fashions, wildly wigged and flashingly beringed. He fainted and vomited a good deal at the ordeal of seeing the body.'

'How vulgar,' commented Sir Gabriel.

'Was he genuinely upset, do you think?' Mr Fielding asked.

John looked thoughtful. 'I'm not sure. It's rather hard to say. The greater the fuss the less the emotion, I always tend to think.'

'Quite. He called his father's betrothed a horrid little whore, by the way.'

'The consensus it would appear.'

Mr Fielding nodded. 'And what of the others? How did they react to the news of Sir William's death?'

'They all seemed saddened, in their different ways. His daughter-in-law Lydia, a somewhat daunting young widow, appeared very anxious that I should hear no family gossip yet hadn't a good word for Amelia Lambourn when I finally drew her out. On the other hand his two youngest children, a delightful pair of twins, disagreed on that point. The boy felt his father could not be blamed, the girl considered the bride a money grubbing harlot. By the way, there is one other odd thing.'

'And what is that?'

'I overheard rather a strange piece of conversation.' And John recounted the words he had heard while he had been concealed in the ante room.

'I wonder, I wonder . . .' said the Magistrate softly.

'What is that, Sir?'

'Whether money *is* the motive for this crime. When is the will to be read?'

'After the funeral, which takes place the day after tomorrow. Apparently the body is being taken to Kirby Hall to lie in state.' He paused, then went on, 'I take it that Lady Hodkin's letter of complaint has reached you by now?'

The Blind Beak chuckled tunefully. 'It certainly has. What an ostentatious vulgarian the woman sounds. She says that you menaced her. Did you?'

'I most certainly did,' John replied guilelessly.

'Gracious heavens!' exclaimed his father, raising an arched eyebrow.

John Fielding chuckled once more. 'What did you say?'

'I told her that refusal to cooperate could be read as a sign of guilt. At that she created such a rumpus, her daughter rushed in to save her.'

'It serves the old woman right, of course. But the situation does present certain difficulties.'

'In what way?' asked Sir Gabriel.

'She has to be questioned, so do all of them who reside in Kirby Hall, but she has refused Mr Rawlings admittance and states that she will not speak to anyone lest they be of her social standing.'

'What arrant posturing!'

'It is indeed, but it causes a problem for all that.'

Sir Gabriel nodded. 'It most certainly does.'

'However, I am sure we will find a way round it.' The Blind Beak turned back to John. 'How did you find the rest of the family, my friend?'

'The eldest female, Sir William's sister-in-law, Hesther, admitted she was in love with him and seemed broken hearted and jealous that he chose to marry a flighty young flap and not herself when he was widowed. Luke Challon, the secretary, appeared anxious to be helpful and murmured that he would see me privately in London. Sir William's office manager, Valentine Randolph, the man who would have acted as bridegroom's witness, spoke highly of his late employer. He was of the opinion that Sir William was entitled to a little happiness. Of the other two, Hugh Hartfield and his wife, Maud, I cannot give an opinion as I did not come across them. However, the twins described them as prudish and prim and made rude remarks about their consequent lack of offspring.'

Mr Fielding laughed again. 'I see. So with the exception of Hugh and his lady you have spoken to everybody concerned?'

'All but Miss Amelia Lambourn herself, and I intend to brave her tomorrow. By the way I was surprised to learn from Mr Randolph that Sir William met her at Islington Spa, where she served the Well water.'

'A fact guaranteed to send Lady Hodkin into a frenzy, no doubt.'

'Particularly if she has been left the bulk of Sir William's fortune.'

The Blind Beak looked thoughtful. 'Have you discovered the name of the dead man's solicitor?'

'Luke promised to tell me when he came to see me.'

'It is imperative that we find out. Someone must learn the contents of the will, and soon at that.'

Elizabeth Fielding spoke for the first time. 'What a shame that you cannot send a decoy into Kirby Hall.'

The Blind Beak turned his bandaged eyes towards her. 'What do you mean exactly?'

'That if someone could go there, someone who would be acceptable to the old woman, that is, yet someone who does not reveal himself as working for the Public Office, then a great deal might be gleaned.'

Her husband laughed. 'You would be ideal, my dear, but alas I cannot spare you from Bow Street.'

Elizabeth nodded. 'I know, I know. It was just a thought.'

Sir Gabriel spoke into the ensuing silence. 'I am prepared to do it if you believe I would be of any use.'

There was absolute quiet in the room as everyone stared at him, the Magistrate bending his head just as if he could see.

'But how would you gain admittance?' he asked reflectively.

'I don't know really. I suppose I could always claim to be an old friend of Sir William's.'

'That might not work,' Mr Fielding answered, and John realised with a shock that the Blind Beak was treating Sir Gabriel's offer seriously.

'Perhaps a coach accident could be contrived,' he continued, still in the same thoughtful tone of voice. 'If a wheel were to come off at Kirby Hall's gates they would be almost duty bound to let you wait there until repairs were made.'

'That's an excellent scheme,' John's father answered with enthusiasm. 'But with the funeral so near, when should I carry it out?'

'You're not in earnest . . .' the Apothecary began, but Mr Fielding cut across him.

'Perhaps tomorrow. With the body lying in state they are bound to give you a tearful explanation as to how the poor fellow met his end.'

'And I could act in a most sympathetic manner and hope that they invite me to dine with them.'

'Really!' John protested, but he was out numbered. Sir Gabriel was warming to his theme, the Blind Beak was nodding enthusiastically, while Elizabeth had clasped her hands in pleasure, delighted that her idea had been so well received.

'A toast,' she cried, raising her glass. 'To the Public Office's newest representative.'

'Hear, hear,' answered John Fielding, and the Apothecary was left with no option but to join them in drinking to what he considered to be an utterly harebrained and somewhat dangerous scheme.

The Apothecary rose particularly early next day and penned a warning note to his father begging him to think carefully about his proposed trip to Bethnal Green. Then, somewhat sulkily, he set off for Shug Lane without eating breakfast. Yet despite the earliness of the hour, John had only been in his shop five minutes before Nicholas arrived, still clad in his worsted suit, obviously the only garments he possessed, but for all that looking very presentable. He seemed slightly surprised to see John in residence.

'I thought you'd be about your business, Sir.'

'No, I've decided to make my visits this afternoon. So, for a few hours at least, we shall be working together.'

'If you're called out this morning may I come with you?' Nicholas asked enthusiastically.

'That would rather negate the purpose of your being here.'

'But how else can I learn?'

'You're not my apprentice, you know,' John said, then wished he hadn't spoken when the boy's expression became utterly crestfallen.

'No, of course not,' Nicholas answered wistfully. He squared his shoulders, obviously used to a lifetime of disappointment. 'Would you like me to make some tea, Sir?' he asked in a different voice.

'Yes please,' the Apothecary answered, feeling quite the most cold-hearted being ever born.

'Very good.' And Nicholas went bustling into the back.

John dusted in silence, thinking about a bastard boy with Muscovy blood in his veins, put into the care of the parish for no sin other than that of having no money or means of support, and how near he himself must once have been to the same terrible fate. That is if it had not been for the intercession of Sir Gabriel Kent. Furious with his own behaviour, the Apothecary put down the ampulla he was holding and called out, 'Nicholas.'

'Yes, Sir?' came a voice from the back.

'You are quite right. Even though you are not apprenticed, I know Mr Fielding sent you here to learn. So if I am called to attend the sick, you may come with me. We can leave a sign on the shop door.'

Nicholas's face, looking positively animated for someone of so pale a countenance, appeared in the doorway. 'Oh thank you, Mr Rawlings. I promise I shall behave fittingly. You see, I used to help the captain with any accidents when I was at sea. We didn't have a ship's doctor other than him.'

'What cargos used you to carry?' the Apothecary asked curiously.

'All sorts really; spices, tobacco, fruit. Once we transported a batch of slaves bound for Liverpool. That was terrible.'

'Why?'

'It was so awful to hear them groaning in the holds below. That's how I got my limp.'

'What do you mean?'

'I was trying to clamber down to take the poor creatures some water but I fell off the ladder and broke my leg. The captain set it, after he'd given me a good flogging that is, but it left me with a permanent defect.'

'What happened to the slaves?'

'Those that survived were sold off in groups, the others were buried at sea. One or two managed to run away. That's all I know. I was put ashore after that because of my injury.'

'And then you came to London to make your way.'

Nicholas's pallid cheeks flushed uncomfortably. 'If you're referring to my thieving, Sir, yes it's true. But I only stole to keep myself alive. I would never, ever touch a penny of yours, I swear it.'

The boy seemed on the verge of tears and John looked at him, a stern expression masking the very real compassion he was feeling. 'If I thought that of you I would most certainly never have agreed to let you work in my shop. Now, where is my tea? I did not have time for breakfast this morning and I am famished for a cup.'

Hearing this, Nicholas insisted on going to a nearby bakery to buy some rolls and so John was alone when the first customer of the day came to the door. Hearing voices outside, he stepped behind the counter so that he could be ready when the bell rang. But the couple, for the Apothecary could distinctly see a man and a woman through the window, were taking their time, standing in his doorway, talking quietly. There was something so familiar about them that John found himself peering. Then he caught the sheen of foxy red hair and could hardly believe the coincidence. Of all the many apothecaries' shops in London, Julian and Juliette Hartfield had chosen his to visit so early in the morning.

Unaware of his covert observation, the twins continued to converse, occasionally laughing but mostly keeping a serious mien. Then, quite abruptly, Juliette, seeing the approach of some chairmen, hailed a sedan, whilst Julian turned in the doorway and entered the shop. Hastily stooping to pick up some mythical object, John took his time before standing upright.

The twin was examining some bottles of physick displayed on a far counter and started wildly as John cleared his throat warningly before saying, 'Good morning, Sir. How may I help you?'

Julian turned abruptly and the Apothecary found himself staring into a pale, somewhat dissipated face, but one of outstanding beauty for all that, indeed almost more so than John had remembered.

The twin's eyes widened to twice their size and Julian's jaw sagged. 'Good God! Mr Rawlings!'

'Yes, Mr Hartfield. Did I not tell you I was an apothecary?'

'You might have done. I really can't recall.'

'Ah well, that is beside the point. What can I get you, Sir?'

The twin gulped audibly. 'A cure for the headache if you have one.'

The Apothecary smiled sympathetically. 'Ah, a hard night, eh?'

Julian gave a light laugh. 'Yes, been at the confounded gaming tables for most of it.'

'Any luck?'

'Precious little.'

John selected a bottle of bright green liquid. 'There, this should help you. Forgive me, but I thought you were at Kirby Hall yesterday,' he continued as he prepared a small glass from which Julian could drink the liquid.

The twin flushed visibly. 'Yes, I . . . we . . . were. But I had to return last evening. I was engaged to play cards and there was no way out of it. Though I suppose I could have pleaded bereavement.' Julian downed the physick and pulled a face. 'Ugh! What a ghastly concoction.'

'But very effective,' the Apothecary said urbanely. 'That will be one shilling, Sir. Why didn't you?'

The twin stared at him. 'Why didn't I what?'

'Make the excuse of your mourning?'

Julian flushed an uncomfortable shade of red. 'Well, the fact is, I adore cards, you see.'

'But surely at a time like this . . .'

'It may seem uncaring but that is not the case. It is simply that Roger and my twin and I are all unconventional. We cannot bear the confines of polite behaviour. We still want to go out and about even though we are grieving,' came the defiant answer.

'And you care not a fig for what the *beau monde* might think?'

'Since you put it like that, no, not a fig.'

'I suppose that indicates courage, to fly in the face of convention.'

'It indicates that we keep our grief to ourselves.' Julian's hands searched his pockets. 'Damnably short of funds, I'm afraid. May I owe you the shilling?' he added in a very different voice.

'Of course.'

'It won't be too long before I can repay you. After all, my circumstances are about to change.'

'You refer to your father's bequest?' John asked innocently.

Julian went from red to puce. 'Well . . . er . . .'

The Apothecary smiled. 'Is there not some saying about an ill wind?'

The twin gulped violently. 'I believe there is,' he said, and bolted from the shop without uttering another word.

Chapter Ten

*I*t being the custom for people to sit down to dine somewhere between the hours of three and five, John, seeing the streets outside his shop begin to clear, handed over the keys to Nicholas Dawkins and went out as planned. The Muscovite, though obviously sad to see him go, for, alas, there had been no calls for John's services that morning and the promised practical experience of tending the sick had therefore not taken place, accepted his fate with resignation and waved the Apothecary a cheery farewell. Wishing he had been able to do more for the boy but making a silent promise that in future he would see to it, John made his way across St James's Park to number twelve, Queens Square, the address given him by Luke Challon for Miss Amelia Lambourn.

Walking through the park, admiring the four lines of trees laid out by Charles II and the landscape contrived by the celebrated French gardener, Le Notre, John wished that his visit was not destined to be so grim. For, or so he reasoned, it would appear that he must break the news of Sir William's death to the girl who only a few days earlier was to have been his bride. That was, of course, unless some member of the dead man's family had had the decency to inform her. Though as none of them seemed to have a good word for the unhappy woman, the Apothecary very much doubted it.

With these thoughts uppermost in his mind, it was almost a relief to see that the door knocker had been wrapped in black cloth and that every curtain in the small but pleasant terraced house was drawn against the intrusive daylight. Adopting his sympathetic face, John tactfully ignored the knocker and rang the bell.

A mob-capped maid answered the summons and bobbed an ungainly curtsey. 'Yes?' she said, revealing by her very attitude that she had scant respect for the caller.

'Is Miss Lambourn at home?' the Apothecary asked, swiftly adjusting his features into his officious look.

'She is but she h'aint receiving,' the slattern replied, giving him an insolent stare.

'I'm afraid I must insist on seeing her,' John continued, beetling his mobile brows at her. 'I am here on behalf of the Public Office, Bow Street, and it is my unpleasant duty to ask Miss Lambourn a few questions concerning her recent bereavment.'

'What?'

'The death of Sir William Hartfield. I want to speak to her about it.'

'Well, you can't. I've got me orders and they is to let nobody in.' And the beastly girl started to close the door.

John inserted his foot into the aperture. 'Obstructing the process of the law is a very serious matter, you know.'

'I can't help that . . .' And the slut would have done his toes a mischief had it not been for a cry from upstairs.

'Betsy, what is it?'

'A Beak Runner's 'ere, Miss. Says 'e wants a word with you.'

There was a shriek, then silence, then finally the voice called again. 'In that case you had better show him up to the salon.'

'Very good, Miss,' the girl shouted grudgingly, and opened the door just wide enough for the Apothecary to squeeze through. 'You'd best come in,' she added, throwing him a malevolent look.

John made a bow. 'Charmed,' he said, and followed her up the stairs to the first floor.

Throwing open a door, Betsy announced him with the words, 'A Beak Runner,' then departed, glaring over her shoulder and saying meaningfully, 'I shall be below if you need me, Miss.'

Making his way into the gloomy interior, John bowed once more. 'The name is Rawlings, Ma'am. John Rawlings. Believe me, I shall do everything in my power to make this interview as easy as possible for you.'

'Oh,' answered Miss Lambourn, and gave a loud sob.

It would seem his fate, John thought, always to see the poor soul either in or on the verge of tears. For Amelia was presently sniffing into a large handkerchief with dark trimming, whilst she herself was clad from head to toe in starkest black.

'May I sit down?' he asked, and in response to a faint nod, took a seat in a chair opposite the couch on which Miss Lambourn drooped supine.

The Apothecary cleared his throat. 'Might I just enquire who informed you of Sir William's death?' he asked softly.

She looked at him with the faintest expression of surprise. 'Mr Randolph sent me a message. He worked for my betrothed.' Amelia gulped. 'I mean my late betrothed.'

John nodded. 'I see. And when was this?'

'When was what?'

'When did Mr Randolph's message arrive?'

'Two days ago, in the morning. I shall never forget that.'

The Apothecary smiled encouragingly, wondering how Valentine had known of his employer's death even before Luke Challon had called at the office to inform him of it. 'Perhaps you would like to tell me,' he said in the same soothing voice.

'His letter came quite early. In fact while I was about my toilette. Why do you want to know?'

'For no particular reason other than that the Public Office is aware you did not enjoy good relations with Sir William's family and it occurred to me they might not have had the courtesy to notify you.' An awful thought struck John and he added, 'I presume Mr Randolph told you how your future husband died.'

'He wrote me that he had drowned in the river. But how, why? William and I were to have been married. The last thing he would have wanted to do was kill himself.'

'I think perhaps,' John said delicately, 'that suicide does not enter the issue.'

'What do you mean?'

'It has come to light that somebody struck your betrothed over the head before he entered the water.'

She drew in her breath with a hiss. 'I might have guessed as much! That poor man was trapped in a nest of vipers. There's not one of 'em would have hesitated to do him ill, including that evil old Hodkin woman.'

The conversation was taking a most unexpected turn and the Apothecary felt his thumbs begin to prick. 'Really?' he said, his voice ingenuous.

Miss Lambourn betrayed her origins. 'Upon the square, Sir. They is the biggest bunch of sham cutters I ever comes across.'

'All of them?' John asked.

'Well . . .' She hesitated. 'Luke was always civil to me, and Mr Randolph, of course. And Roger has very fine manners.'

115

'Oh, you've met him?'

'I've met them all in my time, all but Lady Hodkin that is. William said that to be lashed by her tongue was an ordeal he didn't want to subject me to.'

'Quite right!' said John with feeling. 'But I would be most interested to hear your opinion of the rest of the family. Would you mind?'

'No, I'd like to say what I know. The eldest of 'em, apart from Milady, is Miss Hesther, who is a jealous cat. She's Sir William's sister-in-law and is totally besotted with him. Then there's Roger, one of the biggest bloods in town, so it's said.' She laughed, seeming to find this funny. 'After him comes his brother Hugh, who works . . . worked . . . for William. He oversees the import of goods to this country and often goes abroad to order merchandise. Then there's his wife Maud, an embittered old shrew, just like her sister-in-law, Lydia. The youngest are those stupid twins, arrogant little beasts. There's not one of that family that doesn't wish me dead, I tell you. Afraid that I'll get my clutches on their father's fortune.' Amelia's hand flew to her throat and she let out a sob. 'Dear God, what am I saying?'

'It's perfectly natural to speak so,' John said comfortingly. 'You are doing very well, Miss Lambourn.'

'It's hard to realise he's gone,' she answered in broken tones.

'I hate to put you through this ordeal but if I am to find the person who killed him . . .'

Amelia stood up and began to pace, what light there was reflecting on her face as she strode up and down. His earlier impression of her in the church was now confirmed. She was indeed remarkably pretty, with a beautiful figure and glorious colouring. It occurred to John fleetingly that somebody, somewhere, might well have been jealous of Sir William and that his death could have been at the hands of a man who both coveted and desired his bride-to-be. For no reason he found himself asking, 'Have you met Julian Hartfield?'

'Just once, but I know he's a wastrel,' Miss Lambourn answered vehemently. 'All he wanted was to gamble his father's money away. But Sir William had run out of patience with him and vowed to settle no future debts.' She paused and looked at John with brimming blue eyes. 'You don't think . . .?'

'At the moment I think nothing,' the Apothecary answered,

'except, perhaps, that there were several people who had a reason for wishing your future husband out of the way.'

'He never came to the wedding,' said Amelia, almost to herself. 'I thought at first he had jilted me, until . . .' She stopped abruptly.

'Until what?'

'Mr Randolph's message,' she answered, so hurriedly that she gave John the strong impression she had been about to say something else.

The Apothecary stood up. 'Miss Lambourn, two more questions and then I promise to take up no more of your time.'

She stopped walking and turned to look at him, daintiness personified despite her glistening eyes and damp cheeks. 'What are they?'

'The first is, when did you last see Sir William alive?'

'The night before the wedding. We dined at St James's Square, all the rest of them being out. Lydia saw me, though. She came back early from whist. Anyway, Sir William escorted me into my carriage and that was that. I never set eyes on him again.' She started to weep. 'And he was so full of excitement about it all. It don't seem fair.'

'Was this very late?' John asked.

'No, he had somewhere else to go that evening. Besides I didn't want to be tardy. I was home by seven o'clock.'

'And you did not go out again?'

Amelia hesitated, then coloured up. 'Er . . . no,' she said falteringly.

John decided to let the obvious falsehood pass. 'Where was Sir William off to? Did he say?'

'No, he didn't.'

'Not so much as a hint?'

'Wherever he was going, he was pleased about it. He was smiling a good deal and his eyes were twinkling. Now, tell me your second question.'

'I was simply going to enquire whether you had the details of Sir William's funeral.'

'Yes, it is tomorrow morning in Bethnal Green. At St Matthew's.'

Thinking how very well informed she was and wondering whether Mr Randolph had once again obliged Amelia with the information, John nodded. 'Will you be going?'

'Of course I will. Even Lady Hodkin can't keep me out.'

'My sentiments exactly.' The Apothecary bowed in the doorway. 'Until tomorrow, then.'

'Goodbye,' said Miss Lambourn, and with a sorrowful motion raised the black-edged handkerchief to her eyes so that he could no longer see her face.

It being barely six o'clock, John Rawlings, feeling the need to confide his impressions in the Blind Beak, set off from Queens Square to Queen Street, and thence through a maze of alleyways and cuttings into White Hall. From there it was but a short step to Charing Cross. Striking up St Martin's Lane, the Apothecary wove his way through to Bow Street just as it grew dark. Staring up at the tall façade of the third house on the left, he was delighted to see that candles had been lit in the private rooms, and from this surmised that the family were at home.

In the event, it turned out that they were just finishing their dinner and were still at table, so John was shown into the salon to await the arrival of the Blind Beak, who came in only a few moments later, followed by Mary Ann bearing a tray set with a decanter of port and two glasses.

'I thought you might be coming, my friend,' said the Magistrate, indicating the second glass as if he could see it. 'Nicholas arrived here not long since and said that you had gone to call on the bereaved bride. By the way, when he went to pay in the day's takings to your father, he found that Sir Gabriel had set forth with a travelling trunk. I imagine that the adventure in Bethnal Green must be about to begin.'

John frowned. 'I hope that the scheme is a wise one.'

The Blind Beak nodded to his niece to pour two glasses. 'At the very worst, Sir Gabriel will not be offered hospitality and will discover nothing. At best, he will insinuate himself into Lady Hodkin's confidence and find out everything that we want to know.'

'I suppose so.'

'I hear doubt in your voice. Why is that?'

'Because I am rapidly coming to the conclusion that knowing the contents of the will is vital to this puzzle. And even should they trust my father like a brother, the reading of the last testament is something he will not be invited to attend. Furthermore, Luke Challon is obviously trying to avoid giving me any further information about it because he has not called as promised.'

'Quite true, and with that in mind I have made some enquiries of my own. It turns out that Mr Roger Hartfield, a dandy-cock much intimidated by this office, when asked by Joe Jago to reveal the identity of his father's lawyer, promptly did so. Therefore a request has been sent to the man of learning this very day asking him to disclose the substance of Sir William's will to my representative.'

John smiled into his port glass. 'Request?' he repeated with irony.

The Blind Beak laughed. 'A strong one, admittedly. You are to go and see him tomorrow evening, Mr Rawlings. After the will has been read to the family. Now, what of Miss Lambourn? Is she the horrid whore that Roger described?'

'Possibly she is but she is also very beautiful, and of very humble birth, just the sort of girl that Lady Hodkin would detest. I rather liked her.'

'Is she sincere in her grief?'

'She certainly seems very upset, though whether it is through a broken heart or simply because her provider has gone, it is difficult to say.'

'But she might now find herself very wealthy indeed.'

'Indeed she might. Anyway, three interesting things emerged from our conversation.'

'And what were they?'

'It seems that Valentine Randolph . .'

'Remind me of him.'

'The victim's office manager. A strange individual, not yet recovered from some adolescent love affair apparently. However, it was he who told Amelia Lambourn of her future husband's death but *before* he had been officially informed of it himself.'

Mr Fielding sipped his port and absorbed this information in silence. Eventually he said, 'The sequence of events was that three days after the murder you called at St James's square and told those present of Sir William's death. After which Roger Hartfield wrote to the members of the family residing in Bethnal Green. It was only then that Luke Challon travelled to Wapping and informed Sir William's office staff.'

'Yes, that's correct.'

'And Mr Randolph told Miss Lambourn . . . .?'

'On the morning after I had been to St James's Square.'

'Then presumably somebody from that house was in touch with him.'

'Yes, but I wonder why whoever it was didn't bother to tell Luke that Randolph knew. It would have saved him an akward journey. There's another thing, too.'

'And what is that?'

'A person unknown has given Amelia the time and place of the funeral. For someone supposedly so shunned she is astonishingly well informed.'

The Blind Beak's black bandage veered in John's direction. 'Mr Randolph again?'

'Possibly.'

'Why do you say that? Do you believe it could be somebody else?'

The Apothecary shook his head. 'I don't know, Sir. I really don't. All I do know is that it would be a very interesting exercise to look into the past of Sir William's affianced bride. I think a visit to Islington Spa might be called for. I shall contact Samuel forthwith.'

'A splendid notion. Now tell me the third thing you discovered.'

'Miss Lambourn lied to me about leaving her house on the night before the wedding.'

'Why should she do that?'

'Because it is my belief she was at The Devil's Tavern. The landlord told me that a bride had stayed there on the previous evening and I know instinctively it was her.'

'Then that puts her at the very spot where the body was discovered.' The Blind Beak turned to the fire, just as if he were staring into the flames. 'Go to Islington as soon as you can, Mr Rawlings. I feel there is something that does not quite ring true about Miss Amelia.'

John nodded in agreement. Then, hearing the Apothecary put his glass down and stand up, the Magistrate moved his head to follow the sound. 'Surely you are not off there now, Mr Rawlings?'

'No, I think I might call on the Comte and Comtesse de Vignolles. As my father is away and not expecting me, it seems an ideal opportunity.'

John Fielding smiled. 'I take it you are attending the funeral tomorrow?'

'Yes, and therefore will require Nicholas. Thank you again for that introduction, Sir. I really couldn't have managed without him.'

'I thought the boy might be useful,' the Blind Beak answered laconically, pouring himself another glass of port. 'Good luck, Mr Rawlings. Keep your eyes open. The burial should provide an ideal opportunity to study all those involved.'

'It will be fascinating,' answered John as he bowed in the doorway and took his leave.

It was just as dusk was falling and John Rawlings was making his way into the Public Office that the undertaker's mute posted outside the wrought-iron gates of Kirby Hall nearly forgot his role and shouted aloud in alarm. For out of the gloaming, travelling at quite some speed, came a black coach pulled by an elegant team of snow white horses, which cast a wheel at the very moment it drew level with the portals. In fact so close was it that the mute, an ethereal child with a wistful expression, clad overall in sombre black, was forced to leap to one side in a most energetic manner, a move not at all suited to his general air of having communication only with the other world and knowing nothing of the wickedness of this. Meanwhile, thanks to the quick thinking of the coachman, an accident was avoided and the carriage, though dipping on one side, managed to remain upright. Narrowing his gaze, the mute watched as steps were let down by the postillion and a very fine gentleman of noble stature descended.

'Gracious heavens,' this being said, his eyes taking in the dark wreath upon the gate and the somewhat dishevelled mute struggling to regain his equilibrium. 'I do believe this is a house of mourning.'

'That it clearly is, Sir Gabriel,' the coachman answered cheerfully. 'Still I must disturb them for all their sadness.'

'No.' The fine man shook his head. 'If anyone is to disturb their repose it should be I.'

'Then I'll accompany you, Sir.' And the coachman nodded to the gatekeeper, who had come from his lodge to see what was amiss, to allow them entry, which he did with a grin as Sir Gabriel tossed him a coin.

The mute stared after the departing figures disconsolately, hoping that some mourners would arrive soon, so that he could walk down the drive before them, his gait very solemn, and perhaps earn a tip or two for himself. Meanwhile, without the mute's aid, Sir Gabriel had reached the front door and had allowed his coachman to pull the bell. Then he stood back, wondering which one of the extraordinary family that John had described so accurately on the previous evening, would give permission for him to enter.

In the event, Sir Gabriel was somewhat confused, for a person entered the small salon into which he had been shown who fitted none of the portraits that John's words had so clearly conjured. Nearly as tall as Sir Gabriel himself and without an ounce of spare flesh upon his wiry frame, this man had dark brown hair which curled slightly over his cravat, and eyes of an almost identical shade. His skin, too, was of a brownish hue and John's father took a shrewd guess that this individual had spent a fair amount of time in a hot climate. Wondering if this could possibly be Hugh, the brother that John had not yet met, Sir Gabriel gave a bow that dazzled with its grace.

'My dear Sir,' he said, 'believe me, nobody could be more mortified than I to have thrust myself upon you at a time of bereavement, but the fact of the matter is that my coach cast a wheel at your very gates. I wondered, therefore, if you could tell me where I might find the nearest wheelwright, so that I might be on my way once more.'

Hugh, if it was he, hesitated and at that moment the door to the salon flew open unceremoniously. Gazing round, Sir Gabriel saw a grim faced old woman, a pug whom she closely resembled clutched to her bosom, glaring into the room to see what was going on. Knowing at once who this must be, he gave a low salute which caused the top of his wig to brush against the floor.

'Madam,' he said, 'allow me to introduce myself. Gabriel Kent, Knight, of Nassau Street, Soho. A most unfortunate accident brings me to your house of sorrow and for this I humbly apologise.'

The old snob simpered. 'Cannot be helped, Sir. Cannot be helped. Now, what can we do to assist you?'

'Merely give me the whereabouts of the nearest wheelwright so that he might effect a repair and I can continue my journey.'

Lady Hodkin frowned. 'Who does Sir Gabriel require, Hugh, eh?'

'I'm not too sure but I believe the nearest chap is in Camel Row.'

'In Mile End New Town? That's a fair step, Sir.'

'My postillion could go.'

She looked dubious. 'It's not a safe or easy walk after dark. Can you send a carriage, Hugh?'

'No, Grandmother, not at the moment. We are just about to dine, if you remember. Should we leave it much later we will get caught up with the visitors come to see Father laid out.'

'Perish the thought,' said Sir Gabriel mournfully. 'Madam, I have trespassed on your hospitality long enough. I shall walk to the nearest hostelry and there find rooms for myself and my servants.'

'I wouldn't hear of it,' snapped Lady Hodkin, glaring at Hugh and loosening her hold on the dog which cascaded to the floor like a malevolent waterfall. 'What? Would I have the word go round town that we behave like barbarians in Kirby Hall? Sir, you must join us for dinner. Later, transport will be arranged so that you may find the wheelwright in safety. Meanwhile, direct your servants to the kitchen where they shall be given something to eat.'

'Your humble servant, Ma'am.' Sir Gabriel bowed yet again.

'The pleasure is entirely mine, Sir. Now I shall get a footman to direct you to our facilities, quite the latest thing, you know. Then you must join us in the red salon for sherry.'

Lady Hodkin gave the nearest she could ever get to a coquettish smile and hurried from the room, the pug limping in her wake.

Sir Gabriel coughed deferentially. 'I do apologise for this intrusion,' he said, looking suitably anguished.

Hugh gave a wintry smile. 'It is of no consequence. Now, if you will forgive me, I have much to think about. It is not pleasant to return from a trip overseas to be informed that one's father is dead. One is not prepared, either physically or mentally, if you understand me.'

'Indeed I do and I sympathise deeply. May I ask when this happened?'

'Two days ago. The ship docked at the Customs Quays, I disembarked and went to my father's office in Wapping, only to find his private secretary had been there to break the news of his tragic demise.' Unexpectedly, a sob escaped from Hugh's tight lips. 'D'you know, I think I would have fainted to the floor had it not been for Valentine Randolph.'

'Who is he?'

'The office manager. Fortunately he caught me in his arms as I staggered, then gave me brandy. I would not have retained consciousness if he had not saved me.'

'Mr Randolph sounds just the sort of person to have around in a crisis. Will he be joining us for dinner tonight?'

'No, my grandmother has fallen out with him over some imagined slight. He is to be allowed to the wake tomorrow, but that is all.'

'The funeral is tomorrow! Oh, I am so sorry . . .'

But Sir Gabriel got no further. The door opened once more to reveal a little dark creature so similar to Hugh to look at that John's father instantly took her for his sister.

Not noticing the visitor she flew to Hugh's side. 'I really don't know what this family is coming to,' she said crossly. 'Hesther's in a regular fluster. Lady Hodkin has made her change into her best black and told her to put paint on her face, just like some cheap houri from a harem. Apparently, some man has called . . .'

'Really?' said Hugh, so loudly that the woman jumped. He took her arm and whirled her round. 'Maud, may I present to you Sir Gabriel Kent? His coach met with an accident at our very gates and Grandmama has invited him to dine with us while she decides what's best to be done. Sir Gabriel, this is my wife, Maud.'

Quite amazed by the living proof of the saying that people who dwell together grow to look the same, John's father gave a charming smile.

'Madam, I am most sincere in my apologies . . .'

But yet again he was cut short, this time by the arrival of the footman, come to conduct him to the niche in the hall housing the plunger closet. Somewhat daunted, Sir Gabriel followed him meekly. A quarter of an hour later and much in need of a restorative sherry, he was taken to the red salon where the family, all in black with one glaring exception, was assembled. Testing his skill at remembering, Sir Gabriel looked around him.

Seated in a large chair by the fire was old Lady Hodkin, whilst behind her, standing in a somewhat deferential pose, was a middle-aged woman whom he took to be Hesther. Having heard John remark on her notably plain appearance, Sir Gabriel was aware that tonight the poor creature had indeed made an effort. Rather badly, in a very hit or miss style but there for all that, was a gallant attempt at the use of cosmetics. Admittedly, the cheeks were too rouged, the lips too carmined, whilst the use of patches was eccentric to say the least, but still there was a glow in Hesther's darkened eyes which burned even more brightly when Sir Gabriel bowed in her direction.

Besides these two females there were three others present. Hugh's wife Maud, who made a deep curtsey, obviously keen to make a good impression this time, and a dark beautiful strong woman whose lovely neck revealed her to be Sir William's widowed daughter-in-law, Lydia. Having saluted them, Sir Gabriel turned to the third, the burnished Juliette. Looking as luscious as a fruit with her pale skin and glowing hair, she was studiously ignoring her twin brother, who had moved away from the family group and was presently studying a piece of music over by the harpsichord. Wondering if the siblings had quarrelled over something, Sir Gabriel turned to regard the rest of the company.

Roger was instantly apparent because of his gorgeous clothes and fulsome manner. Tonight, he wore garter blue silk breeches which fitted within an inch of his life, together with a coat of pale purple velvet turned up with lemon colour, the ensemble completed by lilac stockings. Though the rest of the family had already put on mourning, the eldest son was obviously cocking a snook at convention and waiting until tomorrow, Sir Gabriel thought. Roger stared, quite clearly thunderstruck, at Sir Gabriel's starkly eye-catching evening clothes, effected as ever in deepest black and glittering silver.

In stark contrast to the blood's vivid ensemble, a traditionally handsome, serious young man who had to be Luke Challon, stood stiff-legged and clearly unhappy, helping himself unobserved from the sherry decanter. Whilst Hugh, very much as if he were now master of the house, stood directly in front of the fire, warming his posterior and smiling around him urbanely.

So this, John's father thought, was all of them, with the exception of Amelia Lambourn and Valentine Randolph. Was it from these ranks that a killer had risen up and struck Sir William a mortal blow? Or had someone removed from the family been responsible? With a clutch at his heart, Sir Gabriel turned to face the group, introduced himself, made a general speech of apology for intruding at such a sensitive time, then devoted his attention to Lady Hodkin, certain that if she approved of him he would be able to find out much that John had been prevented from doing.

As it happened, he had a stroke of luck he could not have guessed at. Lady Hodkin proved to have a fondness for drink, a fact which combined to make her both irritable and garrulous. Trading on this, Sir Gabriel signalled to the footman every time her glass was empty, meanwhile behaving in so charming a manner that she was soon treating him as a confidant and directing her irascibility towards the others. Poor Hesther, who sat tongue-tied and flushed on Sir Gabriel's other side, came in for her share of scorn from which he rescued her so cleverly that she looked at him from then on with dog-like devotion.

'Foolish frump,' Lady Hodkin was saying. 'Spent all her life mooning after William instead of finding herself a husband. Now she's on the shelf and who's fault is it, eh?'

'It does not behove me to speak ill of the dead, but I would say Sir William's,' Sir Gabriel answered smoothly.

Lady Hodkin glowered at him. 'What's that?'

'I blame Sir William for not observing your daughter's quiet charm,' he continued without faltering.

His hostess hovered on the brink of various emotions, then came down in favour of amusement. 'Oh, that's rich, Sir. Quiet charm, eh? Well, you may be right at that. The old fool made an arse of himself over some whore with a merry smile and an eye on his fortune, so perhaps he didn't like 'em docile. But too late for all that now, Hesther. Somebody's done for him and serve the silly fellow right.'

Her voice rang down the length of the table and everyone stopped eating. There was a horrified silence, then Hugh said, 'Be quiet, Grandmother.'

Lady Hodkin fumed. 'No, I won't be quiet, d'ye hear? Your father begged for trouble when he became involved with that slut from the Spa. Now fate has caught up with him and I for one cannot say I'm sorry.'

'Mother!' exclaimed Hesther, mortified, and it was at that moment that the footman assigned to the front door appeared and announced in ringing tones that the first mourners, come to pay their respects to the body, had arrived.

'Show 'em into the library and tell 'em we'll join 'em shortly,' ordered Roger. His eye ran over Sir Gabriel's garb. 'I'll just go and change into something more fitting. A little jet would not be out of place I think.'

'Peacock,' remarked Lady Hodkin nastily. She turned to Sir

Gabriel. 'Would you oblige an old woman, Sir, and give me your arm when we attend the lying in state?'

'If the gentlemen give me permission,' he answered tactfully.

Before his grandmother could give a snort of contempt regarding what they thought, Roger spoke up. 'We'd be only too delighted, Sir, believe me.'

He spoke with such heavy emphasis that it was all Sir Gabriel could do to conceal a smile, particularly when Juliette let out a barely supressed giggle.

Hugh joined the conversation. 'In view of the fact that the mourners are here, shall we dispense with the serving of port until later?'

There was a murmur of agreement and everyone stood up. Lady Hodkin hooked her full weight onto Sir Gabriel's elbow, Hesther hovering nervously behind, then majestically made her way across the entrance hall into an enormous mirror-lined saloon which lay beyond.

A bizarre spectacle awaited Sir Gabriel's horrified gaze. Yellow wax tapers had been placed in sconces around the room, as had four large candles, each standing at the corners of the coffin. The light from these muted illuminations reflected in the mirrors giving the entire saloon a strangely haunted look. Added to this was the fact that sable cloth had been hung in the spaces between the glass, so as much darkness was imaged there as was light.

In the midst of this unworldly glow stood Sir William's coffin, resting on a trestle table. It was open, the lid lying by its side, so that the dead man's body, surrounded by white silk, was clearly on view to the slow procession of onlookers who now began to file past. Sir Gabriel sniffed delicately. It was the seventh night since John had happened on the body in The Devil's Tavern and no amount of embalming, however skilled the craftsman, could disguise the smell of death which hovered tangibly in the air. Beside him, Hester made a strange sound and Sir Gabriel touched her arm reassuringly. He felt rather than saw her heartfelt look of thanks.

Even in a remote and rural spot like Bethnal Green there seemed an abundance of people come to pay their last respects and Sir Gabriel guessed that every neighbour for several miles around had braved the darkness to attend the lying in state, highly fashionable as this pastime was. Indeed, there were often near riots in London squares when hundreds descended upon a house to go in single line past a coffin, queuing down the street to gain admittance and thus bringing normal traffic to a standstill.

One hour passed, two, and still the winding procession went on. Then, at last, the final mourner traipsed by the deceased, head bowed, and Lady Hodkin spoke, her words slurring slightly. 'There's claret and ale, cakes and biscuits, for you all. Attend me in the library if you would.' And she led the way, still clinging to Sir Gabriel for support.

'One of your relatives?' he heard an acquaintance enquire of Hesther.

'Er . . . no. Just a friend.'

'He seems to be doing wonders with Lady Hodkin. Just the sort of stalwart to have around at the time of a funeral, my dear.'

'Yes,' Hesther answered, swallowing audibly. 'I can only pray that he stays for it.'

'I beg your pardon?' asked the other.

'I said I hope he doesn't go away,' came the faint reply as Hesther, obviously exhausted by all that had happened, gave way to a storm of uncontrolled public weeping.

Chapter Eleven

*A*n evening spent in the company of Serafina and Louis de Vignolles, John Rawlings's closest friends other than for Samuel Swann, was normally that odd combination of being both stimulating and relaxing. Stimulating in the wit of the conversation, the fund of amusing anecdotes; relaxing as was any occasion when good food and fine wine were consumed in convivial company. But tonight all three members of this trio of companions were below their usual level of gaiety. John, very conscious of the fact that he must leave early in the morning for Sir William Hartfield's funeral; Serafina fidgeting as she tried to find a comfortable position in which to sit; the Comte anxiously watching every move his wife made.

She was now in the sixth month of her pregnancy with a hearty, lively baby who danced inside her from morn till night, thrilling yet tiring its charming mother. For much as Serafina loved entertaining and being entertained, the need to retire early was becoming of paramount importance to her as she grew nearer her time. Yet her fondness for the young apothecary who had once played such a key role in mending her marriage led Serafina to delay longer than she should have done, and insist that John sampled the French brandy purchased especially by her husband for their favourite guests, before he left.

'I see so little of you,' she cajoled. 'Stay another hour.'

John looked at her and smiled as she stifled a yawn. 'No, Madam, fifteen minutes is my limit. Tomorrow I have to return to Bethnal Green for Sir William's funeral and must get to bed early tonight.'

'Why are you going? Do you expect his murderer to be present?'

Louis interrupted. 'Serafina, what foolish questions! How would John know if the killer will be there?'

'Because he probably has a fair idea by now who is responsible.'

'Very far from it. Things should become clearer, though, when I have seen Sir William's will,' the Apothecary put in.

'I do hope the poor man has not left much money to that scampish gambling son of his,' Serafina answered, yawning in earnest.

'Do you mean Julian?'

'Yes. The boy with the beautiful face and eyes.'

John paused, his brandy glass half way to his lips. 'Beautiful? Is he? Do you know that idea never struck me.'

'I considered him very much so. But then I have not seen him for a while, having given up the gamester's life.' She smiled ruefully.

'I wonder if Julian is something of a Miss Molly,' the Apothecary said thoughtfully.

Serafina shrugged, her gorgeous shoulders rising in such an expressive gesture that John found himself staring at her with an adoring smile on his face. 'Perhaps he worries not whether he wears kicks or corsets,' she said carelessly.

'You are vulgar,' commented Louis, grinning.

Serafina laughed. 'Quean or queen, it probably makes no difference to him.'

Louis guffawed as only a Frenchman could. 'Who is this poor fellow you are so maligning?'

'The male half of boy and girl twins, son of the murder victim and an habitual, though incompetent, gambler.'

'He sounds as if he has very little to recommend him,' said the Comte still laughing.

'Ah, but that's the puzzle of it,' John replied speculatively, 'he really isn't a bad young man at all.'

'Too much feminine influence from his sister, I dare swear. What we would call in France a petticoat boy.'

'You're probably quite right about that,' the Apothecary answered, and stared into his brandy glass contemplatively as the first faint glimmering of an idea started to come to him.

Frederick Bull, the landlord of The George, that excellent hostelry situated beside the track leading to rustic Bethnal Green, had expected good business to come his way on the day of Sir William Hartfield's funeral, and in anticipation had taken the trouble to make certain preparations. As a mark of respect, the parlour, that part of the inn kept exclusively for the use of people of quality, had been draped with black ribbon. While a terrible drawing of the deceased, executed by the young footman in love with Suky, the landlord's daughter, was hung with black plumes, bought at considerable expense from a draper in Mile End New Town. This, together with a general clean up and an extra polishing of tankards, was as far as Mr Bull was prepared to go, however, in his demonstration of esteem for the dear departed.

None the less, his efforts were to be amply rewarded. The first customer to arrive was Sir William's office manager, Mr Randolph, who rode into the stables on the night before the funeral and promptly took a room. Not long after this, Mr Luke Challon had come up from the Hall to say that a lady would be requiring a chamber for the night and had made a reservation in the name of Miss Lambourn. Mr Bull had been set agog, knowing full well as he did, that this was the name of the young woman Sir William had intended to marry. But there was to be further excitement next morning.

No sooner had the breakfasts been served – Miss Lambourn had a cup of chocolate in her room and nothing further – than the next visitor arrived. The good-looking young man from London, Mr Rawlings, had appeared on horseback and asked if he might book a room in which to change into his funeral clothes. This had duly been arranged and later on, clad in sombre hues, Mr Rawlings had stepped into the parlour for refreshment, only to discover Mr Randolph and Miss Lambourn, firmly ensconsed and talking most earnestly.

Momentarily surprised, the Apothecary had gathered his wits and remembered that the couple had met on the doomed wedding day, and probably several times before that. He had gone to their table and bowed politely.

'Miss Lambourn, Mr Randolph. Arrived early for the funeral, I see.'

'As are you, Sir,' Valentine responded.

'I thought it best to come to The George first and change.'

'A wise precaution.'

'Mr Challon booked me a room here for the night,' Amelia offered. 'He called on me the other day and asked if there was anything he could do to help.'

'That was very kind.'

'He and Mr Randolph have been extremely good to me,' she replied artlessly.

131

Probably because they both have a fancy for you, John caught himself thinking uncharitably.

Valentine squirmed uncomfortably in his chair at Miss Lambourn's words, and the Apothecary took a good hard look at him. The handsome hawkish face was tired, almost drawn, and yet there was a gleam in Mr Randolph's eye that gave its own messages. Aware of John's scrutiny, he looked away. But not before their gaze had momentarily met and a flicker of understanding had passed between them. Mentally raising his eyebrows, the Apothecary stole a glance at Amelia, but she appeared utterly as would have been normal in her wretched circumstances. Pale but determined to present a brave face to the world, she sat with her eyes cast down and her hands folded in her lap, the very picture of unhappy innocence. She was either, thought John, an excellent actress or had spent an entirely blameless night alone in her bed.

'A brandy, Mr Rawlings?' said Valentine, rising. 'I'm going to have one. What about you, Miss Lambourn?'

'Yes, I will,' she said. 'I need to get my courage up.'

John nodded. 'Yes, thank you.' He looked at his fob watch. 'What time is the funeral?'

'At twelve noon,' the office manager answered. 'We'll need to leave here about a half hour before. St Matthew's lies on the road back to town.'

'It's a new church, isn't it?' John asked.

'Ten years old.' Valentine smiled. 'It was built to counter the increase of dissoluteness of morals in the younger and poorer sort.'

'Well, that covers most of us,' the Apothecary said, and laughed at the expression on his companions' faces.

Fortified by the brandy the trio set forth some thirty minutes later. Miss Lambourn, who was travelling in a very smart rig, obviously a gift from Sir William, offered the two gentlemen a ride with her, a proposal which they gladly accepted. Sitting beside her as they bumped over the track, noticing how delicious was her profile, John felt that he could easily understand how anyone, of any age, might fall in love with her, and conjectured again about her relationship with Valentine Randolph, with whom he had caught her conversing in so animated a fashion. And this thought led him on to another. Had she happily decided to enter into marriage with an elderly man, secure in the knowledge that she had a lover in the background to keep her amused? And where, if anywhere, did the helpful Luke Challon feature in all this? As best he could, John decided to observe all three of them.

St Matthew's churchyard was already full of mourners, presumably friends and neighbours, standing together in groups, chattering quite loudly for such a solemn occasion. Attempting to vanish into the background, John allowed Mr Randolph to offer Miss Lambourn his arm, while he stood well away beside a grave stone bearing the stark message, 'He was a candle in the wind, Alas he's been blown out'. Thinking how swiftly the end came for one and all, John shuddered as in the distance, turning off the track and down towards the church, he caught his first glimpse of the funeral procession.

Walking tragically slowly, clad in dark clothes from the top of his small frame to his barely visible boots, came the fragile figure of the undertaker's mute, leading the dead to his final resting place. Behind him followed the hearse, drawn by two gleaming horses the colour of jet, emblazoned with emblems and nodding black plumes, the coffin containing poor Sir William's earthly shell clearly visible through its glass sides. Behind it followed a cortège of unwieldy black coaches, bearing the family who, even at this distance, could be seen sitting bolt upright, an unkindness of ravens indeed. Remembering that he had had this very thought on the day of the wedding that never happened, John felt a sense of familiarity. Coming to a halt outside the church door, the coffin was shouldered out of the hearse and into the house of God by the male members of the family. Roger, white as a sail and sweating copiously, led the way, with a tanned thin crisp individual who could only be Hugh, on the opposite corner. Behind them walked Julian, in tears, and Luke Challon, his expression bleak beyond belief. Two professional pall bearers bore the rest of the load.

John watched the coffin go in, then turned to glance at the bereaved and nearly laughed aloud, an inexcusable action. Escorted by Sir Gabriel Kent, resplendent in a sable trimmed black cloak which swept the ground as he walked, came Lady Hodkin, appearing mightily pleased with herself and more than a little besotted. Hesther, very pink, was her usual step behind and hurrying a little. Yet as she drew level with him the Apothecary thought that sombre colours became her, for she looked more comely than he had ever seen her. Catching his eye, Miss Hodkin gave a tentative smile.

Lydia, a woman whom John presumed to be Maud, and Juliet, the last quite ravishing in a large black hat, followed in next and behind them poured all the other grievers in a body. The Apothecary's heart bled for poor Miss Lambourn who, whatever her faults, whatever her antecedents, would have led the mourners this day had not the hand of a murderer struck her intended husband down. Now she was left like the meanest servant to go in last, a pathetic little figure, already in tears. Even though she was being supported by Valentine Randolph, John took her other arm and walked in beside her.

It truly was the wedding party gathered together all over again and seeing them like this gave the Apothecary the chance to flash that other portrait from St Paul's, Shadwell, into his vivid memory. Comparing the two, he saw that Lydia had not lied, for she had not been present on the first occasion. And though Maud had been in church, Hugh had not, probably telling the truth about being out of the country. As to the rest, they had all been present at the wedding, looking as glum as they did now, with the exception of Lady Hodkin, who on this occasion seemed to be positively cheerful.

John let his mind wander over certain possibilities. Despite her claims to be aged and weak, the old beast was more than capable of wielding a stick, he had seen that for himself. It was Hesther who had received the brunt of that blow, but would Miss Hodkin be capable of striking one herself? Had unrequited love for her brother-in-law driven her into a frenzy, a frenzy which had led to his death? And what of Lydia, so dark and strong and handsome, had she some secret, something he had yet to unearth, which could have caused her to shut Sir William's mouth for ever? Or was it greed with all of them? Had the thought of a vast inherited fortune been the trigger? As far as Maud was concerned, John did not know enough about her to be aware of any other reason. And then he remembered the twins calling her prim. Could she be so fanatically pure that Sir William's adultery had driven her to kill? Or was her prudery a pose? Did it, in fact, mask a life of sin and dissipation?

Reluctantly, John turned his attention to Julian and Juliette. In the young man's case, of course, his addiction to gambling and his debts might well have given him sufficient reason to want his father out of the way. But as for the girl, how could such a shining beauty be associated with anything so brutal as murder? Then the Apothecary mentally took himself to task. It had been his mistake in the past not to equate loveliness with wickedness, yet he knew perfectly well that one did not preclude the other. Perhaps Juliette felt so protective about her twin that she would have killed for him. The two of them certainly acted as if they were in a conspiracy of some kind. But twins were often like that, particularly those born identical, John thought. Yet even though Julian and Juliette were not in that category, being of different sex, they had still shared together the dark secret waters of the womb, a bond between them that no one could ever break.

The service was beginning but John found it hard to concentrate his mind on it, so taken up with the notion that one of Sir William's family had struck the fatal blow and puzzling over which one of them it could have been. And then he heard the door at the back of the church open and a pair of large feet attempt to tiptoe in. Turning to have a look, the Apothecary was both delighted and astonished to see that Samuel Swann had arrived to pay his last respects and was taking his place in a rear pew.

They met at the graveside, or rather in the queue leading down the path towards it, and shook each other most heartily by the hand. 'My dear fellow, how is it all going?' asked the Goldsmith, in the hushed tones of one who is dying to hear the news but simultaneously trying to keep a sense of occasion.

'In the most complicated manner possible. I am supposed to be investigating Sir William's family but have been barred the house by his harridan mother-in-law. Therefore, my father has been sent in, posing as a hapless traveller . . .'

'What!' exclaimed Samuel loudly.

'To try and unravel the skeins of their devious lives. He is here now, even as we speak. Should he pass you, pretend not to know him.'

The Goldsmith rubbed his hands together. 'This is tremendous! I'm so glad I came. If I had not called on Mr Fielding last night I would have known nothing about it.'

John gaped at him. 'Last night? But I was there. What time did you go to see him?'

'About a quarter of an hour after you had left to visit Serafina and Louis. Anyway, the Beak caught me up with as much news as he could. And told me that the funeral was today. I thought as you had found the poor man's corpse it would be only fitting to pay my final regards. But in view of all the intrigue, I am delighted I did so.'

'And well you might be. We stand on the threshold of a great secret, I'm sure of it. Now, how did you get here?'

'By postchaise. It put me down at a place called The George and I walked the rest of the way.'

'I came on Godiva, whom I'm due to take back later today. So I suggest that we return to The George as soon as we can, and meet again later this evening, near the Middle Temple.'

'What will you be doing there?'

'Hearing the details of Sir William Hartfield's will. It is being read this afternoon at Kirby Hall but Mr Fielding has asked the lawyer to reveal the contents to me tonight.'

'Surely the main beneficiary is going to be Amelia Lambourn.'

'That we must wait and see.'

'But if she is, does it give her a motive for murder?'

John looked thoughtful. 'I would have thought not. But there is certainly something odd about the girl. High on my list of things to do is pay a visit to Islington Spa where Sir William originally met Amelia, and find out what is known about her there.'

'And when do you intend to do this?'

'Probably tomorrow afternoon. Is there any chance you could join me?'

Samuel beamed. 'I should be delighted. I feel that I haven't given you my usual help with this latest quest . . .'

John smiled within.

'. . . so I shall leave the shop in the hands of my apprentice and go with you.' He looked anxious. 'But what about you? Do you have an assistant to look after things?'

'I have acquired a young fellow through the good offices of Mr Fielding. My father and I think highly of him but I would like you to meet him and give me your opinion. He is called Nicholas Dawkins and is reputed to be of noble Muscovy descent.'

'How exotic.'

John grinned and nudged his friend in the ribs. 'Did you think I'd choose anyone less?'

But at that point their moment of *bonhomie* abruptly ended. A shriek pierced shrilly from the graveside and looking down the length of the line of mourners, the Apothecary saw that Amelia Lambourn, whose turn it was to throw earth upon the coffin, was swaying in a faint on the very edge of the yawning chasm. Indeed she would have fallen in backwards had it not been for Roger, of all the unlikely people, who with a burst of quick thinking, seized the unhappy girl round the waist and pulled her back to safety.

'How extraordinary,' murmured John.

'What?'

'That he of all of them should have had the presence of mind to save her.'

'Why? Is he a puff?'

'What makes you say that?'

'He looks it, though that means nothing of course. Who is the fellow?'

'Roger Hartfield, Sir William's first-born.'

John continued to stare in the direction of the grave and saw that despite the beau's somewhat feeble ministrations, Amelia had lost conciousness. 'Oh dear,' he sighed, and pushed past the curious crowd to her aid, knocking into his father as he did so and saying, 'Oh, beg pardon, Sir,' in a highly affected voice. At the same time, Luke Challon appeared as if from nowhere, practically hurling people over in his anxiety to get to the fainting woman's side. It was all, John thought, very interesting indeed.

Despite Lady Hodkin's cries of, 'There's that horrible young man!' the Apothecary finally managed to get some sal volatile beneath Amelia's nose and raise her from where she hung limply in the crook of Roger's arm. After a moment her eyes fluttered open and she looked round, saw the greedy-mouthed grave, and swooned once more.

'I'll take Miss Lambourn to her carriage,' offered Luke.

'Permit me to assist,' said Valentine Randolph.

'Really!' interrupted Roger petulantly. 'Allow one member of the family to show a little decency. I'll get her there myself.'

And he minced off on his high-heeled shoes, practically dragging the poor girl with him, leaving the rest of the family to stare at his retreating back, their expressions ranging from downright fury to one of total disbelief.

It was dark when John got back to London and late when he returned Godiva to her stables in Dolphin Yard. But, having hurried into his house to wash the dust of the journey from his face and hands, the Apothecary was out again within twenty minutes, running down into Piccadilly where he hired a hackney coach to take him to the lawyer's office in Middle Temple Lane, the address given to him by Joe Jago before he had left Bow Street on the previous evening.

Afraid that a late arrival might persuade Mr Josiah Bradshaigh, tired by having read the will once that day, to close his office and make for home, none too happy, no doubt, at having to comply with a request issued by the Public Office, John urged his driver on. But in the event he need not have worried. Lights burned in the second floor office and as he made his way up the tottering wooden staircase, he could hear the sound of voices. Somewhat tentatively he knocked on the door with the head of his great stick and was amazed when it flew open straight away.

'John Rawlings, here on behalf of Mr Fielding,' he said, producing his letter of authorisation.

'Come in, come in,' called a voice from within, and John found himself being ushered by the shrivelled clerk who had answered the door, into the inner sanctum.

There were papers everywhere. Standing in piles on the floor, perched precariously on shelves, heaped high on the desk, most of them tied with pink string and nearly all covered with an amazing amount of dust. Behind this mountain of documents, the Apothecary could vaguely glimpse a figure who waved a hand round one of the heaps and silently motioned the visitor to sit. Springing forward nimbly, the clerk cleared the only available chair of yet another heap of parchment and cleaned it off with the bottom of his coat. Very carefully, the Apothecary sat down.

The waving hand pushed several piles round the desk, rather like moving chess pieces, until there was enough room to peer at the newcomer, which its owner then proceeded to do, his eyes the glistening bright brown of those of a fieldmouse.

'Young, eh?' said a voice.

'Rising twenty-four,' John answered swiftly. 'Does that offend you, Sir?'

'Not at all, not at all.' The lawyer growled a laugh. 'We must all start somewhere.' He pushed a pint jug in John's direction. 'Help yourself. I've got another one here.'

Staring down into the contents, the Apothecary saw that it was brimming with claret. 'Do you have a glass?' he asked tentatively.

'Somewhere,' came the answer. 'Coombs, go and look.'

'Yes, Sir,' said the clerk, and begun to hunt round the room, a whistling sound coming from between his clenched brown teeth.

'I'm Bradshaigh,' said the lawyer, extending a hand between the documents which John solemnly shook. 'Did I not see you at the funeral?'

'Yes, I was there. But I can't say I noticed you, Sir.'

'Kept in the background. Could see the family bristling with anticipation every time I drew near, so kept my own counsel until I was forced to reveal all.'

The Apothecary felt a prickle of anticipation, knowing full well how very important the next half hour was going to be, and at that moment another heap of papers moved and John got his first good look at the late Sir William's trusted lawyer.

It was a rubicund face, crimson and jolly, with a shock of silver hair above, which looked quite startling in contrast with the vividness below. The nose was very large, spreading across the features and bearing many pitted pores. While a confluence of broken veins added even more colour to the already reddened cheeks. In the midst of all this glow, the twinkling eyes looked small and somehow out of place.

'Drat that clerk,' said Mr Bradshaigh. 'Can't you drink from the jug, boy?'

'I can try,' John replied, and sipped cautiously.

'That's more like it.' The lawyer drained half a pint at a single swallow, then wiped his hand across his mouth. 'Now, you're here to hear the will, I believe. Do you want it all – or just the main bequests?'

'For the moment, at least, just the bones of it. If Mr Fielding thinks otherwise then we will have to go through it again.'

Josiah Bradshaigh drained his jug then refilled if from a case of bottles standing by his side. 'It's a queer business, this,' he said. 'Very queer indeed.'

'In what way exactly?'

The lawyer slipped a pair of spectacles onto his nose, then peered at the Apothecary over the top of them. 'You *are* acting on the authority of John Fielding as you say?'

'Yes, most certainly. Here is his letter authorising me to carry out enquiries.' With some difficulty, John handed it over the desk.

Mr Bradshaigh examined it. 'Yes, yes, that seems in order. But I had to make sure. For what I have to say to you is not only confidential but assumes a sinister connotation in view of the fact that my late client was done to death.'

'Please continue,' said John, twitching with impatience.

'Sir William was due to be secretly married, as you probably know . . .'

'Yes, I do.'

Mr Bradshaigh drained his jug, then refilled it. 'Well, the fact is, in view of his forthcoming nuptials, my client had asked me to draw up a new will and was due to sign it on the eve of his wedding. It was arranged that he would come to this office at eight o'clock and append his signature to the document before two witnesses. But instead of Sir William one of his footmen arrived bearing a note, a note which I have here.' His hand sought and found a particular piece of paper amongst the dozens on the desk.

'What does it say?'

'That he, Sir William that is, had been called away unexpectedly to attend to some urgent business and would contact me within a day or two. That is the last thing I ever heard from him.'

'Is the letter genuine?'

Josiah Bradshaigh huffed. 'Yes, most certainly it is. I would know my client's writing anywhere.'

John drank from his jug, more deeply than he had intended. 'Are you then stating, Sir, that because of Sir William's nonappearance the old will still stands?'

'Of course. No document is legal without a signature.'

'Then may I hazard a guess that the second will is very different from the first?'

'You may indeed, and you would be right. The second testament left the bulk of Sir William's fortune to his affianced bride, the future Lady Hartfield, while the business was to pass out of the family and into the joint hands of Mr Valentine Randolph and Luke Challon. To his progeny, whom he considered would only fritter the money away, he left mere nominal sums.'

''Sblud!'

'And 'zounds, I feel I might add.' The lawyer smiled at his little joke and his eyes glinted merrily.

'While the first divided everything between the heirs of his body, I suppose?'

'Not quite. The houses and the bulk of the fortune were left to the first Lady Hartfield, with the proviso that should she predecease her husband which, of course, she did, the estate should be divided as follows. The St James's Square house was left to Roger, Kirby Hall to Sir William's sister-in-law, Miss Hesther Hodkin. The rest of the fortune was to be divided equally amongst Sir William's children, with his daughter-in-law, Mrs Lydia Hartfield, receiving an equal share. Lady Hodkin and her daughter were not left money as such but, believe me, can live quite comfortably without a bequest. In view of the fact that the dead Lady Hartfield left most of her personal funds to her husband, this amount will now be added to the children's share. So we are talking about an enormous sum, Sir. A truly enormous sum.'

'What about the others? Servants and so on?'

'Mr Challon and Mr Randolph were each left five thousand pounds. The retainers a few hundred, according to their length of service.'

'I see. How about the business? How was that disposed?'

'Left to the three sons, with the stipulation that Hugh, already a member of the firm as you probably know, became nominal head, and Mr Randolph continued as manager.'

'And Miss Lambourn?'

'Nothing.'

'What?'

'Not one penny piece.'

'But why?'

'Because, my dear boy,' said Mr Bradshaigh, tapping the sheaves of parchment in his hand, 'Sir William did not even know the young woman when this original will was made.'

Without meaning to, John drained the jug in his hand. 'Sir, please think clearly. How many people knew about the second will, were aware that Miss Lambourn was about to become virtually the sole heiress?'

'No one was supposed to but these things have a way of leaking out, of course.'

'Then, by God, we have a mighty motive here.'

'What do you mean?'

'That any member of the family, knowing that he – or she – stood to lose everything if Sir William signed the second will, might do anything in their power to stop him doing so.'

The red face on the other side of the desk flushed an even deeper shade, and the fieldmouse eyes became two points of brilliance as the significance of the words sunk in.

'Including murder?' asked Mr Bradshaigh gravely.

'Oh quite definitely including murder,' John answered with equal solemnity.

Chapter Twelve

*T*o the north of Fleet Street, lying within the shadow of the great church of St Dunstan's in the West, was a cluster of mean little alleyways and festering streets, so jumbled together that to venture into them was like entering a tortuous maze. Here, amongst these hideaways, in the darkness, it was not safe for a man to go unarmed or unprepared. Yet within this squalid labyrinth of alleys, like oases in a desert, lay squares and courts in which respectable citizens lived, though how they picked their way in and out to their dwelling places remained a mystery to the uninitiated. Also concealed in the confines of this tangle was a tavern of repute, a place in which it was possible to dine on an excellent supper, to say nothing of drinking the unusually good wine served to go with it. And it was to find this hostelry, delightfully named The Cheshire Cheese, that John Rawlings bravely headed off into the web of twittens, fervently hoping that he would not lose his way.

The information he had just been given in the lawyer's office had stunned him. For in that surely lay the reason why Sir William had been done to death. And more than that, the time when the victim had vanished could now be pinpointed. Having seen Amelia Lambourn into her carriage at about half past six, following their wedding eve dinner together, the bridegroom had received a message which had caused him to alter his plans and meet somebody other than Josiah Bradshaigh. And that somebody had to be the last person to see him alive. Wondering if the note Sir William had received might still be in existence at St James's Square, John decided to go there as soon as possible and make a thorough search. Meanwhile, though, he must locate The Cheshire Cheese and get some food, for various messages from his stomach were reminding the Apothecary that he had not eaten since midday, when he had hastily snatched a piece of mutton pie, consumed at The George following the funeral.

Turning down a blind alley, John cursed and retraced his

143

footsteps, then heard a burst of laughter coming from his left. Light fell across the cobbles and there was more noise, including a clatter of plates. A door opened and the pungent smell of unwashed bodies, tallow, roasting meat, tobacco, ale and cheap perfume, attacked his nostrils. John hurried towards it. He had found his destination.

Samuel had not only already arrived but had downed a pint of ale and secured a tavern chair, luxury indeed. After some searching, the Apothecary managed to locate a stool, the only seating left, and thus, squeezed in by a table, the two friends ordered a large meal consisting of dressed meats carved by the landlord, capons in pastry and various custards, all for the price of three shillings.

'And what,' asked Samuel, with his mouth stuffed full, 'did you learn?'

John rolled his eyes, unable to speak. Then gave a convulsive swallow and said, 'What did I not! It was only Sir William's death that prevented him from signing a new will in which Amelia was named as principal legatee. Everyone else's portion would have been reduced to a minor share, and the business was destined to pass into the hands of Luke Challon, the secretary, and Valentine Randolph, the man we saw at The Devil's Tavern.'

'Hare and hounds!'

'Precisely.'

'Then that means one of the others murdered the old chap in order to stop him signing.'

'Probably, unless . . .'

'Unless what?'

'Unless that is too easy a conclusion to come to. Suppose, just for a moment, that nobody other than the lawyer was aware of the new will. It is said that ignorance is bliss. If that is so, why kill Sir William?'

'To get their hands on the inheritance sooner?'

'Why risk the rope when the money will come eventually?'

Samuel shook his head. 'I've no idea. You've foxed me with that.'

John took another mouthful and chewed it thoughtfully. 'Do you know, it occurs to me that this might yet be a crime of passion.'

'Really? Why?'

'You saw Amelia Lambourn at the funeral. She is remarkably pretty, is she not?'

Samuel bit into a capon. 'Glorious creature,' he mumbled.

'Well, one can't help but notice that both Luke Challon and Valentine Randolph show a great deal of interest in her. So perhaps the business of the new will is a mere coincidence. Maybe the motive was jealousy all along.'

'If that is the case, Amelia herself must be free of guilt.'

'Not if she had a lover in the background. Perhaps the pair of them plotted to kill her elderly bridegroom before the ceremony ever took place.'

Samuel's face, full of food though it was, assumed a totally bewildered expression. 'This is all too convoluted for me. I can't follow the twists of it.'

John grinned. 'Neither can I, to tell the truth.'

'So what will you do?'

'Try to probe each possibility. Now, are you still on for tomorrow?'

'Islington Spa, you mean . . .?' John nodded. 'Yes, I most certainly am. What time do you want to go?'

'I think I should visit Bow Street first thing and tell Mr Fielding about the second will. Could you come to Shug Lane at noon?'

'Certainly.'

'Good. Then you can inspect young Nicholas.'

'I look forward to it.'

A serving girl appeared at their table to remove the empty plates but was restrained by Samuel, who asked, 'Would it be possible for the landlord to carve me another helping of beef?'

She smiled at him saucily. 'You're hungry, ain't yer?'

The Goldsmith gazed at her seriously. 'It's all this thinking. It plays the very devil with my appetite.'

'Then you'll have to give it up,' the girl answered cheerfully. 'Cos wiv men it's either brains or ballocks, ain't it?'

And off she went to get some more meat, leaving Samuel to whisper hoarsely, 'Dear God, I hope that isn't true!' before both he and his companion guffawed till their eyes streamed.

The candles were still lit when John returned to Nassau Street by means of a hackney. Too many to be merely a welcome. With the sudden hope that his father might have come home, the Apothecary paid off the driver and rushed within.

'Sir Gabriel is in the library, Master John,' said the footman who answered the door.

'Then I'll join him.'

'He has waited up in the hope that you would.'

Feeling more than delighted, the Apothecary made straight for his favourite room, only to find that Sir Gabriel had already changed into a nightrail and turban, and was dozing in his chair by the fire. Suddenly acutely aware of his father's advancing years, John would have crept out again, had not his parent said, 'Ah, there you are, my dear. I was not asleep but had merely closed my eyes. After all, it has been rather a tumultuous day, has it not?'

'It certainly has,' John answered, collapsing into the chair on the other side of the fireplace. 'I could not believe my eyes when I saw you with Lady Hodkin on your arm, for all the world as if you were head of the family. Tell me what miracle you wrought to bring that about.'

Sir Gabriel smiled and raised his lids. 'No miracle, my child. Merely the exercising of a little tact and charm.'

John snorted and his father continued, 'Pray do not make that inelegant sound. Such behaviour does not become you.'

'Sorry,' the Apothecary answered, compressing his lips to hide a smile. 'Now, Father, if you have time to listen, I have a great deal to recount.'

And he repeated almost word for word, drawing on his excellent memory, the conversations he had had with both Josiah Bradshaigh and Samuel.

Sir Gabriel remained silent after his son had finished giving his account, the tips of his long fingers together, the index pair resting lightly on his chin. Then eventually he said, 'Well, even though the situation seems more convoluted than ever, it is obvious that a great deal of progress has been made.'

'In a way, yes,' John replied pensively. 'But, as I said to Sam, I am not certain that gain was the entire motive for this crime, though most probably a major part of it. However, I do think we can now be safe in assuming that Sir William was killed either late on his wedding eve or early next day.'

'Oh, indeed. Those are the vital hours.' Sir Gabriel poured two glasses of port and sipped his slowly. 'I think,' he said, his voice reflective, 'that in view of all this I should take Lady Hodkin up on her invitation sooner than I had intended.'

'She has asked you back to Kirby Hall?'

'At any time. I do believe it is her fond hope that I am going to take Miss Hesther off her hands at last.'

'And are you?'

'My dear boy, please don't be frivolous! No, my initial plan was to infiltrate myself into their confidence, which I have succeeded in doing. Now I feel I should enter the second phase, namely to try and discover as much as I can about all of them. With particular concentration on where they were – and by they I mean every member of the household – on the night before Sir William's wedding.'

John gave him a delighted smile. 'My clever Papa, if you can do that for me you will rise even higher in my esteem, if such a thing were possible.'

'In that case I must leave at once.'

The Apothecary laughed. 'I think tomorrow will be quite soon enough.'

'Splendid. Then I shall return to Kirby Hall making the excuse of having left something behind.' He stared at John closely. 'And now, my child, I suggest that you go to bed. Are you aware that your eyes are actually closing?'

'More than aware,' his son replied with a yawn, then before he could say another word fell fast asleep in the chair, where Sir Gabriel, having covered him with a rug and called a servant to stoke up the fire, left him to doze in peace.

Despite the fact that he should have woken with an aching back and tender limbs, the Apothecary rose feeling fresh and well at about six o'clock the following morning. Considering that he smelled of horseflesh and lawyer's offices, he washed very thoroughly and in view of his proposed visit to Islington Spa later that day, dressed in a fine suit of plum satin with a pink embroidered waistcoat to go with it. Then John went downstairs and partook of a substantial breakfast before going into the street and summoning some weary homegoing chairmen to take him to the Public Office as quickly as they could. Hoping that he would tip them generously, the poor souls put their backs into the task and the Apothecary arrived at Bow Street just as the Blind Beak was rising from table, his napkin still in his hand.

147

'Mr Rawlings,' he said with pleasure as John was shown into the morning room and announced, 'will you join me in some coffee?'

'I would be delighted, Sir.'

'Then do have a second repast here. Nicholas has already left for Shug Lane so you have nothing to fear.' And the Magistrate sat down again to show that he meant what he said. 'Now tell me about the will,' he went on as the Apothecary refilled Mr Fielding's cup and poured another for himself.

'There are *two* wills, Sir. One of them unsigned.'

'Can you explain that?'

'Certainly.'

The Blind Beak turned his head, listening intently, as John told him everything he had heard on the previous evening. 'So that might be one reason why a man was put to death,' the Magistrate said eventually.

'You believe there could be others?'

'It's possible. Gain alone might not be the cause. But on the other hand it might. There's a tangled mesh here, my friend.'

'And several people with something to hide.'

'One of whom is Miss Lambourn?'

'I think so. Anyway, I shall know more shortly. This afternoon Samuel and I are due to visit Islington Spa and there find out a little more about her past.'

'Meanwhile,' said John Fielding, emptying his cup and wiping his mouth, 'I have a very busy day in court. By the way, Mr Rawlings, is it your intention to try and find the note that was sent to Sir William on the night before his wedding?'

'It most certainly is. I shall go to St James's Square tomorrow.'

'Be sure to take your authorisation. Servants are always much more difficult to deal with than their masters.' The Blind Beak chuckled. 'If that fails, try a *douceur*. Greased palms have always opened locked doors.'

'Alas, that I should encourage such lack of morality!'

'But encourage it you will.'

'Of course,' said John, and bowed to Mr Fielding as they left the room together.

First fashionable in the late seventeenth century, when a spring had been discovered in gardens growing opposite the New River Head in Clerkenwell, the Islington Spa had originally been known as

Islington Wells, then New Tunbridge Wells, whose health giving waters it claimed to rival. However, in order to avoid confusion with its more famous neighbour, the Wells owned by Mr Sadler close by, the pleasure garden had finally changed its name to Islington Spa, though the earlier title still tended to be used.

In addition to its chalybeate spring, its shady lime trees and romantic arbours, Islington Spa also possessed the more sinful attractions of a dancing room and a raffling shop, where the pursuit of gambling could be enjoyed by those of such a mind. There were also the Walks, where beaux strutted with scarlet ribbons on their great sticks and ladies surveyed one another coldly, tearing reputations and fashions to pieces as they paraded. Yet perhaps the greatest attraction was the dancing, held daily after the public breakfasting, from eleven to three.

Mindful of this draw, John and Samuel left Shug Lane shortly after noon and hired a hackney in Piccadilly to take them to Leicester Fields, then across various alleyways to Long Acre, then up Drury Lane towards Holbourn. From there the driver headed northwards, going up Hatton Garden, these days establishing something of a reputation for its jewellery, then picked his way via Clerkenwell Green to St John's Street which led directly to the Spa. Tipping the man generously from the expenses he had drawn at the Public Office before he left, John bought two tickets costing eighteen pennies each, and he and Samuel made their way immediately to the ballroom. There they found themselves amongst very mixed company, the Spa having a reputation for allowing in the lower orders. Highborn ladies and good wives mixed with seamstresses and prostitutes, dressed to the hilt in their tawdry finery. Whilst country gentlemen and minor knights rubbed shoulders with lawyers' clerks and shopkeepers, to say nothing of members of the criminal class, skulking amongst the crowd to see what pickings might be had.

Much intrigued by this great social mix, the two friends decided to make the best of the hour and a half left before dancing ended and tea began, and whirled about with whoever would have them as partners. Fortunately, all the dance figures were of the country variety, either longways or rounds, constructed to a formula, and it was relatively easy to pick up any unfamiliar steps. Sweating and laughing and forgetting all about murder and violence, John and Samuel threw themselves into Rufty Tufty, Row Well Ye

Marriners, Sellengers Round and finally Graies Inne Maske, a longways set dance for four couples which ended in a kiss, a salutation which Samuel very much enjoyed. Then it was time for business again and mopping their brows, the Apothecary and the Goldsmith strolled down one of the Walks towards the Well.

With Amelia long since departed, the water was currently being served by a pert little creature with flaming red curls perched on top of her head beneath a pinner. While next to the Well sat a beldame taking the money, threepence a glass. Huddled as she was in a folding chair, there was still something familiar about the old woman and John turned to Samuel, suddenly wild with excitement.

'It's her, Sam. The one I saw in church. The person who was with Amelia on her wedding day.'

'Is it really? Do you think she could be Miss Lambourn's mother?'

'Yes, I believe she very well might.'

The Goldsmith clapped his hands. 'How extremely fortunate.'

'Let it be hoped that she agrees to speak to us.'

'I'm sure she will,' Samuel answered, rubbing his thumb and fingers together in the age old sign for money, and simultaneously winking an eye.

Ahead of the friends straggled a queue of elderly people, suffering with gout, nerves, weak knees, stiff joints and ineffectual bladders. Most of these tottered down the steps to the Well, which was surrounded by a grotto of shells supported on stone pilasters, groaning with every movement they made. As each one approached, the pretty server dipped a cup on a long handle into the brownish water, mixed the contents with ordinary water, then gave the sufferer a glass of the resulting concoction.

'Why is she doing that?' whispered Samuel.

'It's supposed to be too strong otherwise. It has a reputation for making the drinker giddy or sleepy.'

'I hope it doesn't kill anyone. They all look fit to drop.'

'Now, now,' said John severely. 'You'll be like that one day.'

'No I won't,' his friend answered stoutly. 'I intend to emulate Sir Gabriel Kent when I grow old.'

Hearing his voice, raised with enthusiasm, the water server looked up and shot a ravishing glance in Samuel's direction.

'My goodness!' he exclaimed.

'I thought your heart had been captured by Miss Verity, at least it was last Christmas,' John said, smiling.

The Goldsmith looked sad. 'It still is really. But, alas, my passion is unrequited. She is a dedicated business woman and has engaged her affections with another, more established than I. A better prospect all round than someone just making his way in the world.'

'How fickle of her.'

'I thought so.'

The queue slowly moved on until it was John's turn to take the waters. This he did with much relish, pouring a little of the undiluted original into a phial which he carried in his pocket.

'Why are you doing that?' asked the server, clearly astonished.

'I want to analyse it. Water and its composition fascinates me.'

'Oh,' she answered, none the wiser.

John lowered his voice to a whisper. 'That old lady sitting beside the Well, would she be Mrs Lambourn by any chance?'

'Yes, Sir.'

Putting the phial away, John produced five shillings from his pocket, an enormous sum to a poorly paid individual. 'Thank you for your help,' he said.

'But I haven't done nothing.'

'Yes you have, you told me her name. And anyway you look charming. That's enough.'

She blushed delightfully and a woman waiting her turn behind, called out, 'Now, now, young man. There are people of condition here this season. We don't want none of your lewd behaviour on these premises.'

The Apothecary swept off his hat and bowed low. 'Madam,' he said, 'might I suggest a purgation of hellebore, excellent for dull and heavy persons.'

'How dare you?' she huffed.

But John had beaten a tactical retreat to where Mrs Lambourn sat, counting the money before she put it in a leather bag attached to her belt. He bowed again.

'Mrs Lambourn?'

'Yes?'

'I have a message from your daughter Amelia,' he lied pleasantly.

'What is it? Is she poorly?' she asked, her voice anxious.

Thinking quickly, John decided on a businesslike approach. 'Madam, you are aware that Sir William Hartfield is dead?'

'Yes, she wrote to me. I couldn't read the letter, mind, but the Spa's pastry cook did. Is it true the poor soul was done away wiv?'

'I fear so.'

The old woman's chest heaved. 'Oh my poor gal. How will she fare wiv no one to look after her?'

The Apothecary decided to take a chance. 'Oh come, she's hardly on her own, now is she?'

Mrs Lambourn shot him a look of immense cunning. 'Well, that depends.' Her eyes narrowed suspiciously. 'Who did you say you were?'

'The name's John Rawlings. I'm a friend of Valentine Randolph.'

'Who?'

So either the office manager was not Amelia's lover or her daughter kept a close secret, John thought.

'Also of Luke Challon,' he added.

He hit home this time. 'Oh, Sir William's secretary. Oh well, that's all right then. He always treated her decent did Luke. A very nice young man. The others called my girl names because she had relations with her intended before they was wed.'

'Weren't the insults because he was married to someone else at the time?'

She flared up at him. 'Yus, to a bedbound invalid wiv no use of her legs or parts! What was a proper man like Sir William supposed to do?'

'I'm not criticising, believe me,' John said soothingly. 'I have every sympathy with them. And for Amelia in her hour of grief. I only hope that there is someone on hand to console her at this terrible time.'

The old hag glared at him. 'You think I'm going to tell you something, don't yer? Well I ain't, so there.'

The Apothecary bowed. 'On the contrary, Mrs Lambourn, you have told me a great deal.'

She looked aghast, frightened almost, then the situation was saved by the arrival of Samuel, who came up wearing a besotted expression that John knew well.

'Sorry I've been so long,' he said. 'I've been strolling about admiring the view.'

'Admiring the girl more likely.' The Apothecary bowed and handed over his second five shillings of the day. 'Thank you for your help, Madam. May I wish you good day.' And putting his hat back on his head, he strolled away.

'Well?' said Samuel.

'She's hiding something. Amelia definitely has a lover and the old woman knows all about it.'

'Is it Luke Challon?'

'Probably.'

'Do you think that's why he hasn't been to see you? Afraid you might discover something?'

'It's no use conjecturing about his absence. The only way is for me to ask him direct. Now, let's enjoy the rest of our time here. What would you like to do, other than elope with the water server?'

Samuel chortled. 'Let's look round, then take afternoon tea.'

'A good idea.'

Perambulating slowly, the friends set off to make a tour, peering into the pretty arbours where lovers could meet and acquaintances chat, to discover who from the *beau monde* was at the Spa that day. Eventually, though, they found that their footsteps had led them to the raffling shop, where they stood in silence listening to the roll of the dice.

'Serafina should be here,' said John with a smile.

'Does she miss her old pastime?'

'She confessed to me that now and then she longs to return to it.'

'Then let's see who is in there so that we can report back to her.'

'Very well.' And they stepped within.

Staring round, John's eyes widened at the sight which greeted him. For seated at the board, dressed to the teeth in purple satin stitched with brilliants, despite custom his mourning clothes already cast to one side, was Roger Hartfield, throwing the dice with a great flurry of lace cuffs.

'Good God,' said Samuel, following the Apothecary's gaze. 'Who the devil's that?'

'The prodigious beau I told you about. He was at the funeral. The one who saved Amelia from falling into the grave.'

'Roger Hartfield? He looks very different.'

'He was probably on his best behaviour that day.'

'Teaze and tackle, he's much worse than I remembered!'

'Keep your voice down,' hissed John. But it was too late, Roger had looked up and was waving a large white hand.

'Mr Rawlings! God's life, what are you doing here? Is this fate or coincidence?'

'Quiet!' ordered another gambler, at which Roger, with much swishing of his coat skirts, petulantly rose from his place.

'My dear,' he said, grabbing John by the elbow. 'How fortuitous. I have been meaning to come and see you. My sister Juliette told me you had an apothecary's shop in Shug Lane and I intended to come in for a consultation. I've been having such trouble since the funeral. Cannot keep a thing down. Billious is simply not the word for it.' His wide-eyed gaze took in Samuel's powerful stature. 'Oh, *quel homme*. Won't you introduce me?'

'This is my friend Samuel Swann,' said John, and almost laughed aloud at the expression on the Goldsmith's face. 'Samuel, may I present Mr Roger Hartfield?'

'Charmed, charmed, charmed,' Roger gushed. 'Now why don't we all leave here and go back to my club? They don't serve anything stronger than ale in this place and I feel like a bumper or two of champagne. Meeting new friends – and old ones as well of course.' He flickered his eyelashes.

'Wine is very bad for you if you're suffering from sickness,' John said sternly. 'Best that you go home and take a Cotiniat of Quinces, that should do the trick.'

Roger made a truculent mouth. 'You sound just like my father.'

'I'm sorry about that. I was only trying to give you my professional advice.'

Samuel gulped noisily. 'John's right, and as it happens I have an urgent appointment this evening. But thank you anyway.'

'Another time then. As you can see, I can't bear to incarcerate myself indoors but as soon as I am officially out of mourning I intend to give a little supper party for my friends, start entertaining again. You two must come.'

John bowed. 'It will be a pleasure. Meanwhile, Mr Hartfield . . .'

'I have told you before. It's Roger.'

'. . . Roger . . . will it be in order for me to visit St James's Square tomorrow? There are one or two questions I would like to ask your servants.'

Did he imagine it, or did a wary look momentarily appear in the beau's pale and protruberant blue eyes?

'Of course. What time will you be coming?'

Instantly on the alert, the Apothecary answered, 'I really have no idea. If I might just call.'

Roger's gaze was suddenly covered by heavy lids. 'Very well. I shall tell them to expect you.'

'Many thanks.' John found that he and Samuel were bowing simultaneously. 'Goodbye, Mr . . . Roger.'

The beau recovered himself and threw an extravagant kiss. 'My dear John, until we meet again.'

Chapter Thirteen

*D*uring the night following his visit to Islington Spa, John Rawlings woke abruptly, certain that he could hear Samuel's voice. But having sat bolt upright and listened, he realised that he had been dreaming, that his friend had long since gone home and that there was no one other than Sir Gabriel and the servants in the house. Yet the feeling persisted, and something at the back of John's mind kept telling him that part of the conversation shared by himself and the Goldsmith in the pleasure gardens had contained a vital fact, a fact which he had overlooked and was continuing to ignore. A fact which, if he could only bring it into his consciousness, would have an important bearing on the mystery surrounding Sir William's death. Quite unable to sleep with such an idea weighing on his mind, the Apothecary eventually got up and made for his shop in the dawning.

Unbelievably, Nicholas Dawkins, who had now been issued with his own set of keys as a mark of trust, was already there, pale-faced and yawning, but none the less making tea and tackling the dusting.

''Zooters!' he exclaimed on seeing John come in, 'I never thought you'd be here, Sir. I imagined you'd be about Mr Fielding's affairs.'

'I will be later,' the Apothecary answered. 'But first I felt I should visit the sick. Did anyone call for me yesterday afternoon?'

'Several people. I made a list of them.'

'Was anyone too ill to wait?'

'Two. I sent them on to the nearest apothecary as you instructed.'

'Very good.' John poured himself a cup of tea. 'Tell me, Nicholas,' he said, removing his coat and putting on his long apron, 'what in your opinion would be the best time to visit servants in order to catch them alone?'

The Muscovite screwed up his pallid features. 'Well, not early, that's for sure.'

'Why?'

'Because their masters would all be abed but would wake and demand to know who had called, lest it be a tailor or a debt collector or another of that ilk from whom they must hide.'

John grinned. 'I see you are a keen observer of human frailty. Go on.'

'I'd rule out the morning, too, Sir. A beau or belle could well take a good three hours to effect a toilette so would probably be at home until well past noon. Then, of course, there are the dining hours, which occupy the time between three and six, or even seven.'

'So when then?' the Apothecary asked with a sigh.

'I should think early afternoon, Sir. One or half past. They will all have perambulated forth to show their fashions by that o'clock and, with luck, will have met cronies and not be returning home for a while.'

'I think you're right,' John answered thoughtfully. 'That is the moment I will choose. Now, my Muscovy friend, let me show you what things to take when you are visiting the poorly.'

'I am to come with you?'

'I promised that you would. Anyway, I want to see you put to the test.'

'What?'

'You told me that you did not faint at the sight of blood or wounds, that you had seen it all aboard ship. Now is your chance to prove your claim.'

Colour blossomed in Nicholas's cheeks. 'You can rely on me, Sir.'

'I already do,' said John. 'I'm sure you must have noticed.'

In the event there were no really exciting cases to see: a child with croup, for whom John prescribed a decoction of the leaves and roots of coltsfoot, picked and dried in the previous year; a bibulous gentleman, not yet fifty but already a sufferer from chronic gout, who was given a brew of angelica and asparagus roots, lemon balm and chopped centaury, to name but a few ingredients. A third patient who had loose teeth and dared not go out for fear of losing one, came next. The Apothecary, glad that for some reason he had put this somewhat unusual cure in his bag, gave the poor woman a decoction of boiled bramble leaves, honey, allum and a little white wine. Finally, he and Nicholas both set to, rubbing oil of ripe olives into the joints of a rheumaticky cleric who had not been able to hobble from his bed for days. He pronounced himself feeling greatly restored and was able to go downstairs and take tea. This done, John went back to Shug Lane to change his coat, then set off for St James's Square.

Fortunately, the footman who answered the door turned out to be Gibson, the servant who had identified Sir William's snuff box and who had been present when Roger had crashed to the floor in a faint. Silently thanking his luck, John put on his most pleasant expression and asked if he might have a few private words on behalf of the Principal Magistrate.

'In what regard, Sir?' Gibson asked cautiously.

'I would like to know a little more about the night when Sir William left the house for good. Can you help me with that? A great deal depends on somebody telling me what transpired.'

'I can indeed assist, Sir,' the footman answered, such a strange expression on his face that John guessed at once the man was longing to unburden himself.

'Everything you say will be treated in the strictest confidence,' the Apothecary continued in a low voice. 'Mr Fielding must be told, naturally. But as to your master . . .'

'Whoever that might be.'

'Quite. Anyway, rest assured that none of the family will get wind of this.'

'I trust your discretion, Sir.' And with that they stepped into the anteroom, Gibson having checked carefully first that nobody had observed them.

John cleared his throat and opened his mouth to ask a question, but was forestalled. The footman launched into speech as if the Hound of Hell was baying at his heels and he had only a few moments in which to relay his story. And probably a very good thing, John considered, in view of the fact that somebody might return at any moment.

'That was an odd night, Sir, and I remember it vividly as a result,' Gibson began in a hoarse voice. 'Miss Lambourn came here to dine. They were to be married the next day though nobody was supposed to know it. Naturally, it was the talk of the servants' hall, though none of us let on.'

John got a word in. 'What time did she come - and go?'

'Early, Sir. Four o'clock and left again by six. You see, Sir

William was meant to go out later and had ordered his coach for half past seven. Then, at about seven, a hackney driver came bearing a note addressed to the master – the old master, that is. I took it to him and waited to see if there was to be any reply for the man to take away. Anyway, Sir William flew into such a rage when he read it, went white as snowdrops and shook from head to toe. Then he said to me, "Tell the driver the answer is yes, I'll be there." Then he asked me to call Oliver, the youngest footman, to take a letter to Middle Temple Lane cancelling his appointment.'

The Apothecary managed another question. 'That note, the one that came by hackney coach, it isn't still here by any chance?'

Gibson shook his head vigorously. 'Most definitely not, Sir. Sir William threw it on the fire and watched it go up in flames. Then he went upstairs and came down a short while later with a travelling bag.'

'Good gracious! Had he intended to go away?'

Somewhat surprisingly, Gibson answered, 'Yes, I think he had. His valet had packed his best clothes for him and it was our belief in the servants' hall that Sir William was going on from Middle Temple Lane to spend the night somewhere near the place where he was to be wed.'

John digested this thoughtfully. 'What happened next?'

'Sir William scribbled a letter which Oliver took off in the coach, then the master went out.'

'Without his carriage?'

'Yes, Sir. He must have hired a hackney to take him to wherever he was going.'

'And you have no idea where that was or who wrote the note which made him alter his plans?'

'No, Sir, to both.'

John's expressive eyebrows rose. 'What a curious tale.'

'Yes, Sir.'

Gibson hesitated and the Apothecary, reacting quickly, said, 'There's something else, isn't there?'

The footman dropped his eyes. 'I don't want to get anyone into trouble and it might only be a coincidence . . .'

'Yes?'

'But it seemed to me that Mrs Hartfield followed him out.'

'Mrs Hartfield? Which one?'

'Lydia. She was standing in the hall when Sir William left.

Wearing a dark cloak and with her hair so black, it wasn't easy to notice her. Anyway, I'd swear that she followed him.'

'What for?'

Gibson shook his head. 'I don't know, Sir. All I can tell you is that Miss Lydia left the house within a minute of her father-in-law, walking stealthy as a cat.'

'And what time did she come back?'

'That's just the point; she didn't.'

'What?'

'Her maid told me that Mrs Hartfield did not return until late the next day.'

''Zounds!' said John with much feeling, and sat down on the little sofa, the breath quite gone from him.

But there was to be no period of quiet contemplation for at that precise moment the front door opened and voices could be heard in the hall. Gibson shot him a look of pure panic but the Apothecary raised his finger to his lips, then said in a loud voice, 'Thank you. I'll wait in here.'

'Very good, Sir,' the footman replied, and made as dignified an exit as he could in view of the fact that he was trembling from head to toe.

There was the sound of murmured conversation and then the door opened once more. The man whom John believed to be Hugh Hartfield put his head round. 'How may I help you?' he said coldly.

The Apothecary rose to his feet and withdrew his letter of authorisation from an inner pocket, handing it over in silence. Hugh read it, then looked up, his brown eyes hard as marbles. 'Well?' he enquired.

'Sir, I have been asked by Mr Fielding to aid him in the search for your father's murderer. I take it I am addressing Mr Hugh?'

'Indeed you are. However, I don't think I can be of any assistance. I was abroad at the time of my father's – death.'

'So I believe,' John answered soothingly. 'But perhaps you would be good enough to tell me when you went and when you returned. A mere formality, I assure you.'

'Well . . .' But Hugh got no further. The door opened yet again and the woman whom the Apothecary had identified as Maud came in. She stared at John in surprise.

'Oh!'

'My wife,' said Hugh. He turned to her. 'Dearest, may I present Mr . . .' He glanced at the paper still clutched in his hand. '. . . Rawlings, here on behalf of the Public Office. Mr Rawlings, Mrs Maud Hartfield.'

John made an extremely flowery bow. 'Madam, I am honoured.'

She cast him a suspicious look and dropped the sort of curtsey reserved for people of the lower orders. 'How d'you do.'

'Mr Rawlings is here to ask questions about Father's death.'

'Does he have any right?' Maud said nastily.

'Yes, Madam, I most certainly do,' John answered, hardening his features. 'As Principal Magistrate Mr Fielding is within his jurisdiction to enquire into any mysterious death. Therefore I must request both of you to tell me what you know of this crime.'

'How would we know anything?' Maud continued in the same snappish tone. 'Surely you can't imagine that Sir William was murdered by his own kin?'

John assumed his severest look. 'On the contrary, Madam. The facts gathered so far seem to indicate just that. Now, pray tell me where you were on the days leading up to the thirteenth of March. Were you in London or at Kirby Hall?'

'I won't stand for this,' she stormed angrily, only to meet with a glare from her husband.

'For Heaven's sake, Maud, don't make such a show. Simply answer Mr Rawlings's questions and then we can forget all about it.'

She bit her lip furiously, reminding John of a lap dog chewing on a biscuit. 'Well, I was in town until the third of the month, when my husband sailed for France. Then I went to join my grandmother-in-law at Kirby Hall. She is Lady Hodkin, don't you know?'

'Yes,' said John acidly, 'I was aware of that.'

'I was still there when Roger's letter arrived saying there had been a fatality. I remained to give comfort to the family and to await the return of my husband.'

'You went with Lady Hodkin to the church in Shadwell where Sir William intended to get married I believe?'

Maud looked thoroughly startled. 'How did you know that?'

'The Public Office is cognisant of most things,' the Apothecary answered grandly. He shot her a penetrating stare, wondering

162

whether his idea that her puritanical façade might disguise a sinful interior could by any chance be correct. 'And did you leave Kirby Hall during that time, Madam? Did you return to town to shop or attend a play?' he added.

Maud looked uneasy. 'Once or twice, yes, though not to visit a playhouse, let me hasten to assure you. I went to London to call on my aged mother, nowadays very deaf and almost totally blind.'

'You did not come to this house to see Sir William?'

'No, indeed I did not.'

She was too flushed and vehement to be telling the truth, John thought, and considered the fact that even a boring little woman like her might have a lover, probably just as dull and uninteresting as she was. However, with her husband present he was obviously going to get nothing further out of her on that score. So the Apothecary merely looked wise, nodded, and turned to Hugh, thus intercepting a most peculiar glance that Sir William's third son was giving his wife.

So he is wondering, too, John speculated, and questioned how many more threads were waiting to be uncovered in the search for Sir William's murderer.

'Tell me, Sir,' John asked pleasantly. 'Were you close to your father?'

He watched Hugh debating his reply and deciding to come down on the side of truth. 'To be perfectly honest with you, no,' he answered hesitatingly. 'I am a compassionate man, Mr Rawlings, and it fair tore my heart from my body when my mother not only had to endure the anguish of a stroke but also the heartache of knowing that her husband was engaged in an adulterous affair.'

Maud made a strange sound which John could not interpret.

'Oh yes,' Hugh went on, 'she may have been bedridden but she had not lost her wits. I think my father behaved in an atrocious fashion, yet I had to hold my tongue, more's the pity.'

'Oh? Why was that?'

'Because I worked in the family firm. I depended upon Sir William for my livelihood. It was not an easy situation for someone like myself, used to speaking his mind.' Hugh smiled ruefully, his spruce brown features relaxing somewhat.

'Very difficult I imagine,' John answered sympathetically. 'Tell me, what is it exactly that you do?'

'I am in charge of importing goods from foreign climes. As Maud told you, I have recently been in France, in Burgundy to be precise, seeing to the shipment of some extremely fine wines.'

'How very pleasant. When did you return?'

Hugh grinned disarmingly. 'It was damned hard work, let me assure you. Two weeks of extremely busy graft. Anyway, I came back on the seventeenth. We had some goods aboard so our ship joined the queue for the Legal Quays, then I came ashore and went to my father's office in Wapping. It was there that I first heard the news, told me by Valentine Randolph. I regret that I was unmanly enough to faint.'

'Quite understandable,' John murmured. He looked Hugh straight in the eye. 'I believe that under the terms of Sir William's will you now become head of the entire business.'

'Nominally so, yes. My brothers will be running it with me, however.'

Wondering just how much interest Roger and Julian would have in work of that kind, the Apothecary merely raised his brows.

Hugh looked uncomfortable. 'Why do you ask?'

John answered the question with another. 'Were you aware, Sir, that your father had made a new will, a will that he never signed? And that in that will the running of the business passed out of family hands? Have you any idea why he should have done that?'

Hugh looked wretched. 'No, I know nothing of it, and I have no notion why he should have wanted to take control away from us. Who *was* going to inherit the firm, tell me that?'

'I'm afraid I can't.'

'But I can,' interrupted Maud, 'it must be that vile Luke Challon. Always pandering to Sir William's lustful ways, and just as bad himself. As to why my father-in-law wanted to cut us all out, I know the reason. Because I told him he was steeped in sin and that no good would ever come to him while he consorted with a whore.'

'Strong words,' said John, his tone bland.

'Not strong enough,' answered Maud, and flounced from the room.

Hugh stared after her, his expression anguished. 'My wife is deeply religious,' he stated apologetically. 'My father's : . . er . . . relationship with Amelia Lambourn was as repugnant to her as it was to me.'

'But she told him so.'

'Yes. And so did other members of the family. That is why he was about to disinherit us I imagine.' Hugh paused. 'Why didn't he sign the new will, Mr Rawlings?'

'Because,' John answered harshly, 'somebody decided to summon him to his death instead.'

There was little custom about that afternoon, probably because of some unexpectedly warm sunshine which shone on the flowers in London's splendid parks, bringing out those members of the *beau monde* able to face the brilliance without sustaining injury to eyes more used to twilight. Rather wishing he could close the shop and walk to Bow Street, John passed the time by discussing the virtues of various herbs with Nicholas, who seemed very interested in the efficacy of love potions.

'Why do you want to know?' asked John, much amused.

'Because my grandmother always swore that her mother gave one to the Russian who fathered her.'

'Why should she do that? Surely she didn't want to bear his child?'

Nicholas's face creased into a naughty grin that the Apothecary had not been aware he possessed. 'Perhaps she thought he would marry her and take her back to the snowy wastes.'

'Just to think, if that had happened you might be a sycophant at the court of the Empress Elizabeth Petrovna.'

'I might even be her lover.'

'Nicholas, you are getting out of hand,' said John firmly. 'Your fiery ancestry is beginning to show. Where is the timid young man whom first I met?'

'He's beginning to go away. Do you mind, Mr Rawlings?'

'On the contrary. I'm delighted. Now, as I was saying . . .'

But there their discussion of herbs was brought to an abrupt halt as the shop doorbell rang unexpectedly. Pleased to have a customer at last, John left his compounding room and went to stand behind the counter, only to stop short at the sight which greeted him. Juliette Hartfield, looking almost edible in her mourning clothes, had just come in.

'Miss Hartfield!' he exclaimed with pleasure.

'Mr Rawlings,' she replied. 'I heard that you had called round this morning and thought that as I missed you I would come here instead.'

'How very kind. Did you want to consult me professionally, or is this a social visit?'

'A little bit of both. I am not sleeping at all well, dreaming too much about my poor Papa. But that aside, I wanted to talk to you.'

'I'm flattered.'

Juliette smiled at him, just a little sadly. 'How are you getting on with the hunt for the killer?'

'We are making slow progress, but steady for all that.'

'Will you catch him?'

'Why do you say that?' John asked. 'What makes you think that a man is responsible?'

His visitor looked uncomfortable. 'It was just a figure of speech.'

The Apothecary nodded. 'It is not easy to equate women with violent crime, I agree. But believe me, Miss Hartfield, they can be just as desperate as men when their passions are aroused. And it seems to me there is a lot of passion in this case, of one kind or another.'

Juliette did not answer and John turned to take a bottle of physick from the shelf behind him, the main ingredients of which were valerian roots and wormwood leaves, guaranteed to get anyone off to sleep. In the mirror that ran along the wall behind the shelf he could see his visitor's gorgeous face reflected, and spinning round he said his next words impulsively, inspired by her charm.

'Miss Hartfield, it seems to me that your family is not in conventional mourning. Am I right?'

She bridled a little. 'What do you mean, Sir? I am wearing black.'

'I was referring to the fact that since your father's death I have seen both you and your brother, to say nothing of Roger, out and about the town.'

Juliette's eyes suddenly twinkled. 'Yes, that is true,' she said demurely. 'We consider ourselves enlightened and believe that private grief is what counts, not public display.'

John took heart. 'In that case, I wonder whether you might consider accompanying me to the first assembly of the season at Marble Hall? Mr Napthali Hart himself is to act as Master of Ceremonies.'

Juliette frowned. 'I am not certain. Do you not think it might appear indecorous?'

'In what way?'

'Well, I am involved in the sad affair which you are currently investigating. John Fielding might not approve of our meeting socially.'

Everything that was impetuous and scampish in the Apothecary bubbled to the surface. He leaned across the counter and took one of Juliette's hands in his. 'I've no intention of telling him. Have you?'

'No, of course not, but . . .'

'You feel perhaps you should have a chaperone?'

She sighed. 'I'm afraid I would already have one. Julian has booked to go there with . . .'

'Yes?'

'His secret love.'

John's smile hid a strange leaping of the heart, partly caused by the fact that Juliette was giving him a glance which said she would enjoy going dancing with him, partly because another, hidden, aspect of her twin brother was about to be revealed and might prove interesting.

'We can pretend we don't recognise them,' he answered lightly. 'Everyone is to wear masks.'

'Then I accept your invitation, Sir.'

'In that case I shall collect you at eight o'clock tomorrow evening.'

Juliette cast him a ravishing look. 'I shall be waiting, Mr Rawlings.' She turned to go, then came back. 'Oh, I nearly forgot my sleeping draught. How much do I owe you?'

'Consider it a token of my great esteem.'

'Oh, I will, I will,' she said liltingly, and wafted into the street, leaving behind a lingering trace of her perfume.

'Was that flirting?' asked Nicholas, emerging open-mouthed from the back of the shop.

'Mind your business,' answered John, and gave him a friendly cuff on the ear to show him that advantage must never be taken.

It was just as they were about to close for the night that Luke Challon came in out of the dusk, his squarish handsome features perturbed, his hands clenched into fists.

'My dear Sir,' he began without preamble, 'whatever must you be thinking? I have been meaning to call on you for days. Surely you have taken it that I have something to hide from you, but that is most certainly not the case. No indeed.'

Still thinking about Juliette, John gave him a civilised smile. 'Mr Challon, please do not upset yourself. You are here now and that is all that counts. Pray step into my compounding room where we can be private. I shall get the lad to lock up.'

'You are about to close. I fear I am encroaching on your personal time.'

'Not at all, not at all. Now sit down, do. I shall only be a few moments.'

Having organised Nicholas into shutting the shop for the night, the Apothecary blew out the candles and lamps that lit the interior, then placed a lantern in each of his windows, partly to light the pavement outside and partly to deter gangs of window breakers. Shug Lane, minor thoroughfare that it was, had only the wretchedest form of street lighting and to illuminate the shop was a safe precaution. Having done this, he went into the back.

'Now, Mr Challon, I can offer you tea, coffee, or some excellent Bordeaux. Which is it to be?' he asked cheerily.

'The wine if you please.'

The Apothecary removed his apron, took a bottle and two glasses from a cupboard, put them down on the compounding table, then sat down on a stool opposite his guest, wondering how best to broach the subject of Sir William's second will. In the event, Luke did it for him.

'I expect by now that you have discovered the name of Sir William's lawyer.'

'Not only that, I have been to see him.'

Luke digested this information in silence. 'Then you will probably be aware that he was due to sign a second will on the night before he was to be married,' he said, swallowing the contents of his glass rapidly.

'Yes. I also know that Amelia Lambourn, you and Valentine Randolph would have all stood to gain had this taken place.'

Luke flushed. 'Yes, Randolph and I were to be left the business. While Amelia was to become her husband's principal heiress.'

The Apothecary refilled his visitor's glass. 'I take it that Sir William had fallen out with his family over his love affair.'

Luke nodded. 'Very much so. They hated the fact that he made her his mistress while he was still married to their mother. And they despised Amelia for being from the lower class.'

'The first reaction is understandable, I suppose. The second is a characteristic of the society in which we live.' John paused, then went on, 'What did *you* think of Sir William's betrothed?'

'I liked her very much,' his visitor answered thickly.

'Were you in love with her?'

'How dare you, Sir?' Luke protested, jumping to his feet.

'Look,' said John, laying a restraining hand on his arm, 'we are both young, in fact I doubt whether there is much more than five years between us. You must believe I know only too well what it feels like to desire someone. I am in the throes of such an emotion even now. Mr Challon, if you truly want me to find your employer's killer, then talk to me as you would one of your friends. I am not here to sit in moral judgement.'

Luke emptied his third glass. 'Of course I'm in love with her,' he said forcefully. 'Who wouldn't be? She's a beautiful little thing and I've adored her from the moment I first met her.'

'Does she reciprocate your feelings?'

'No, God damme. She was Sir William's mistress and besides there's . . .' he stopped abruptly.

'There's what?'

'Nothing.'

'Not nothing, something.' John took a wild chance. 'There is somebody else, isn't there? Somebody other than Sir William. That pretty creature has a lover, hasn't she?'

'Yes, yes, yes,' hissed Luke, then poured himself a glass, emptied it and pounded the table with his fists.

'Who is he?'

'I don't know.'

'Oh, come now . . .'

Luke raised his head, his eyes blazing. 'I don't know, I tell you. If only I did.'

Feelings were running high and the Apothecary fought to keep control. 'Calm yourself, Mr Challon, nothing can be achieved by getting perturbed. Love rarely plays fair with any of us.'

'That's for sure,' said Luke bitterly.

'Tell me one thing, though. How long has Miss Lambourn had this attachment?'

'I'm not certain; quite some considerable time.'

169

'Surely not as long as she has known Sir William?'

Luke gave a miserable nod. 'It could be.'

'Um,' answered John, considering.

'I'd best be off,' said his visitor abruptly, making as if to go.

'Help me finish this bottle,' answered the Apothecary. 'You see, there's one more thing I have to ask you.'

'What is it?'

'Did Miss Lambourn spend the night before her wedding at The Devil's Tavern? And, if so, did you take her there?'

Luke gave him a strange glance. 'Yes, to both questions. Sir William booked a room for her. He wanted his bride to be near the church where they were to wed.'

'And where did he stay? Do you know?'

'No, he kept that location secret, even from me.' Luke stared into John's face, his expression utterly dejected. 'Do you realise, I've been through years of hell. Loving Sir William – and I truly did – and being in love with his mistress as well. The number of times I have just wanted to die.'

The Apothecary sighed. 'I pity you, my friend. I think the best thing you can do now that Sir William is gone, is to turn your back on the whole sorry business.'

'I could never do that.'

'Not even if Miss Lambourn betrays you and marries her secret love?'

'If she does that,' answered Luke, his words slurring very slightly, 'I swear to God I shall be forced to kill them both.'

Chapter Fourteen

*T*here could be little doubt that Marble Hall was one of the most attractive spots for entertainment in London. Lying within the shadow of the famous Vaux Hall Pleasure Gardens and sharing their waterway access, it was most pleasantly placed on the banks of the Thames, whereas its celebrated neighbour lay further inland and did not enjoy such a splendid position. The gardens themselves, though small, were beautifully laid out and illuminated by many lamps, some of which hung from the trees. But the crowning glory of the establishment was undoubtedly the Long Room, which faced the river and was used for assemblies and balls throughout the spring and summer. When the warmer months ended, the proprietor, Mr Napthali Hart, undaunted by the changing seasons, occupied the winter with teaching music and dancing at Hart's Academy in Essex Street, just off The Strand.

John had been much intrigued by one of Mr Hart's advertisements in the newspaper which had read, 'At this Academy grown gentlemen are taught to dance a minuet and country dances in the modern taste, and in a short time. Likewise gentlemen are taught to play on any instrument, the use of the small Sword and Spedroon. At the same place is taught Musick, Fencing, French, Italian, Spanish, Portuguese, High German, Low Dutch, Navigation, or any other part of the Mathematicks. A sprightly youth is wanted as an apprentice.' Thinking that Mr Hart must indeed be a Jack of all trades and something of a character into the bargain, John had let his mind wander over the interesting future that lay before the apprentice.

Hoping, perhaps, to steal a march on its competitors, Marble Hall was opening the assembly season of 1755, and taking into consideration its peerless location, John felt sure there would be a great demand for tickets. With this in mind he had sent Nicholas Dawkins to Essex Street to buy two almost as soon as Juliette had left his shop. So, it was feeling very pleased with himself for having organised such an exciting occasion so quickly, that John went to call for Miss Hartfield at St James's Square on the following evening as arranged.

Dressed to the hilt in midnight blue and silver, John was somewhat disappointed that he was forced to lower the tone and travel by hackney carriage. But true to his word, Sir Gabriel had already departed for Kirby Hall and the coach, which his father would have been pleased to lend him for such a stylish engagement, was therefore not available. Wishing that he had his own equipage with which to make an impression on such a gorgeous young woman, John paid off the driver and went inside.

Juliette was already waiting for him in the library and immediately saved the Apothecary from any embarrassment by saying, 'I do hope you came by hackney because Julian has decided to take one of the carriages. Do you mind if we travel with him?'

'Not in the least,' John answered, inwardly breathing a sigh of relief.

'Then I'll tell him you are here.' And she pulled the bellrope.

Unconventional though she might be about mourning, Juliette was none the less wearing black taffeta, the skirt drawn back over two enormous hoops to reveal a silken petticoat below. Discreetly woven into this were tiny flowers, the faces of which were represented by little winkers which sparkled as Juliette moved. On her head, Miss Hartfield wore a most unusual cap, formed in the shape of a black butterfly with outstretched wings, these edged in brilliants to match those on the petticoat. Taken as a whole, the entire ensemble was one of the most eye-catching John had ever seen.

He bowed. 'Miss Hartfield, you look exquisite, if I might be permitted to say so.'

'Please call me Juliette, Mr Rawlings. And yes, you are permitted to pay me compliments, the more the better.'

'Really, you are quite shameless,' said a voice from the doorway, and they both turned to see that Julian had come in.

'Do hope you don't mind me joining you,' he said.

'Not at all. It will be a pleasure.'

'Once there I shall go my own way. I have an assignation, d'ye see.'

'Of course,' the Apothecary answered, and thought that whoever the lady was she was certainly going to get a handsome escort, for Julian, also in deep black, his satin waistcoat trimmed with jet, looked better than John had ever seen him.

'Then shall we be off?'

'Certainly.'

During the high season the *beau monde* travelled to Vaux Hall and Marble Hall by water, it being considered *de rigueur* to do so. But on chilly nights carriages were taken to the rural area beyond Lambeth Palace leading to the pretty village of Kennington, where coaches could be left at the corner of Kennington Lane. From there it was but a short distance on foot to either destination. Aware that she would have to walk, Juliette had taken the precaution of carrying her dancing shoes with their four inch heels, in a box under her arm.

As soon as they were within sight of the pleasure garden, Julian put on his mask and strode ahead of the other two, obviously eager to get there. Intrigued, the Apothecary wondered who was the object of the twin's affection and whether the answer might possibly shed any light on the matter of Sir William's death. So once inside, having handed his cloak to an attendant and covered the upper part of his face with a mask, John took a good look round. And it was then that his heart stopped beating, or he thought it did. For in the corner of the room, gazing directly at him, incapable of being disguised by any domino ever made, was the woman whose effect on John he did not care to admit, even to himself. In the company of the Duke of Richmond, Miss Coralie Clive, the young actress in David Garrick's company whose star was most certainly in the ascendant, had come to the first assembly of the season.

Thinking that at any moment Juliette would rejoin him from the Ladies Retiring Room, where she had gone to change her shoes, John felt momentarily flustered, afraid that Coralie might assume the beautiful twin to be his sweetheart. Then he took himself to task. After a certain closeness at the end of the previous year, a closeness that had not gone far enough for John's liking, the actress had made it clear that she wished to concentrate on her burgeoning career. They had ceased to see one another, and this coolness had been followed by rumours that Richmond was keen to make Coralie his Duchess.

'Hang an arse!' swore John forcefully, aware at that moment that the actress's merciless attraction for him had not diminished over the passage of time as he had hoped it might.

She had recognised him, mask or no, that much was clear, for Coralie waved a hand and smiled, then turned to Richmond and muttered something. The Duke looked across the room and grinned hugely, and John realised to his horror that they were coming over to speak.

'Isn't that the Duke of Richmond?' said Juliette's voice from beside him.

'Yes.'

'And who's that with him?'

'Coralie Clive, the actress.'

'Oh, is it? I saw her in *La Belle Espagnole* last month at Drury Lane. I thought she was very good.'

'Yes, she is.'

'I think they're coming to talk to you,' Juliette continued. She shot him a sideways look. 'How intriguing.'

But further discussion was out of the question. With a hoot of laughter, Charles Lennox, Duke of Richmond, was upon them, his face disguised by a mask representing a grinning red devil, his own mouth lengthened with crimson paint beneath. The Duke seized John in a bear hug.

'Rawlings, my favourite man of herbs,' he bellowed. 'Haven't seen you since Christmas. Where have you been hiding yourself, my dear fellow?'

Acutely aware that Coralie was running her eyes over Juliette, assessing her from top to toe, and that the actress's glance kept switching from him to his dancing partner in a manner that could only be described as icily curious, John forced a smile.

'My lord . . .'

'Charles, please. By God, we've been through enough together to be on friendly terms, I believe.'

Coralie broke into the conversation. 'All of us have. Good evening, John. How are you?'

He bowed and kissed her hand. 'I am well but extremely busy. And you?' Before she could reply, the Apothecary continued, 'May I present Miss Juliette Hartfield? Juliette, this is His Grace the Duke of Richmond and Miss Clive of Drury Lane.'

They saluted one another respectfully but through the peepholes of the cat's mask that Coralie was wearing, John could see her green eyes glinting. It occurred to him that she was none too pleased to find him with such an attractive girl and instantly decided to play the situation for all it was worth.

'Indirectly, I met Miss Hartfield through Mr Fielding,' he went on conversationally.

'Are you working for him at the moment?' Coralie asked.

Juliette answered on John's behalf, cooing like a dove. 'Mr Rawlings has been investigating a crime that has brought much sadness to my family. However, the presence of so charming and delightful an enquirer, has done much to alleviate our suffering.' She slipped her arm through John's in a companionable way.

Did he imagine it, the Apothecary thought, or did Coralie's eyes actually flash?

'Well, it sounds like a fine business all round,' said Richmond. 'If I had to assist John Fielding and met such charming persons as yourself, Madam . . .' He bowed to Juliette who shot him an impish smile from behind her mask, shaped like a butterfly to match her cap. '. . . I'd consider myself damnably lucky. Now champagne all round, for who could be in the company of two such charming ladies and not propose a toast to love?'

And he had whisked them off to the refreshment room before anyone could argue.

Within half an hour, Mr Hart was calling for the first dance of the evening, a formal minuet to start the proceedings off graciously. He then insisted that the custom of the ladies throwing down their fans upon a table, the gentlemen advancing and taking one up, then inviting its owner to be his partner, should be performed.

'Though only for the opening two dances, ladies and gentlemen, so that the company may become thoroughly introduced.'

This remark was greeted with groans and laughs, but everybody set about enacting the ritual with much good humour. Watching carefully, John saw Julian pick up a golden fan which he obviously recognised. Then, suddenly, it was his turn. The Apothecary advanced to the table and could hardly believe his luck. For there, on top of a pile of others, was the black feathered fan belonging to Coralie Clive. Without hesitation he snatched it up and went to join the other gentleman forming into a line, holding the fans above their heads so that the ladies might see and identify their property.

Mr Hart clapped his hands. 'Are we all done?'

'Yes,' came the general reply.

'Then ladies forward if you please.'

There followed several minutes of general scurrying about and giggling while the females went in search of their fans.

'Mr Rawlings, what a surprise,' said Coralie, as she curtsied to him.

'Miss Clive, I had no idea,' John answered, bowing politely. 'I presume you have no objection to my leading you out?'

'None at all,' she replied cooly, putting her hand in his.

Though they were both gloved, the touch was enough to set the Apothecary's blood pounding. 'I've missed you,' he said, as the opening bars of music played.

'Really? I would have thought you had found yourself a very pretty companion and thus been preoccupied.'

'Miss Hartfield is the daughter of a man who has been brutally killed. I invited her here this evening to take her mind off the tragedy. But what of you? Is it true that you are to marry Richmond?'

Coralie burst out laughing, despite the fact that they had started to dance. 'I am married to the theatre, Mr Rawlings,' she said grandly.

As had sometimes happened in the past, he suddenly lost patience with her. ''Sblud, Coralie, you sound like some prating school marm. Tell me, will the theatre warm your bed for you? Will it tell you how fascinating you are? Would the theatre die for you if it had to? Do me the honour, please, of answering a straight question. Are you and Charles betrothed?'

'No, we're not,' she replied angrily, 'and we have no intention of becoming so. He and I are great friends and there's the beginning and end of it. And how dare you lecture me when you come here with one of the prettiest girls in the room.'

'She is very beautiful, of course she is. But Juliette and I are as I described to you. Both involved in a savage case of murder.'

'Are you trying to say you have not flirted with her?'

'Spare me, I beg you! Of course I have. I thought you had decided not to continue our acquaintanceship. What else did you expect me to do?'

'Poor John,' said Coralie.

'Don't patronise me, please,' the Apothecary answered furiously.

From behind her mask, he saw the brilliance of the actress's emerald eyes regarding him. 'I would never do that,' Coralie said softly. 'I hold you in too high a regard.'

He pulled her close to him, following the steps of the dance. 'Do you mean it?'

'Of course I do.' The tension between them was tangible.

'You are not trifling with me?'

She moved away from him very slightly, even more than the sideways steps called for. 'That is the difficulty,' she answered quietly. 'I find myself unable to do so.'

'What are you saying?'

'That though you may scoff, in one sense I *am* wed to the theatre.' The glowing gaze was looking at him earnestly through the cat mask. 'I love my profession, Mr . . .'

'You know my name is John,' he said harshly.

'And I have no wish to let anything come between me and my chosen path.'

'Are you implying that I would?'

'Shall I simply say that I could never deal with you lightly, as I do Charles Lennox. That is why, for the time being at least, I feel it more sensible to see less of you.'

Not knowing whether to weep or laugh, John bowed low as the dance ended. 'It seems we are committed to a second bout,' he said, 'or would you prefer to step into the gardens?'

'But what about Richmond and Miss Hartfield?'

'They are dancing together, did you not notice?'

Coralie smiled. 'No, to be perfectly honest with you, I didn't.'

'Then if you have not seen them, surely they won't see us. Come, the company is forming up for the next dance.'

Outside it was cold, a March evening wind blowing in across the Thames. Coralie shivered. 'Do you remember the circumstances of our first meeting?'

'Vividly. You saved my life as I recall.'

'And a girl died in the dark waters out there. I shall never forget that.'

'Nor I. Strangely, I haven't been back to Marble Hall since.'

The actress smiled in the faint light. 'I, too, have kept away till now.'

'Perhaps it was fate that we should both be here tonight.'

'It certainly seems significant that our paths continue to cross.'

'Despite,' said John, taking her hand in his, 'your strenuous efforts to avoid me.'

'Obviously not strenuous enough,' Coralie answered as they simultaneously swept each other into an excitingly carnal kiss. For a long moment their passion and their wildness mingled together, then they drew apart, well aware that should they ever finally make love, it would be the most profound experience of their lives.

'It really is getting rather chilly, my dear Miss Hesther,' said Sir Gabriel in a tone of concern. 'Do you not think we should return to the house?'

From beside him came a small sad sigh. 'I would rather not, Sir. Mother is particularly tetchy this evening and, quite truly, the longer I can keep out of her company, the better it will be for me. Are you, then, getting cold?'

'No, but I noticed you shiver just now. At least let us go and sit in the little pavilion. That will get you out of the breeze if nothing more.'

Hesther gave him a grateful glance and Sir Gabriel bowed and offered her his arm. Then they walked together, the fitful moon throwing their shadows upon the ground, his enormously tall, the three-storey wig upon his head lengthened out of all proportion. Hers, short and dumpy, like a jolly mechanical doll. Judging his companion's mood, Sir Gabriel walked slowly and easily, then, when they had finally reached the summerhouse, settled Hesther into a garden chair which was stored there. Finally, he sat down beside her and gave her a kindly smile.

'You must miss Sir William,' he said reflectively.

'I suppose I always will,' Hesther answered with a sigh.

'It really is a most tragic affair. One simply cannot credit who would commit such a crime.'

'Yet somebody did, and the Public Office seem convinced it was not the work of a common cutpurse.'

'I am certain they are right,' Sir Gabriel replied. 'What thief would leave such valuable items on his victim's body?'

Hesther's voice lowered to a whisper. 'Do you really think it could have been someone William knew?'

'It would seem very likely,' Sir Gabriel murmured dramatically. 'Tell me, Miss Hesther, where were the family and staff on the night before Sir William's wedding? Can you remember? It might be of enormous help to Mr Fielding if you could.'

She shifted in her chair and he wondered why Hesther was so uneasy. Then, after a pause, she said, 'Roger, Lydia, and the twins were in London, of course, and Hugh in France.'

'So who was staying here at Kirby Hall?'

'Mother, myself, Maud and Luke. At least he was meant to be, though he never came back that night.'

'What do you mean?'

'He left in the morning saying he would return, but did not do so. The next I saw of him was at the church.'

'I see. What about your mother and Maud? What did they get up to?'

Hesther gave an extraordinary little laugh. 'Surely, you don't think . . .'

'No, of course not. But it is a good mental exercise to remember such things. I believe it keeps the brain agile.'

'Oh! Well, then I'll try. Mother had, unusually, taken the carriage and gone out. She had arranged to play cards with some neighbours in Bethnal Green and was due to take a light supper with them. As I recall it, she was very late back and in a profoundly strange mood.'

'What sort of strange?'

'Elated and exhausted all in one. She went straight to bed without saying a word to anyone. She didn't even snap at me.'

Hester gave an apologetic laugh and Sir Gabriel squeezed her hand in the darkness, an action which caused her to tremble slightly.

'Go on, you have a wonderful memory. Tell me about Maud.'

'She was in a regular fidget, simply couldn't sit still during dinner. Picking at her food, gulping her wine. Anyone would think she was anxious about something. Then, later, when I came back . . .' Hesther stopped abruptly.

Sir Gabriel chuckled. 'So you left the house too, my dear?'

'Well, yes. I did go out in the small carriage for a spin.'

'Anywhere in particular?'

'I went to Camel Row in Mile End New Town,' Hesther answered defiantly. She paused but Sir Gabriel remained silent. 'Aren't you going to ask me why?'

'I had not intended on doing anything so rude.'

'Well, I went to see someone. A woman, a gypsy with a sailor husband, renowned hereabouts for reading the future.'

'How very brave of you. Did she say anything interesting?'

'As a matter of fact, she told me that William's wedding would never take place, though she did not explain why.'

'Gracious heavens, how extraordinary! You must give me this woman's address. I should like to consult her.'

'I'll write it down for you,' said Hesther, somewhat unwillingly.

'Anway, you were saying . . .' coaxed Sir Gabriel.

'What?'

'That when you came back you saw Maud.'

'Oh yes. She was pacing about in the garden as if she were possessed. Then, when she heard my carriage, she hid behind a tree. I saw her quite distinctly.'

'How very strange. What conclusion did you draw from this unusual behaviour?'

His companion hesitated and Sir Gabriel felt that Hesther was weighing her words very carefully. 'I got the impression that she was waiting for someone – or something – to arrive,' she said.

The first assembly of the season was over, the masquerade done. At midnight everyone had removed their disguises and enjoyed a rousing dance which ended in a kiss. John's group of four couples had claimed the wildness of youth and all the gentlemen had saluted all the ladies so that, once more and very briefly, he had been able to brush Coralie's mouth with his. It had also given him a chance to get as close a look as he could at Julian's sweetheart, who turned out to be of small physique, and to possess finely chiselled features, an extremely knowing expression, and a mop of daffodil coloured hair.

But John, acutely aware that he was at Marble Hall to find things out as much as anything else, had still found it hard to concentrate on anyone other than the actress. He had come back from his few ecstatic moments in Marble Hall gardens certain of three things. The first that between he and Coralie Clive there existed something so electric, so highly charged, that its culmination could only lie in commitment or catastrophe. That they aroused in one another such powerful feelings, an immature flirtation would never suffice for either of them. He also knew that because of this fact Coralie might decide an affair with him would be too intrusive and bid him farewell for ever. The third thing of which John Rawlings was certain was that whatever happened in the future, which ever way the chess pieces moved, he would never escape from Coralie's spell. Women might come and women might go in his life, but she would always remain his ideal, the one being with whom he could fit perfectly in every aspect of a partnership between two people.

So it was with sadness that he said goodbye to Charles Lennox and Miss Clive, uncertain when he would see her again, then climbed into the coach with Juliette, bound for home. And it was with a great deal of astonishment that, even while he sighed, John spied through the window Julian going off with his sweetheart in a very grand equipage with a coat of arms on the door.

'Good heavens!' he exclaimed. 'I hadn't realised your brother's lady love was so well connected.'

Juliette laughed. 'She's Lady Almeria Noel, the Earl of Gainsborough's daughter. But you're not to say a word. Her father considers Julian far too low down the social scale for one of his highborn offspring. The whole affair is completely clandestine.'

'So where is Julian going now? Surely he won't be allowed inside the Earl's house?'

'Oh, those two have a way of managing these things,' Juliette answered mysteriously.

'I wonder what it can be,' said John, but in the darkness of the coach's interior he was smiling.

Chapter Fifteen

'**B**ut I simply can't interrupt your breafast a second time, Sir,' John protested vigorously as a servant showed him into John Fielding's morning room a mere seven hours after the masquerade at Marble Hall had ended.

'But, equally, I insist that you must,' answered the Blind Beak, chewing upon a piece of pickled pork and washing it down with a great draught of tea. 'There is obviously much to tell or you would not have called so promptly.'

'There certainly have been developments.'

'Then sit down, my young friend, and apprise me of everything that has transpired.'

'You may speak in front of Mary Ann,' said Elizabeth Fielding, who was sitting opposite her husband, picking at a little fruit. 'She long ago learned to be discreet.'

Their niece nodded her head and rolled her eyes, her mouth stuffed too full with a piece of toast and a large helping of eggs to speak. Not for the Fieldings the delicate breakfast of the *beau monde*, a fashion which the Apothecary despised heartily, but rather the veritable feast with which all working days should be started, at least in John's opinion.

'This is very kind of you,' said the Apothecary, taking a seat opposite the child. 'As a matter of fact I have not yet eaten, my father being on his travels once more.'

'In that case help yourself,' said the Blind Beak, and accurately stabbed another piece of meat with his fork.

Half an hour later the tale was told and the Magistrate was drinking his final cup of tea, the women long since gone about their daily affairs. 'So Lydia has something to hide,' he said, wiping his mouth with a large linen napkin.

'I find it more than strange that she followed Sir William from the house and did not return till next day,' the Apothecary answered.

'Particularly as it was the night on which the poor chap was probably done to death.'

'And what' asked John, spreading conserve on one last piece of toast, 'do you make of Luke's story that Amelia has always had a lover in the background?'

The black bandage turned, just as if the Beak were staring into the middle distance. 'I find that fascinating. Indeed significant.'

'Could the man have murdered Sir William in a fit of jealous rage?'

'The trouble with this enquiry is that there is an abundance of motives, would you not agree?' Mr Fielding said slowly. 'Perhaps, when the truth comes out, we will find that it was a combination of things which finally drove the perpetrator to deliver the fatal blow.'

Not waiting for a reply to that remark, the Magistrate once more appeared to gaze at the wall, sitting so still that John, as he had sometimes done before, wondered whether he had briefly dropped off to sleep. But the Blind Beak was speaking again, this time with urgency in his tone.

'Mr Rawlings, I have just been seized by a powerful idea. Are you able to act upon it?'

'If it is at all feasible.'

'It is. I would like you to call upon Amelia Lambourn, now, this very next half hour. Make some excuse about telling her the contents of the will, which indeed she may well already know. Be that as it may, I want you to surprise her in her early morning boudoir. It strikes me forcibly that she might very well not be alone.'

'You mean her lover may have spent the night with her?'

'Indeed I do. If you go now you stand a good chance of catching the rogue with his kicks down.' The Magistrate rumbled a laugh at this minor vulgarity.

John grinned. 'In that case should I take some treatment for shock with me?'

The Blind Beak slapped his thigh, obviously a devotee of schoolboy humour. 'Can you picture his face? And certain other parts of his anatomy, come to that?'

'Vividly,' said John, and burst out laughing.

Mr Fielding dabbed at his sightless eyes. 'Best be off then, my friend. Take a hackney. If you walk for your health you might miss the gentleman in question.'

'Is there really a good chance he will be there?'

The Magistrate grew serious once more. 'I cannot be certain, of course. But with Sir William out of the way and none of the family in touch with her, it occurs to me that Amelia might have become careless.'

John pushed back his chair and stood up. 'Then I'll leave straight away. Thank you for my breakfast, Sir. I shall report to you soon.'

'Very good. And now, Mr Rawlings, if you would be so kind as to send Joe Jago up to me.'

'I certainly will.'

Placing his hat on his head, the Apothecary ran down the stairs, had a brief word with the foxy-faced clerk, then hurried into the street, his heart pounding at the thought that he might meet Coralie Clive on her way into the Theatre Royal, Drury Lane. But there was nobody about and John easily picked up a hackney carriage and directed it to the other side of the park and the house where Amelia Lambourn resided.

It was still only eight o'clock, not the sort of time when lovers leave their bed, and as John pulled up outside twelve, Queens Square, he wondered whether Mr Fielding's instinct had been right. Staring around for a conveyance of some kind, the Apothecary saw none, though that in itself proved nothing. Determined that this time he would stand no nonsense from the slatternly servant, John pounded the black wrapped knocker.

A window on the first floor opened. 'Yes?' demanded the girl, sticking her head out.

'I've come to see your mistress and to do so right away,' John thundered.

'Well, she h'ain't receiving so be off with you.'

'And you mind your tongue. I am here on behalf of Mr Fielding and I shall summon extra Runners to help me break your door down if you don't do as I say. Now, open up. I'll give you five minutes.'

The head withdrew and John took his watch from his pocket to check how long the process took. Exactly seven minutes later he heard the sound of bolts being drawn back and a key turn in the lock. The girl, very flushed and angry looking, stood in the doorway.

'Mam says you're to wait in the downstairs room while she dresses. You've disturbed 'er from a nice sleep, you 'ave.'

The Apothecary flashed his eyes. 'I'll wager I have at that.'

Betsy tightened her lips. 'Now, go in there.' And she opened the door of a tiny anteroom and practically threw him in.

Acutely aware that he had not been shown to the first floor as on his previous visit, John hovered on the threshold and listened. A few minutes elapsed and then in the distance he heard a door open and close, this followed by the sound of stealthy footsteps coming down the stairs. Without hesitation, the Apothecary put his eye to the keyhole but the key was in place and the crack by the hinges was too small to allow any vision at all. Throwing caution to the winds, John flung the door open just in time to see a pair of lavender breeches and two stockinged feet swiftly disappearing through the main entrance. Muttering an oath, the Apothecary hurled himself towards the window, but to no avail. The man had hared off down the road and was out of his line of sight. Whoever it was who had spent last night in the arms of Amelia Lambourn had managed to escape without his identity being revealed.

Yet there had been something vaguely familiar about those legs, encased in their lavender kicks. And who was it who had worn a suit of that colour only recently?

'Valentine Randolph,' said John aloud. 'By God, it was him!' And without further ado he rushed down the hallway, raising his hat to Amelia who was just descending the stairs, his final vision her astounded face as, unable to resist, he bellowed 'Tally ho!' before he shot into the street.

As it transpired, John had decided against heading straight off for Wapping. A few moments' deliberation convinced him that Valentine would be making for his office and obviously there would be little point in trying to talk to him there. Instead, the Apothecary went home to Nassau Street, packed a change of clothes in a bag, then walked to Shug Lane where he worked alongside Nicholas until five o'clock. Then he set off for Hungerford Stairs to hire a wherry, instructing his assistant to lock up for the night.

'Are you on the trail, Sir?' the Muscovite asked, his pinched features animated.

'I'm following a thread, yes. But the trouble is, Nicholas my boy, there are so many strands in this pattern that I really don't see how I am going to sort them all out.'

'I expect the moment will dawn on you.'

'I only hope it does,' John answered with feeling.

He reached Pelican Stairs, situated beside The Devil's Tavern, just as darkness began to fall over the river, turning the water deep purple with slashing ribbons of light reflected in its shimmering surface. The dying sun, suffusing the sky with shades of lilac and pink, harmoniously echoed the colours of the river at dusk. Just for a moment, the Apothecary stood on the top step, staring out over the Thames, his eyes absorbing every detail of the breathtaking prospect before him.

It was low tide, so low that he had had to walk over the muddy shore to reach the bottom rung of Pelican Stairs. One great ship was out of the water, leaning to one side, waiting for the river to flood, while three others, jostling close, lay helpless in the shallows, like sea creatures plucked from their element. Everywhere was that strange salty smell which John thought of as the breath of the river, filling the air with its scent and the mind with visions of wild grey oceans and distant shorelines. In mid-stream, the ships that braved those unfriendly depths appeared almost motionless, reminding the Apothecary of caged greyhounds, forced to inactivity but longing to be set free.

Looking over his shoulder, he saw that lights were appearing in The Devil's Tavern, at the window of the room in which Sir William's body had been put for the night, in the attic where he had stayed. They shone comfortingly, softening, though only a very little, the haunting, mysterious atmosphere which the river at sunset seemed to conjure. Then a wind whipped across the water's surface and the dangerous beauty of the scene caused John to shiver, before he turned and went into the warmth and conviviality of the inn.

Having secured himself a room, the Apothecary returned to the bar to sit quietly in a corner and observe the pageant of waterside life being played out all around him. A fishwife and a pedlar were in noisy argument, a cutpurse was knocked senseless by a member of the *beau monde* with faster reactions than most of his kind, a dog being fed a sailor's beer became inebriated and fell asleep beneath a table. But of Valentine Randolph, the person John most wanted to see, there was no sign.

An unpleasant thought struck the Apothecary. Supposing his quarry had gone straight home, had rowed himself across the river to Redriff and was not going to call into The Devil's Tavern that night. Or, even worse, had put his head round the door, seen

John, and made a hasty exit. Not knowing quite what to do, the Apothecary went to the bar to enquire whether anyone had seen the office manager. And it was at that moment, with John leaning comfortably against the rail, chatting to the landlord as if he were a regular patron of the establishment, that the man he was seeking walked in.

What happened next was very strange. For instead of looking hunted and haunted, Valentine Randolph approached the Apothecary with a beaming smile.

'My dear Mr Rawlings,' he said, clasping him by the hand and shaking it warmly. 'How very nice to see you. What are you doing here? Or am I not allowed to ask?'

Every instinct John possessed told him that he had made a mistake, that the owner of the vanishing legs had not been the office manager. None the less he decided to proceed with caution.

'Well actually,' he said, adopting his friendly face, 'I was hoping to run into you. There are just one or two points I'd like to go over, that is if you have no objection.'

'None at all. Shall we sit at a table?'

'Certainly. Let me get you something to drink.'

They chose a bottle of claret to share between them and managed to find room in a dark corner, as private a place as any in an inn teeming with riverside life.

'I'll come straight to the point,' said the Apothecary, having raised his glass to his companion. 'It seems that Sir William made two wills, the second of which was never signed. Have you heard about this?'

'Yes, Luke told me.'

'Did he also tell you that under the terms of the second will, you and he were to have been left the business?'

'He did. And that the bulk of the inheritance would have passed to Amelia Lambourn.'

'Um,' John replied thoughtfully. 'As you've mentioned her, may I ask you a question?'

'Yes.' There was no doubt that Valentine's voice was cautious.

The Apothecary cleared his throat. 'How close are you to the lady?'

Valentine stared at him. 'What do you mean by close exactly?'

John felt himself starting to flounder. 'Well, you know . . .'

'No, I don't. If you mean am I fond of her, the answer is yes, in a way. She was my employer's mistress, soon to be his wife. It was not my place to disagree with his choice. Anyway, I felt sorry for the girl, reviled by the family as she was.'

'And that is all?'

'What exactly are you hinting at?' asked Valentine, his hawk features dark.

'I'll be honest,' said John resolutely. 'When I met you at The George on the morning of Sir William's funeral, there was a certain look about you. I concluded that as Miss Lambourn had also spent the night under the same roof, she might be the cause of it.'

Valentine flushed violently, drained his glass, then stared at the floor. 'You're bloody observant,' he muttered.

'I'm sorry. I didn't mean to cause offence. It is just that so far Sir William's killer is eluding me and, strange as it may seem, every little detail, however unrelated to the crime it might appear, is of vital importance. Mr Fielding taught me that originally, and I can only state that events have proved him right.'

The office manager raised his head and his sombre eyes regarded John thoughtfully. 'Is that the truth?'

'It is, believe me.'

'Then I think there are certain things you should know.'

The Apothecary felt the familiar prick of his thumbs which told him something important was about to be revealed.

'You are right, of course,' Valentine said softly. 'I had spent that night with a woman. But it was a woman who came to The George late that evening. It was not Amelia Lambourn.'

'May I know the lady's identity?'

'No,' the office manager answered violently, 'you may not.'

Someone I know then, John thought. Aloud he said, 'Very well.'

'Anyway, she was long gone before morning, so there's no more to say.'

'Quite. Now, what else did you want to tell me? Was it about Sir William's whereabouts on the night before the wedding by any chance?'

Valentine's flush turned pale. 'How did you know that?'

'I didn't. It was just a lucky guess. Though it did occur to me that you of all people might be aware of where he went.'

'I suppose you realise that Amelia spent the night here? Luke was in charge of those arrangements.' The Apothecary nodded. 'Well, it was my task to book a room for Sir William on the south bank, at The Angel, a waterside inn not far from where I live in Redriff village. Anyway, the agreement was that I was to meet my employer in The Spread Eagle, have a celebratory bottle there, then row him the short distance to the inn.'

'Wasn't that rather an odd arrangement? Why did he not go straight to The Angel?'

'Simply because he liked the other place. I think he had fond memories of it from his boyhood in this area. Anyway, the rendezvous was late because Sir William had business to conduct in London first. Accordingly, I arrived at The Spread Eagle at half past nine. But Sir William did not come, even though I waited till eleven. By that time I began to wonder what was wrong and went to The Angel, where they told me that Sir William had not been seen. Then I . . .'

His voice trailed away and Valentine stared into the depths of his refilled glass.

'Then . . .?'

The office manager collected himself. 'I went home.'

'It must have been very late.'

'It was. Anyway, early next day I returned to The Angel to collect the bridegroom, only to find that he had not been there. At that I panicked slightly, wondering whether to leave the office in the hands of the clerks and go to St James's Square. In the end, though, I decided against and so worked all the morning, expecting him to appear at any second, then changed into my best suit and went to St Paul's. The rest you obviously know.'

John poured himself another glass of wine. 'Mr Randolph, I cannot thank you enough for telling me this. I think I can now be certain exactly when Sir William was killed. You see, it was his intention to visit his lawyer and sign his new will that evening. But a note arrived, obviously asking him to go somewhere else, which prevented him from doing so. He left the house in quite a fury, so I am told. It is clear that wherever he went after he left St James's Square was, alas, his final destination.'

Valentine did not answer, emptying his glass in a single swallow, then he said, suddenly and violently, 'He got as far as Redriff.'

John gazed at him in amazement. 'Did he? How do you know?'

'Because somebody saw him.'

'Who?'

The office manager pulled his watch out of his pocket. 'God's

190

life, is that the time? I must be off. Thank you for the wine. It was pleasant to talk to you Mr Rawlings. Good night.' And he was gone before the Apothecary could say another word.

How very very interesting, thought John. I wonder exactly who he is protecting.

But the evening of contemplation he had hoped for was not to be.

'Like any fresh oysters, Sir?' said a voice close by, and John looked up to see that somebody else he knew was about to join his table.

'Well, well,' he said, and got to his feet to greet Miss Kitty Perkins, the shellfish girl, pretty as ever, and even more strongly redolent of the tangy, unmistakeable stink of the sea.

Chapter Sixteen

*R*esisting Kitty's offer of a bed, repeated several times and accompanied by the most ardent glances and gleams from her spectacular blue eyes, John avoided temptation and climbed the attic staircase alone, feeling both virtuous and pleased with himself. The thought that it might have been the strong smell of fish rather than his adoration for Coralie which had given him the strength to resist so delectable a maiden, he absolutely refused to countenance. Instead he looked at himself in the mirror and said, 'Well done,' before pushing up the lower sash of the window and leaning out to gaze at the river.

The tide was in fully, and the beached barges and ships were afloat once more. John could hear the slap and suck of water against their hulls, though to see them was more difficult. For a mist had come up over the river, rolling amongst the rigging of the great vessels, allowing only the occasional glimpse of a masthead or spar through its ghostly veil. A mist which draped itself over the smaller craft so that they vanished into its vaporous depths, and which wreathed over the water's edge like the phantoms of all those who had drowned in the dark reaches of the waterway. Looking up, the Apothecary saw that the sky had been transformed into a nether world of fog, and was seized by the strange fancy that the inn itself was afloat, adrift in a sea in which time and place no longer existed. Suddenly cold and in need of his bed, he pulled the window down and hastily retired for the night.

He woke to a morning which belied the fact that his odd notions could have ever existed. The sun was coming up, burning the mist as it ascended, transforming the river to a blue jewel and the sky to a rose. The tide had been out but was now on the turn, so that the ships waiting with great courage to sail to the remotest parts of earth, began to feel the heave of the sea. Dirty boys, who appeared bright and burnished in the early light, played on the receding shore, grinning upwards as they heard the noise of an attic window flying up. One waved an old shoe he had found and John threw them a coin, for which they scrabbled in the mud.

It was a morning for devouring a severe breakfast, such as The Devil's Tavern was known to serve, and John more than did justice to the fare set before him, gladly paying for the privilege. With this happy lining to his stomach, he settled his account and went to the top of Pelican Stairs to see what was going on.

The tide was rising fast and there was a great deal of activity aboard the ocean going vessels, sailors clambering up the rigging to unfurl the sails and passengers excitedly walking the decks. Distantly, across the expanse of waterway, the Apothecary could see the south bank, and about a mile to the right, the spire of St Mary's Church. It was at that moment that a rowing boat with a solitary oarsman appeared at the bottom of the steps.

'Want a ride, my rum duke?' he called up.

'Can you take me to The Spread Eagle?' John shouted back.

'Bit early ain't it?' the fellow responded cheerfully.

'Damme, not a moment,' the Apothecary answered, as he clambered aboard the precariously rocking vessel.

They set off upstream, keeping inshore for a while, then pulling across to the middle of the river and hugging the south bank, before finally mooring at some steps. Beside these stood an inn, the signpost of which read The Spread Eagle, beyond them and slightly to the right loomed the spire of a church.

'Church Steps,' said the boatman, 'and there's the tavern.'

'And that I take it,' John answered, 'is Redriff.' And he pointed to the cluster of houses and cottages centred round St Mary's, as pretty a riverside village as he had seen for a long time.

'Yes, that's it.'

'And where's The Angel?'

'Upstream. Between Elephant and Princes Stairs, immediately opposite Execution Dock. My father told me Judge Jeffreys used to go there to drink and enjoy the view of the hanging corpses. It's said his ghost still haunts the balcony where he sat.'

'Not one that I'd particularly care to come across.'

'Nor I.'

These pleasantries exchanged, John paid the man his fare and went ashore, going straight into the hostelry. At this hour of the day the place was empty except for a few sailors speaking some exotic tongue and a handful of slatternly women accompanying them, all of whom sat glazed eyed but smiling stiffly, unable to understand a word their companions were saying. Moving as far away from them as possible, the Apothecary took a seat and looked round for any sign of a local, the sort of person who might have been present on the night that Valentine Randolph waited in vain for Sir William Hartfield. There was no one to be seen, indeed there appeared to be nobody serving, and John was just about to go to the bar and call for the landlord when there was a loud clatter of pots and the sound of gasping. A door, presumably leading from the kitchens, flew open and a boy appeared, laden with tankards, some of which still dripped water onto the floor.

'Sorry,' he panted. 'Just been below. Was you waiting long?'

'Are you the potboy?' John asked.

'Yes, Sir.'

'And do you work here all the time?'

The child looked suspicious. 'Mostly I do. Why?'

'No reason,' answered the Apothecary affably. 'Now, my lad, I'll have a jug of ale. And what about yourself?'

'Not supposed to on duty. But seeing the landlord and Betty is out, I'll join you, duke.'

'Very good,' said John, and thought to himself that if anyone had seen anything it would be this child. For, if he was not mistaken, he was looking at a mudlark, those robust little creatures who dwelled by the river, all scavengers and thieves, many of them orphans, totally ragged and wretched, yet strong and healthy, every one, because of their vigorous outdoor lives. This boy, if the child was indeed one of that cheerfully dishonest fraternity, would be slightly different in that he had been able to find work and did not rely solely on stealing in order to feed himself.

'What's your name?' asked John, as the potboy returned with two tankards of ale.

'Fred, Sir. After the late Prince of Wales.'

The Apothecary supressed a smile. 'And you live in Redriff?'

'Not exactly, but nearby.'

'Are you a mudlark?'

'I was, but I saw the error of me ways. I come up before the Beak, you see, and he wanted me to go to the workhouse for me own protection. But I got out of that . . .' Fred's freckles appeared to glow as his colour came up. 'Anyway, I give up thieving and took up work instead. Now I can live me own life and no fear of someone coming after me.'

'That all sounds very commendable.'

Fred sighed. 'These days I just scavenge,' he said wistfully, making it quite clear that he sorely missed his past criminal activity.

He was a bluff, hearty child, as were all of his kind, his freckles myriad, his hair a shock of orange, standing totally on end as if he had just had a fright. In body, Fred was wiry and tough, and the Apothecary could imagine him taking to the water like a rat. Momentarily, John mused on these children of the river, the very own offspring of the Thames, living beside the waterway in empty barges or uninhabited hovels. Subjected to every kind of neglect and privation, still they emerged robust and fit, the true descendants of their implacable father.

Staring Fred straight in the eyes which, strangely, were the colour of clear water, almost without tone except for a mossy green reflection, John produced a coin and held it between his thumb and forefinger.

'My friend,' he said trenchantly, 'I need your help.'

The mudlark looked somewhat alarmed and it occurred to the Apothecary that the boy might think he was making an indecent proposal.

'Let me explain,' John added hastily. 'I am looking into the matter of a mysterious death which occurred in this area some twelve days ago. A gentleman's body was retrieved by watermen and put in The Devil's Tavern overnight. It transpires that the poor fellow was done to death, and it has also come to light that he was to have met a friend here, in The Spread Eagle, but never kept the appointment. Now the friend was Mr Randolph who lives in Redriff. Do you know him by sight?

Fred squinted his crystalline eyes. 'Are you one of them London Beak Runners, duke?'

'In a sense, yes, I am. But please don't let your early brushes with the law prejudice you against me. My task is to bring a cruel killer to book. Mr Randolph will not be harmed by your answers, I assure you.'

The mudlark looked uncertain. 'He's a good chap, is that gentleman. He's always very kind to me.'

'He and I are friends, believe me. Now, can you cast your mind back and recall that evening? Mr Randolph came here late and must have sat alone for a good while. Do you remember the occasion?'

Fred wiped his hand across his mouth and said, 'Thirsty work, this.'

John handed him the coin. 'Get yourself another and keep the change.'

There was a burst of laughter from the sailors, at which the dollscommon in their company looked even more stony faced. In the interval Fred disappeared, then returned with another tankard, brimful.

'Yes, I do recall that night,' he announced, having swigged.

'Tell me about it.'

'Well, it was as you said. Mr Randolph come in about nine or half past. He sits down, orders himself a drink, just as if he was waiting for somebody, but nobody appears. Then he goes again, about eleven or thereabouts.'

John felt a vague sense of disappointment. 'Is that all?'

'Yes, duke. True as I stand here.'

'Did nothing else happen? Didn't you see anything strange? Had anybody come in earlier, then left again before Mr Randolph arrived?'

'No, nuffink like that. It was all as usual. Unless you count the drunks.'

'What drunks?'

'Well, we usually get a few. That was what struck me as peculiar.'

John's thumbs twitched. 'What do you mean?'

'That night we didn't get none.'

'So?'

'So, just as I was washing the last of the pots I hears summink and I looks out onto Church Stairs, where the sound come from.' The boy quaffed from his tankard and paused, obviously aware that John was hanging on his every word. 'And there I sees two chaps, drunk as drumbelos, weaving their way down to the water. One so far gone in his cups that he clung to the other to keep standing.'

'Not an uncommon sight, surely?'

'That's just the point, duke. They hadn't come from here, that I'll swear to. So where did they hail from? It couldn't have been The Angel. They would never have got that far.'

'Perhaps they were drinking privately.'

197

'They weren't from Redriff, I know everyone hereabouts.'

'Somebody's guests?'

Fred shook his head violently. 'I don't think so. There was summink rum about them. Summink that didn't look quite right.'

'Umm.' John fingered his chin. 'You're sure they were two men? One of them couldn't have been a woman, by any chance?'

The mudlark looked thoughtful. 'I suppose it's possible. It was very dark and they both wore a cloak and hat. It just *could* have been a lady dressed to deceive, though I'm not saying it was, mind.'

'And they were coming from the direction of the village?'

'That I didn't see. But where else could it have been? Either Redriff or the church, had to be.'

'Yes,' the Apothecary said pensively. He took ten shillings from his pocket, a very handsome reward, but before he gave it to the broadly smiling mudlark, asked one more question. 'Did you by any chance notice a stranger around on that night, a woman, tall, dark and striking?'

Fred shook his head. 'No, I didn't, Sir. No one like that come here. Have you asked at The Angel?'

'No, by God, I haven't. But that's a very good idea. Is it far to walk from here?'

'No, Sir. A mile at most.'

'Thank you for your help,' said John, standing up. 'If you think of anything further can you get word to Mr Valentine?'

'I'll do me best. Will you be down this way again, Sir?'

'Oh, I am absolutely certain that I will,' the Apothecary answered resignedly.

The full title of the parish church of Rotherhithe or Redriff, as it was more commonly known, was St Mary the Virgin, Parish of St Mary with All Saints. And it was towards this imposing building that John purposefully made his way, having come out of The Spread Eagle into the harsh morning sunshine. The hostelry stood almost directly opposite the back gate to the churchyard, a mere stone's throw away, and the Apothecary went in through this entrance, walking amongst the graves and approaching the church from the back.

It was a relatively new building, having been erected some forty years earlier, in 1715, to replace the old church, which had become a victim of the constant flooding experienced by Redriff, and slowly rotted away. Rounding the corner, John saw a pillared entrance with steps leading up to the doorway, and guessed that before these stone columns ships masts had once stood in their place. Deciding not to go inside directly and hoping that the occupant would not take it amiss, John sat down on the grass beside a grave, his arms resting on his knees, and stared at the tombstone in front of him. 'Elizabeth Wells,' he read, '1715–1730. Beloved daughter of Louisa and David Wells. A rose plucked in the dawning.' Then, even while he was thinking how sad it was that a maiden of fifteen should have been taken from life, the Apothecary's eyes were drawn to something else. Staining one side of Elizabeth's tombstone was a reddy brown mark, a mark that had trickled downwards, then dried, a mark that looked for all the world like congealed blood.

Suddenly alert, John got up, then went down on his haunches and scraped a little of the substance into his hand with his herb knife, touching it carefully. It was most certainly blood, and blood that had turned hard, indicating that it had been on Elizabeth's tombstone some considerable while. But what had caused it? Had someone walking through the churchyard tripped and fallen, striking his head on a gravestone as he fell? Or was there a more sinister explanation? Could this be the place where Sir William had been mercilessly beaten about the skull by a cane bearing a fox's head for handle? John bent even closer, wishing he had got his magnifier with him. And then he saw them, fluttering in the river breeze and reflecting the sunshine, a few white hairs, clumped together and stuck to the gravestone before the blood had dried. Very carefully extracting his find, John wrapped the hairs in his handkerchief and put them in his pocket. Then after having looked round Elizabeth Wells's grave most thoroughly and retrieving from the site a serviceable and rather boring button, which he also carefully stored, the Apothecary left the churchyard, frowning, deep in thought.

Nor did the walk by the riverside help to clear his teeming brain. Striding along by the wharves and warehouses, then through fields and market gardens, John hardly saw the colourful scenery, and remained oblivious to his surroundings until he practically fell over the entrance to The Angel. He stepped back to look at it.

Just as the mudlark had told him, this ancient den of thieves and smugglers stood directly facing Execution Dock and did, indeed, have a balcony running along its water frontage. Furthermore, the size of the building indicated that it was a place where travellers stayed. Hoping that he was about to get the information he so desperately needed, John went in.

Like all others of its kind, The Angel had reserved a parlour for gentry folk but John headed for the other bar, certain that this was where he would hear gossip. But even his stout spirit quailed at the sight of the custom already present. So rough a bunch of rogues was gathered there that the Apothecary doubted anyone could put up much of a fight should the mood turn ugly. Raising his hat politely, he beat a tactical retreat and ended up sitting by a pleasant fire in the snug, alone but for a jolly young fellow who introduced himself as a general workhand.

'And will you be requiring a room for the night, Sir?' this bright spark enquired, having fetched John a meal and some claret to keep him going.

'Alas, no. Not on this occasion. Perhaps next week.'

'I take it you come from London, Sir?'

'Yes, but my business brings me here from time to time.'

The workhand was obviously not that interested but said politely, as he had no doubt been taught, 'Oh? And what business might that be, Sir?'

'I,' John answered dramatically, 'am a Runner, acting on behalf of Mr Fielding.'

The young man's face underwent a series of interesting changes. 'You're not going to investigate them as sometimes comes here, are you, Sir? You see, I really wouldn't advise it. We keep them well away from the other folk because that's best all round.'

Deducing that he was talking about the smuggling fraternity, John answered, 'No, I haven't come about them. As a matter of fact I'm here to ask about somebody else. I just wondered if you might have seen either, or both, of these people.'

And he launched into an accurate description of both Sir William and his daughter-in-law, Lydia, ending with the words, 'Their family name is Hartfield, by the way. And I believe they might have stayed here about twelve nights ago.'

'I know Sir William,' the workhand answered promptly. 'But I never saw him on the night you mean. He was booked to stay here but didn't appear. His bed was not slept in and it was Mr Randolph, he works for Sir William and is a resident of Redriff, who settled the bill in the morning.'

'And the woman I described? What about her?'

'Oh yes, I'm sure she was here. She came in late, very disturbed and flustered, said that a hackney had dropped her in Redriff and she had no idea where she was. She walked to The Angel apparently, alone and in the darkness.'

John's eyebrows danced. 'Did she and Mr Randolph come across one another? He called here that particular night, didn't he?'

A shutter came down over the workhand's face. 'I really wouldn't know about that, Sir. I was busy serving food and drink and saw little of those who were staying. The girl dealt with them, and she's gone to market.'

John nodded slowly, an idea taking shape. 'I understand,' he said. And he thought he did – a great deal. He drew his watch from his waistcoat pocket. 'Two o'clock. I must get back to London. What is the tide doing?'

'Coming in, Sir.'

'Then I'll be off. Thank you for your help.'

'I'm sorry I couldn't tell you more.'

The Apothecary smiled. 'Please don't apologise. I can assure you that one way or another I feel I have learned a very great deal.'

Chapter Seventeen

*D*espite the fact that it was six o'clock in the evening, John was amazed to see that light was shining from the courtroom attached to the Public Office in Bow Street, and there was a general air of bustling activity about the place. Realising that the court must be in late session, the Apothecary crept inside, only to find to his amazement that all seats reserved for the public were full and there was standing room only. Even though it was a fashionable pastime amongst members of the *beau monde* to come and watch a blind man administer justice, John would have thought that this clash with the dining hours might have emptied the place, though clearly not. Then he looked towards the dock and saw that over thirty people stood there, surrounded by Beak Runners, all severely armed, and realised that something untoward must have occurred.

'What's been going on?' John whispered to the Runner who stood guarding the courtroom door.

'A riot at Drury Lane last night, Sir. The galleries got out of hand. It took every man we had to quieten 'em down. You're seeing the tail end of it.'

'Just as well I was out of town,' answered John wryly.

'It was an ugly scene,' the Runner replied with feeling.

'Shush,' said somebody close by, and both of them stopped speaking as they realised that John Fielding was about to pass judgement. Joe Jago shouted, 'Silence,' and there was a ripple of response as the Magistrate cleared his throat.

'It is my solemn duty to pronounce sentence in this case, though before I do so I would like to make certain comments. Of late, several persons have been detected at both the Theatre Royal and Covent Garden Playhouse, scandalously throwing things out of the galleries into the pits, not only contrary to law, but to common sense, nay to common humanity. These actions have contributed to the disturbance, annoyance and danger of the rest of the audience. Last night, being authorised by the management of the Theatre

Royal to put an end to such rumpus, certain members of its staff did enter the galleries in order to restore order. Thereupon, those persons who had been responsible for this injurious comportment set upon those who had come to calm the situation in a manner that can only be described as barbarous. Further, those foolish and immature enough to make capital of the situation, responded with equal bad behaviour, and I refer in particular to young Lord Dartmouth. This last was seen to jump from a stage box and assault an actor when the fighting began. I therefore have no hesitation in committing the prisoners to Newgate for the term of a whole year. Let me make it quite clear that I will spare no pains to punish to the utmost extremity of the law, all those who shall be found guilty of thus distressing fellow members of the audience.'

There was a huge murmur of support from the *beau monde*, quelled by Joe Jago shouting, 'All rise.' Everyone shuffled to their feet as John Fielding, the switch he used to guide him into court twitching before him, left the premises.

'He'll be very tired,' murmured a voice in John's ear, and he turned to see that Elizabeth Fielding had slipped into the back of the court and was standing directly behind him.

The Apothecary kissed her hand. 'Should I not call to see him?'

She smiled. 'No, no, John would hate that. Come now, this very instant. While he is still fired by the day's proceedings, fill his mind with your story and ask him any question you like. Later, when all he wants to do is rest, it would be cruel to disturb him.'

'Are all wives as splendid as yourself?' John asked.

'Very few,' Elizabeth answered, laughing.

'Then remind me to find a model made in your image, Madam.'

'Flatterer,' said Mrs Fielding, and they proceeded out of the courthouse and into the main body of the building.

A few minutes later, seated in the upstairs salon, cosy against the cold as ever, John heard the footsteps of Joe Jago preceeding those of his superior up the staircase, and was glad that the brain of this remarkable individual, who conversed as easily in cant as he did in everyday tongue, was to be added to the discussion of events. Indeed, so pleased was he, that the Apothecary sprang from the chair in which he sat opposite Elizabeth, and shook the Magistrate's clerk warmly by the hand.

'My dear Sir, I am so glad to have a chance to talk to you.'

'Rum affair, Mr Rawlings, rum affair.'

'You mean the riot at Drury Lane?'

'I do, Sir. I do. There were agitators in amongst 'em, if you want my view.'

'You mean that the gallery mob was encited?'

'Oh yes. Small doubt of it.'

'But by whom?'

'A certain Mr Wilkes, Sir. Young yet but bound for trouble ahead, mark me.'

'I do not know the name, Mr Jago.'

'You will, Sir. You will. A man who lacks good birth, who lacks looks, humility, kindness. A man who lives a life on the edge of politics. We will hear more of him, there's no doubt of it.'

'Why was he not tried in court today?'

'I did not say that he lacked cunning, Sir.'

'No more did you,' answered John, and they both turned as John Fielding entered the room.

For once, and probably the only time, the black bandage was pushed up from the sightless gaze, and the Apothecary had a moment to study the Blind Beak's face in its entirety. Despite the ardent mouth and large strong nose, the closed eyes gave his features a look of vulnerability, almost of tranquillity, as if their owner slumbered. It was unnerving to see a mask of such calmness concealing a brain so alert, so alive, that it was virtually impossible for its owner to rest. Strangely moved by what he observed, John fought against an urge to embrace John Fielding and tell him how much he respected him.

Realising from the sounds in the room that he was in company, the Blind Beak slipped his bandage back into place. 'Mr Rawlings, is that you?'

'It is, Sir.'

'Good, good.' The Magistrate rubbed his hands together. 'There is much to discuss, I feel sure of it. Elizabeth, my dear, if you would be so kind.'

She nodded and pulled the bellrope but did not leave the room, obviously keen to contribute to any open discussion that might be about to take place.

'So,' said the Beak, taking his seat by the fire, 'you were in court today?'

'I came in late and stood at the back. The *beau monde* had filled all the seats.'

'And so they should. There was much in my sentencing that was to their advantage. As you know, Mr Rawlings, the upper gallery is filled with servants, the lower with tradespeople. But last night there were those in Drury Lane of an infinitely more sinister stamp. On their way in, ladies had had their dresses slashed, gentlemen their cloaks. There were disruptive forces at work which I had to be seen to put down ruthlessly and at once.'

'You certainly did that.'

Mr Fielding sighed. 'But, alas, I am but stemming the tide. There's worse to follow, I feel sure of it.'

'You mean this man Wilkes?'

'He is but a fart in a thunderstorm at the moment, but he will grow into a hurricane, I feel sure of it.' He took a glass from the tray brought in by a servant. 'Elizabeth, gentlemen, are you served?'

'We are,' they chorused.

'Then let me propose a toast to the downfall of Wilkes and all his kind.' Everyone murmured approval and drank, then the Blind Beak moved his head in the direction of John's voice. 'Now, Mr Rawlings, tell me everything that has transpired since you went in search of Amelia Lambourn's lover.'

The Apothecary, anxious to hear other opinions, launched into his account with relish, reducing his audience to laughter as he described the legs disappearing through the young woman's front door. After that, though, they listened carefully and grew silent when John handed Joe Jago the specks of congealed blood and the white hairs he had so carefully retrieved. Finally the Blind Beak spoke.

'It seems to me that there is much still to be discovered about the whereabouts of various persons on the night Sir William was killed.'

'There is lying and subterfuge, no doubt of it,' John answered. 'And when I catch up with my father I feel certain he will have more to tell me about the activities of those in Kirby Hall.'

'Yes,' said Mr Fielding thoughtfully. He turned towards his clerk. 'Joe, what do you think our next move should be?'

'Call them all together and challenge them with the information you have, Sir. Otherwise you might remain buffle-headed, for they sound a bunch of rum maunds, and clever into the bargain.'

The Magistrate nodded slowly. 'Yes, I think that is a good plan.'

'And why don't you,' put in Elizabeth, 'ask them to bring their great sticks with them? Somebody must own one with a fox's head, though he'd be too clever to show you, I suppose.'

'My mind has been running on those lines,' John added. 'I keep wondering where that stick is now?'

'Disposed of into the Thames alongside the body, I imagine. Too bloodstained to carry away from the crime.'

'You know,' the Apothecary said thoughtfully, 'I have a strong suspicion that Sir William was murdered in the churchyard, then dragged to Church Steps and thrown in.'

Joe Jago, who had been examining John's finds carefully, nodded slowly. 'Then the lurching drunkards that the mudlark saw could have been the victim and his killer, the body pulled to the river in the least suspicious way of all.'

'You're right,' said John, 'It's possible.'

'Everything fits in, certainly,' the Blind Beak agreed. 'Joe, could you get letters to the Hartfields out tonight?'

'Yes, Sir.'

'Then call them to a meeting at St James's Square on the day after tomorrow. Say that failure to attend will have the most serious consequences. Tell them, also, to bring all the sticks and canes that they possess.'

'Are you going to include Lady Hodkin in this?' asked John in awe.

'I most certainly am. She is as answerable to the law as anybody else, as I shall take great pleasure in pointing out to her.'

'Do you want me to be present?'

'I expect both you and Joe to accompany me. He shall be my writing hand. And you, Mr Rawlings, as always, my sharp pair of eyes.'

'Thank you,' said John, touched by the great man's faith in him.

Just as had been the case at Bow Street, the Apothecary saw lights on at number two Nassau Street as he rounded the corner from Gerrard Street, and guessed at once that Sir Gabriel had returned from his adventures in Bethnal Green. Hurrying in, he found his father partaking of a cold collation in the dining room and joined him with enthusiasm, not only delighted to see Sir Gabriel again but equally pleased to fill his stomach, by now rumbling with hunger.

Chewing his way through a large chicken drumstick, John asked with some difficulty, 'And did you find they had all been up to no good?'

'On the night before the wedding which, I presume, is considered to be the time when Sir William died . . .?'

John nodded but did not speak.

'. . . Lady Hodkin was out, so was Hesther, while Maud paced the garden as if waiting for someone. Luke Challon, who was supposed to return, did not do so. The rest remained in London.'

'And did the two ladies say where they were?'

'Lady Hodkin was engaged to play cards with neighbours, Hesther went to consult a gypsy fortune teller.'

'No doubt to discover her future with you.'

Sir Gabriel shot his son a reproving glance. 'Really, how you do run on! Anyway, tell me of your findings.'

John did so between mouthfuls of chicken.

'So,' said his father eventually, 'if Valentine Randolph is not Amelia's lover, who is? Luke?'

'I don't think so. His performance as a man who loved his employer yet nursed a hopeless passion for the employer's intended wife, convinced me. No, I believe we must look elsewhere.'

'I think the meeting at St James's Square might well reveal something previously hidden,' Sir Gabriel said reflectively.

'I sincerely hope that you are right,' answered John in heart-felt tones.

In view of the speed with which the gathering of the Hartfield family had been called, there had been no time for a response from any of them. Therefore, it was uncertain as to whether he would be speaking to one or a dozen people that Mr Fielding, complete with his entourage, set forth from Bow Street on the day arranged.

Roger, somewhat grudgingly, had given permission for the grand salon to be used as the conversation room, whilst those waiting to go in could take their ease in the library. Accordingly, Mr Fielding, John, and Joe Jago, went into the salon first and stationed themselves behind a large table drawn up before the window, its sole purpose, apparently, to bear a display of flowers. Joe took out paper, pen and ink from a small case, John produced a list of questions which he had written the previous evening. Mr Fielding, who sat in the middle, turned to his colleagues.

'Are you ready, my friends?'

'Yes, Sir.'

'Then let's see what we can do to trick a villain.'

Joe pulled the bellrope and asked the servant who answered to show in Lady Hodkin, should she be present.

'She *is* here, Sir,' the footman answered, 'but says that she will not be interviewed by anyone who does not have a title. Despite the protests of Miss Hesthers, she is demanding to see Lord Suffolk.'

The Blind Beak chuckled. 'The Secretary of State, no less.' He turned to his two companions. 'What shall we do with her?'

'Frighten the old mort,' answered Joe crisply. 'Tell her she'll see the inside of Newgate if she refuses to cooperate.'

'I agree,' said John. 'It's high time that tyrant was given a lesson.'

Mr Fielding stood up, putting out his hands. 'Take me to her, Joe. Mr Rawlings, you wait here.'

'May I listen at the door?'

'Of course.'

As it transpired, the conversation was well worth overhearing. From the library, the Apothecary could clearly catch the Blind Beak's booming tones and Lady Hodkin's disgruntled replies.

'If you do not agree to speak to me, Madam, you will leave me no option but to take you to Bow Street, by force if necessary, and there charge you with impeding the course of justice, for which several months' imprisonment is the usual punishment,' thundered the Magistrate.

'How dare you . . .' the hag huffed in reply.

'I dare because I'm right,' retorted Mr Fielding. 'Now, which is it to be, Madam? Will you talk or will you go to Newgate?'

A chorus of cajoling voices could be heard, all trying to persuade Lady Hodkin to behave herself. Then there was the sound of stamping feet crossing the hallway. Rushing to his post behind the table, John attempted to look calm and unruffled as the door was flung open and Lady Hodkin appeared. She gazed at him angrily.

'I will not utter a word in the presence of that horrible young man.'

John Fielding loomed large behind her. 'You will not refer to my assistant in that derisory manner, Madam. And you will speak in front of him as I instruct you. By God's wounds, do not try my patience any further or you will rue the day.'

'I feel faint,' she answered, grasping her heart.

'Then Mr Rawlings will attend you. He is an apothecary.'

Lady Hodkin glared from one to the other. 'What is it you want to know?' she said between gritted teeth.

'Where you were on the night before your son-in-law was to have married. That is all.'

She sat down heavily. 'How would I remember after all this time?'

Mr Fielding took his seat. 'Let me help you. You went to play cards with neighbours – or say you did. You returned home very late. Did you, in fact, I wonder, go to Redriff in your carriage and there put Sir William Hartfield to death?'

The old beast exploded. 'How can you say such a thing? I played whist with Lady Dimity Thrush. She will vouch for me.'

'It has been said that you came back in a strangely excited mood. Why was that?'

'Because I had won,' Lady Hodkin answered defiantly.

'So you tell us,' snarled the Magistrate, looking thoroughly ill-tempered. 'Jago, make a list of all those persons whose whereabouts need to be checked and put Lady Hodkin at the top of it. Now, Madam, Lady Dimity's address if you please.'

Probably for the first time in her life, the elderly creature became suddenly subdued and gave the information about her neighbour quite meekly.

'Now you may go,' said John Fielding. 'And be so good as to send in your daughter. Good day, Madam.' He bobbed up from his chair as politeness decreed. 'No time for discussion,' he continued in a hiss, 'we will talk over all they say when we return to Bow Street.'

Hesther came in almost at once, as if she had been waiting by the door. Without preamble, the Blind Beak asked her exactly the same question as he had her mother. She coloured a little.

'I went out on my own to consult a fortune teller in Mile End. I took one of the carriages and went straight there and back. The gypsy can confirm this, as can the coachman.'

'I see,' said Mr Fielding expressionlessly.

Hesther drew in a breath. 'I expect you want to know why I did such a thing and there is no point in beating round the mulberry bush. I have been feeling unsettled, more than a little unhappy, and I wondered if she could be of any help to me.'

'I believe you were very fond of the late Sir William. May I ask if that fondness had recently turned to hate?' the Magistrate enquired calmly.

'In a way it had,' Hesther replied. Her eyes suddenly filled with tears. 'I could not tolerate his association with that wretched girl. But since his death I have realised that it is pointless to carry a hatred beyond the grave.'

'Did you kill your brother-in-law?' Mr Fielding asked, as casually as if he were enquiring the time of day.

'No,' Hesther answered levelly.

'Then tell my clerk where the gypsy can be found, and you may go. Good day, Madam. Could you ask Mrs Maud Hartfield to step inside.' And in this businesslike manner, Mr Fielding dismissed her.

Hugh's wife entered the room almost unassumingly, her eyes cast down and her hands clasped in front of her. Looking at her hard, picturing her pacing in the gardens of Kirby Hall, John wondered just what thoughts teemed behind her docile facade and whether her demeanour concealed a guilty secret. However, Maud's calm manner was abruptly shattered by Mr Fielding's opening gambit.

'I have received certain information, Madam. Information which leads me to believe that on the night of your father-in-law's murder, which is also the night before his proposed wedding, you were seen in the grounds of Kirby Hall behaving in a most suspicious manner. As if you were expecting someone or something, so it was related. Would you care to explain your actions.'

Maud's cheeks flushed and her mild expression vanished. 'And who told you all this, may I ask?'

'I'm afraid you may not,' the Magistrate answered. 'Intelligence received at the Public Office is always treated as confidential.'

'Then all I can say is that your informant was mistaken. I was merely taking the air after supper. It is my habit to get a little exercise before I go to bed. It helps me to sleep better.'

'So what of the statement that you hid behind a tree when a carriage came up the drive?'

'Fiddlesticks is my reply, Sir.' She was a tough little creature, there could be no doubt about that.

'Lying to a magistrate is a serious offence, you know,' the Blind Beak said, trying to alarm her into telling the truth.

'So I am aware.'

'Then I will give you one more chance to reconsider your words.'

'Your informant needs spectacles,' Maud snapped back sharply.

'Good day,' snarled the Blind Beak, losing patience.

She stared at him. 'Am I finished with?'

'For the time being, yes. Send in Mr Roger,' John Fielding answered tersely.

The beau's story was somewhat garbled. Apparently, he had been away from home for several days, staying with friends, and had not returned to St James's Square until the morning of the wedding.

'And these people will vouch for you?' the Magistrate asked.

'Well yes, but the matter is a little delicate.'

'Why?'

'Actually it's a friend, in the singular. I would not like to cause this person any harm.'

'Mr Hartfield,' said the Blind Beak, a note of exasperation in his voice. 'Do stop mincing words. Are you talking about a married person and a possible scandal?'

Roger nodded, looking suitably repentant.

'I can assure you that if we need to contact the lady concerned it would be with the utmost discretion.'

'It isn't quite like that. You see, my friend is her husband.' Realising that he might be treading on dangerous ground, Roger burst into a torrent of explanation. 'I mean, there is nothing untoward between us, my dear Sir. It is all in the mind of this jealous creature he took as wife. However, I would not like to get him into difficulties. People might jump to the wrong conclusion even though our friendship is completely innocent.'

Joe Jago let out a growl that could have been a laugh. Mr Fielding, however, remained calm and John, to his credit, kept his features impassive.

'My dear Sir,' the Magistrate said. 'I'm afraid that I must insist that you give my clerk the name of your intimate. His wife need never know anything about it provided people behave discreetly and do not become hysterical. Now, Mr Hartfield, are your sticks and canes in the house?'

'I have put them with the others brought by my brothers.'

'Very good, a neat rhyme. We will examine them later. Now if you would be kind enough to send in Mr Hugh.'

A moment later the third Hartfield brother came into the room, his tanned face bearing a miserable expression.

'What's all this about Maud?' he asked in a low voice.

'I don't understand you, Sir,' answered Mr Fielding.

'She's up to something, isn't she? There's another man involved, I feel certain of it. I've had my suspicions for quite some while. Every time I go abroad on business I come back to find things are not quite as they should be. Why, even my own father hinted as much.' Hugh stopped abruptly.

'Go on,' the Blind Beak said softly.

There was a moment's silence, then Hugh answered, 'It is of no importance.' He cleared his throat and continued a little nervously, 'There's nothing that you know about Maud, is there? Nothing that might prove me right.'

'Mr Hartfield,' said the Magistrate weightily, 'what is told us in confidence remains so, you must realise that. But let me just say that I believe your fears regarding your wife are most likely unfounded.'

The two sharp lines above Hugh's eyebrows eased considerably. 'Thank God,' he murmured. He looked round brightly. 'Now, gentlemen, what can I do for you?'

'Simply tell us the names of the ship's Captain and officers who accompanied you on your recent trip to France, Sir,' said Joe Jago.

'Certainly. Anything else?'

'No, that will be all for now. Will we find them at the Legal Quays, these men?'

Hugh nodded vigorously, appearing to be much relieved. 'Yes, you most likely will.'

Joe smiled affably. 'Thank you, Sir. Now if you could just tell me who they are.'

Hugh began to dictate and John, out of the corner of his eye, saw the clerk making one of his famous lists. He turned to Mr Fielding. 'May we save Lydia till last?' he murmured. 'There are several questions I would like to put to her.'

'By all means,' answered the Blind Beak. 'But now let's have Luke. Mr Hartfield, would you ask your father's secretary to step in please.'

Hugh bowed politely and left the room and a minute or two later, the secretary came in, looking thoroughly wretched, John thought. Mr Fielding did nothing to help by adopting his sternest tone.

'Mr Challon, I know a great deal about your movements on the night that Sir William died, so please do not deny what I am about to say. I am aware that you had been at Kirby Hall during the day and were meant to return there that night, which you did not do. I also know that you fetched Miss Lambourn from her home in Queens Square and took her to The Devil's Tavern in Wapping where she was to spend her wedding eve. May I ask what you did with your time after that?'

'Having seen her comfortably settled I went into the bar and got blindingly drunk,' Luke answered miserably.

'Is that because you were in love with the bride?'

'Partly. And partly because I was heartily sick of the whole damnable situation.'

'Did you speak to anyone during this time?'

'No. I sought my own company.'

'That is a great pity.'

'Why?'

'Because, Mr Challon, we now believe that Sir William was murdered in Redriff, a short row across the river. What could be easier than to slip across the water, kill your employer, then return to The Devil's Tavern and play the part of drunkard?'

All the colour drained from Luke's face and he shot to his feet. 'That is the vilest accusation I have ever heard. I'll not stand for any more of this.' So saying, he slammed from the room, crashing into Julian who was waiting outside the door.

'Oh dear,' said the twin, gazing at Luke's departing back. 'Am I about to be upset like that?'

'Not at all,' answered Mr Fielding jovially. 'All you have to do is tell me where you were on the night before your father's wedding.'

'Oh, out and about the town,' Julian replied cheerfully.

'Did you go anywhere specific?'

'No, I can't say that I did. I called in various taverns and clubs. Went to see Freddie Framlingham late. That sort of thing.'

'Was he at home, your friend?'

'No, gone to White's, lucky devil.'

'So there's no one who can vouch for your whereabouts?'

'No, not really.'

'Then you must go away and think hard, Mr Hartfield,' said the Blind Beak seriously. 'Try and remember where you went and whom you saw there. It is very important that you do.'

Julian grinned. 'That's all right. I'll ask Jul . . .' He stopped speaking abruptly, then added after a pause, '. . . iette to come in.'

John and Joe Jago exchanged a glance and Mr Fielding shifted in his chair. 'Yes, please do.'

'What was that concerning?' asked the Beak as soon as the door closed.

'I think I know,' answered John, and told the others his idea.

Mr Fielding frowned. 'I've a mind to inform his twin that we don't want to see her. That should give them something to think about.'

'Good plan,' said Joe firmly. 'There's no call to be bamboozled by a pair of gemini gigs. Such a game as they play could be dangerous.'

'Then let us call Lydia,' said the Magistrate, and John picked up his list of questions.

In the event he did not use it, so determined to get the truth out of her at last that he had no time to refer to notes. Having asked the widow to take a seat, the Apothecary started to speak.

'Mrs Hartfield, certain facts have emerged and it is only fair that I tell you exactly what they are. Firstly, it is known that you followed Sir William from this house on the night he was killed. Secondly, you were seen at The Angel in Redriff later on that same evening. Thirdly, you claimed that you walked alone and unaided from Redriff village to the inn. Do you realise that puts you in the very spot where it is believed Sir William was slain? And at the right time?'

Lydia stared at him coldly. 'What do you want me to say?'

'You can tell me if it's the truth.'

'Of course it is, every word. With one exception.'

'And what is that?'

'Somebody guided me to The Angel from Redriff. I was not solitary.'

'I thought as much. Was it anyone you knew?'

Lydia gave a bitter laugh. 'What ever I say, you're bound to discover the truth, so I may as well confess. The man who walked with me was my lover.'

'Or destined to become so later.'

'What do you mean?'

'It is my belief, Mrs Hartfield, that the night your father-in-law died was the first time you and Valentine Randolph shared the delights of the bedchamber together, though that, of course, does not clear either of you from the suspicion of murder.'

She looked at the three men defiantly. 'Yes, it was. The first – but certainly not the last.'

'That, of course, is a matter entirely for you,' John answered without censure. 'But there is still one vital matter we have not yet discussed. Tell me, why did you pursue Sir William to Redriff that night?'

'Because,' said Lydia, speaking very clearly, 'I wanted to come face to face at long last with the wretch who had been making my father-in-law's life a living hell.'

'Who do you mean?' John asked, thoroughly startled.

'I am referring,' the widow answered icily, 'to the man – or woman – who had consistently and without mercy been blackmailing him.'

Chapter Eighteen

'*T*he trouble with this entire affair,' said John reflectively, 'is that everyone seems to have something to hide. I have never known such a devious bunch of people.'

'Tell me,' answered Samuel.

'Well, the men are all strange. Hugh is clearly ambitious, Roger does not know whether to pursue dolly or molly, Julian is playing some pretty little game of his own. Luke is in love with Amelia and unrequited passion gnaws him up. While Valentine, whose heart was broken by a childhood romance, has once again found desire in the arms of the black-haired widow. As to the women, Lady Hodkin is a secret tippler, Hesther is frustrated, Maud is hiding something, Juliette is involved in her brother's jest, Lydia is lecherous, and Amelia, pretty though she might be, has the scruples of a Covent Garden whore. And to add to all their other delights, one of the family is probably a blackmailer.'

Samuel groaned. 'What a charming crew!'

'Quite.'

'John, remind me about those two wills again.'

'The first one still stands and benefits everyone except Amelia. The second, unsigned and therefore not legal, leaves the bulk of the estate to her, small bequests to the family, whose extraordinary ways Sir William must have discovered long ago, and the business to Luke and Valentine.'

'Why was that do you think?'

'Taking the family firm away from his sons?' The Goldsmith nodded. 'Because he must have been heartily sick of the lot of them, I suppose.'

Samuel sunk his chin into his hand. 'Whoever killed Sir William must have known that they were about to lose everything.'

'Unless it was an unpremeditated act of violence. Let us suppose, for argument's sake, that Luke Challon, so sick with love that he lost his reason, went to Redriff and begged Sir William not to marry

Amelia. The old man, quite naturally, refused to listen and Luke struck him with a stick, inadvertently killing him. Now it benefits Sir William's secretary not at all, because the second will hadn't been signed and he is only left a small amount under the terms of the first, but rage overcomes all other considerations. As I said to you before, the will alone proves nothing.'

'Oh good, London Bridge,' said Samuel, visibly brightening.

'Hang on tight,' answered his friend, and removed his hat as a precaution.

It was early evening, the day after the gathering of the Hartfield family at St James's Square, and John, for one, had been relieved to leave London and take to the river once more, hoping to clear his thoughts. At the meeting at Bow Street following the interrogation by the Blind Beak, he had been forced to admit that, if anything, he was now more confused than ever.

Lydia had told them everything – or had purported to do so. According to her, she had followed Sir William's hackney coach to Redriff but by the time she had alighted and paid off her driver, had lost her quarry. 'Just as if he had vanished from the face of the earth,' she had said in rather a chilling phrase. Then, so the widow's story had continued, she had wandered around looking for her father-in-law and had eventually run into Valentine Randolph, leaving The Spread Eagle and making for The Angel along the riverside path.

'So you still do not know the identity of the blackmailer?' John had said.

'There was no one about at all. Redriff was like a deserted village. I cannot imagine where Sir William and the person he was meeting could have got to.'

'A rum tale,' Joe had said thoughtfully.

'Do you believe it?' John had asked.

'I'm not sure. You see, it occurs to me that the blackmailer might not exist,' Mr Fielding had said harshly.

'But why should Lydia make that up?'

'What cleverer way to throw dust in our eyes than to invent an evil extortionist who has his being only in the mind of a murderer.'

'So you think she might have killed Sir William herself?'

'She and her lover between them.'

'What we need now is a stroke of good fortune. To come across something that will lead us straight to the killer,' John had said.

'What we need now is to find that great stick,' Mr Fielding had answered. 'It is a unique piece of evidence, the importance of which cannot be underestimated. Obviously, it didn't show up today – but then I hardly thought it would.'

'Reckon it's been done away with,' Joe had put in forthrightly. 'Burnt to a cinder fit for a garbler.'

The Magistrate had shaken his head. 'I'm not so sure. When would the killer have had time to consign it to flames? No, if it's anywhere, it's either gone out to sea or ended up on a mudflat.'

'I think I'll have a search round,' John had answered.

'The traditional needle in a hay stack, I fear. Yet a hunt would certainly do no harm.'

'Samuel and I will go tomorrow.'

So now they were on their way, in a small wherry, about to enjoy that dangerous pastime known as 'shooting the bridge'. Laughing uproariously and temporarily dismissing the complexities of finding Sir William's murderer, Samuel and John bobbed like corks as their craft mounted a cataract and cascaded down the other side, soaking all three of its occupants to the skin. The Goldsmith guffawed, the child in him never far from the surface. While John removed his coat and dabbed at his shirt with his handkerchief.

They had entered the Pool of London and a forest of masts, reminiscent of a scene in Amsterdam, spread before them. Amongst these great ships, many queuing at the Legal Quays to unload their dutiable cargo, buzzed the bumboats which serviced them. All craft vying for space with the barges bearing produce and colliers carrying coal.

John stared round, his eyes reflecting the blue of the river. 'I would like a house by the water one day.'

'With Coralie Clive also in residence?' Samuel asked saucily.

His friend smiled sadly. 'Did I tell you that I saw her recently?'

'Yes.'

'She still exerts a powerful hold on me, Sam, and I have a strange feeling that she always will.'

'So what are you going to do about it?'

John shook his head. 'There's not much I can do. She is determined to become as famous an actress as her sister Kitty, if not more so. At the moment men feature in her life only as companions.'

'Can't you remain that until she is ready for more?'

'No, I don't think I can,' John replied seriously. 'I'd be wanting to sweep her off to bed, take her to the church on the hill, laugh and cry with her, get her with child. I don't think Coralie and I are cut out for friendship.'

Loyal Samuel said, 'Then she's a fool not to realise what she's missing.'

The Apothecary sighed. 'One day, perhaps, something will happen to bring her to my side.'

'I hope so, if that is what you want,' the Goldsmith answered.

It had been John's plan to spend a pleasant evening in The Devil's Tavern, where he and Samuel would then stay the night, before devoting the whole of the next day, dressed in extremely servicable clothes, to a search of the riverbank and mudflats for the great stick with the fox's head. This idea his friend had agreed to with alacrity, so it was with the prospect of an enjoyable time ahead that the two of them climbed Pelican Stairs and made their way to the, by now, familiar confines of the riverside hostelry.

It was still early evening but already the bar was beginning to fill with the vivid flotsam and jetsam of waterside riff-raff. A sailor with two crimson parrots in a wooden cage was pestering a lady of quality for a sale; a blind man with a begging bowl wandered from table to table asking for alms; two blisteringly large seamen, obviously candidates for the bare knuckle fight, glared at one another pugnaciously. While a pedlar with one eye, a terrible scar in the cavity where the other had been, exhibited a tray of strangely carved objects brought from the Indies.

'What a place!' said John in admiration. And it was then, as he looked round for somewhere to sit, that he saw the three Hartfield brothers, together with Valentine and Luke, occupying a settle and two chairs by the fire. 'Well, well,' he murmured to Samuel.

His friend followed the direction of John's eyes. 'Here to discuss the future of the business?'

'More than likely. Oh dear, just read their faces.'

Samuel grinned, for Roger was stifling a yawn and Julian examining his fingernails, while Hugh held forth. Valentine, on the other hand, was attempting to look interested, though Luke was not bothering, glaring at the floor as if it had done him a diservice.

'I wonder if we can get near enough to listen without being seen,' John continued in the same low voice.

'The settle where they're sitting has another backing on to it. If we squeeze into that . . .'

'*If*! Have you seen the size of the man occupying it?'

'He must weigh at least a ton and a half.'

'I don't think I could stand the strain,' said the Apothecary, but at that moment the man they were staring at, an enormous Oriental complete with pigtail and long trailing black moustaches, heaved himself to his feet and waddled away. Under cover of his more than adequate screening, John and Samuel took their seats.

'. . . can leave the day-to-day running to me,' Hugh was saying. 'I mean, I was practically in charge while Father was alive.' Someone cleared his throat, and the speaker added, 'With Valentine's help, of course.'

'Well, I couldn't bear to go into the beastly place too often,' Roger's voice replied. 'You can take over the entire administration as far as I'm concerned, Hugh.'

'One moment,' put in Julian. 'I don't think we should release too much control, Roger. I think we should see all the documents daily.'

'That would cause an unwarrantable delay,' Hugh answered cuttingly. 'By the time you'd recovered from a night's gambling and were sober enough to look at the papers, we would probably have lost a day's important business.'

'Decisions are hardly that quick,' Valentine remonstrated. 'A twenty-four-hour deferment would make little difference.'

Hugh started to protest but Julian shouted him down. 'Listen, Hugh, the company belongs to all of us under the terms of Father's will. You were given the management, not total authority.'

'You've become a regular tongue-pad, young man, if I might say so.'

Luke spoke for the first time. 'This is just the sort of thing Sir William dreaded might happen.'

'Which is no doubt why he made a new will. But he never signed it, did he? Much to your regret, my dear Luke.'

'Yes, I do dislike the fact that Miss Lambourn has been left penniless,' the secretary answered angrily. His tone was decidedly nasty and John hazarded a guess that Luke had consumed a great deal of alcohol.

'Oh, you've always had a soft spot for the silly slut,' Hugh remarked carelessly.

'Oh dear!' muttered Samuel, as there was the sound of a chair scraping back and somebody jumping to his feet.

'Don't insult the lady,' growled Luke, between gritted teeth.

'For the love of God . . .' shouted Valentine. But too late. There was the crunch of a fist making contact with bone, followed by an angry roar and the crash of two bodies as they hit the floor.

It was like a signal. Instantly, every inhabitant of the long low room stopped what they were doing and looked over in the direction of the fight, while the landlord, with simply amazing agility, leapt clean over the pewter bar and advanced on the argument. As he did so, the two enormous sailors grappled and started to knock hell out of each other, while the seaman with the parrots put down his cage and hit the man standing next to him. Deciding that discretion was the better part of valour, John and Samuel climbed up onto the settle from where they had a commanding view of the entire proceedings.

Immediately in front of them, Luke and Hugh were rolling on the floor, punching furiously, Hugh getting by far the worst of it. Valentine and Julian, meanwhile, were attempting to separate them, while Roger had slumped in a faint into a large oak chair. The lady of quality had also risen to stand on a table and was busy throwing plates at the fighting sailors, while her escort seemed on the point of drawing his sword.

'Cor,' said a voice beside John, 'what a lovely mill.' And a small hand was thrust into his as Kitty Perkins, the oyster girl, clambered up to join them. She peered over the back of the settle. 'What's happening?'

'Do you remember me telling you about Sir William Hartfield, the man who was killed on the night we first met? And how I found his body?'

'Yes, may his soul rest in peace. He always said good day whenever he saw me. A proper gentleman he was.'

'Well, that's some of his family down there.'

'Yes, I know. I've seen them before. Not that they come to this part of the world very often. Too lowlife. They're fighting over the money, I suppose.'

'Something like that.'

Kitty peered closely, taking everything in, then her expression changed. 'That's funny,' she said.

'What?'

'I saw that one the other night and thought at the time he didn't ought to be there . . .' And she pointed vaguely in the direction of the fight.

In her excitement her voice soared over the general rumpus, clearly audible to all. But Kitty got no further. The vast Oriental had returned from wherever he had been and was now laying about him with a series of strange throws and kicks that sent anyone who approached him flying through the air. With a grunt, he picked up the settle, shaking off its occupants as if they were so many rag dolls. Lying in a heap where he had landed on the floor, John saw the massive piece of furniture whirl high then crash down onto Hugh and Luke, stopping their fight for good and all. A violent desire to laugh was strangled at birth by the sight of all the missing teeth and blood which covered the flagstones right next to where he lay. Searching madly for his bag, John staggered to his feet in order to do his duty and tend the wounded.

An hour later he was finished and the scene in the Devil's Tavern had changed yet again. The Oriental sat by the fire like the Emperor of China, plied with drink and congratulations. The warring sailors had removed with their various entourages to the room upstairs, where they could punch in peace. Valentine had taken Roger and Luke away, or so John was informed by Samuel, while a very angry Julian, not looking in the least effeminate and scowling thunderbolts, had removed Hugh. The man with the parrots had made a sale at last, the lady of quality and her beau were drunk, and the pedlar well content, having disposed of the entire contents of his tray.

''Zounds!' said John, wiping the blood from his hands and face. 'Have you ever seen the like of it?'

'Wasn't it exciting though!'

'Well, yes.'

'Do you think Luke will be dismissed from his post?'

'I'm certain he will. Poor soul. And all for love of an amorous jade who wouldn't look twice at him.' The Apothecary gazed down at his bloodstained clothes. 'I think I'd better go and change.' He stared round. 'Where's Kitty gone?'

'She had to leave with the tide. She asked me to say farewell and that she'll see you tomorrow. There's something she wants to tell you.'

John lowered his voice. 'Yes, she recognised one of the scrappers from somewhere.'

'Do you mean Hugh and Luke?'

'Either them or one of the other three. I don't know which.'

'I wonder what she wants to say.'

'I have simply no idea.' John straightened himself. 'Come along, Samuel old friend. I shall clean myself up and then I suggest a brisk row across the river. I think it's high time you met that merry imp, the mudlark.'

They borrowed one of the boats belonging to the inn, the landlord considering himself heavily in John's debt for services rendered on the battlefield, and set off across the darkening Thames in the direction of The Spread Eagle. Samuel, built like a windmill and pleased to show his superior strength, did the rowing while John leaned back and let the delights of watching the river at dusk, flow over him. Yet even the Goldsmith, strong as a shire horse, found the going a little hard and the negotiation of a small craft through the lines of great ships not as easy as it looked. Somewhat relieved but refusing to say so, Samuel was delighted when John shouted out, 'Those are Church Steps,' and he was at last able to ship his oars and bring the boat neatly to the bottom stair and tie it to one of the many mooring rings provided.

It seemed that by some most mysterious means, news of the sensational fight in The Devil's Tavern had crossed the river to the south bank, and as John and Samuel walked into The Spread Eagle somebody bellowed, 'That's him. That's the duke what patched them up.' And a small cheer was raised.

'So much fame,' said John, attempting to look modest.

'So much affectation,' countered Samuel, as only an old friend could.

There was a tug at the Apothecary's elbow and he looked round to see Fred, the mudlark, a broad grin splitting his face, a frothing tankard in each hand.

'The landlord says you are to have these on him, Sir. Remember the riverman with the bleeding nose what you seen to? Well, that was his brother.'

John relieved him of the ale. 'Thank him very much from me. Samuel, this is Fred, former mudlark. Fred, I'd like you to meet my friend, Samuel Swann.'

'Happy to do so,' said the potboy.

'Former mudlark?' queried Samuel. 'I thought you were still very much a river lad.'

'Oh, I am, I am. It's just that I've given up me dishonest ways. But I still live by the water, up on the bank. Under an old wherry.'

The Goldsmith looked astonished. 'Under a wherry?'

'Yes, duke. It's overturned, see. I made a little door in it and it's big enough for me to stand up in. It's a better home than most of the mudlarks have round here.'

'I'd like to see it,' said John.

'Well, it's about two hundred yards downstream, just beyond Redriff. You can't miss it. Come when I'm not working.'

'How about tomorrow?'

Fred frowned. 'No, I'm busy. Make it the day after.'

'I will if I'm still in the area.'

There was a loud call of 'Boy, boy,' and the mudlark glanced furtively over his shoulder.

'I'm wanted. Best be off. Come and see me if you can.' And he disappeared into the heaving throng.

Samuel stared after him, amazed. 'Are there many children like that? Living by the river, completely on their own?'

'There certainly are. Ragged, filthy, surviving on what they can thieve, ill-educated, neglected, and stronger than almost any other child in the kingdom.'

'One could almost envy them.'

John looked thoughtful. 'There's certainly a lesson to be learned from it all.'

'In what way?'

'Consider the mortality rate amongst the pampered offspring of the aristocracy, then look at these healthy little water rats.'

'Surely you're not suggesting that rich but sickly children should be heaved bodily into the Thames?'

'It might not be such a bad idea at that,' answered John, and smiled at the incredulous expression on his old friend's honest face.

Chapter Nineteen

*M*uch as John had feared, the search of the riverbank had proved fruitless. He and Samuel had risen surprisingly early after an enjoyable evening in The Spread Eagle, from which, thankfully, one of the water people had rowed them back to The Devil's Tavern. Then, having consumed a gallant breakfast, they had set forth armed with stout boots and even stouter gloves, to seek the implement which had ended the life of poor Sir William. Yet though they had found many things washed up by the tide, which had been high when they set out but was now steadily falling, nothing resembling the great stick had come to hand. By midday, with the water level still going down, and by dint of covering different areas separately, the friends had reached Ratcliff Cross, the point from which mariners of an earlier time had sailed forth for the unknown.

Samuel, having come across yet another dead dog, straightened his back. 'This is hopeless. The thing could be anywhere.'

John sighed. 'I know.'

'So what do you suggest?'

'Let's get someone to row us across to the other bank and work our way back to The Spread Eagle. That will probably occupy the rest of the daylight hours.'

'Oughtn't we to stop for a little refreshment soon?' asked Samuel hopefully.

'Yes. But I think we should get over the river first.'

In this way, fortuitously having run into Fred, who had somehow acquired what John could only think of as a coracle, a flimsy and dangerous craft which provided an extremely nerve-racking journey, the pair found themselves on the south bank, in Jamaica Inn in Jamaica Street, still officially part of Redriff though a considerable distance from the village.

'Samuel,' said John, remembering something that he had been meaning to ask but had forgotten until this moment. 'Can you cast your mind back to the day we visited Islington Spa?'

'Yes. Why?'

'What was it you said about Roger on that occasion?'

The Goldsmith stared blankly. 'I don't know, what did I say? That he wore cutting fashions? That he looked worse than I remembered him?'

'Yes, that was it! That he seemed changed. What did you mean exactly?'

Samuel frowned. 'Just that when he caught Amelia, stopped her falling into the grave, he appeared quite forceful. But when he came flapping over, all frills and flounces, he was exactly the opposite. It was odd.'

'Yes,' John answered slowly. 'Very odd. And you're quite right. He was different at that moment.' The Apothecary sat in silence.

'What are you thinking?' Samuel asked.

'I'm not quite sure yet. There's something bubbling inside my brain but it refuses to rise to the surface.'

'It will,' his friend answered confidently. 'Now come on, sup your ale. There's work to be done.'

The river reached its lowest point at about two o'clock that afternoon, so that many of the things that had been thrown or fallen into its watery recesses now lay on the banks. Scavenging their way through all the extraordinary objects, which ranged from chamber pots, their contents, thankfully, long since washed away, to a rather valuable ring, John and Samuel still found nothing relating to the murder. Then, with the river at flood and the late March sun beginning to dip, they gave up the task as The Spread Eagle came into sight.

'Hopeless,' the Apothecary admitted. 'I feel a fool.'

'Why, for heaven's sake?'

'Because I told Mr Fielding that we'd be sure to find something.'

'Well, we've done our best. My back is breaking, to say nothing of my knees.'

'Let's get back to The Devil's Tavern. Kitty is probably looking for us.'

'Yes. I wonder where she's got to.'

But though John and Samuel waited for the oyster girl all the evening, staring round every time the door opened, there was no sign of her. Somewhere deep in the Apothecary's consciousness an alarm bell rang.

'I expect she's gone up to Whitstable and still isn't back,' said Samuel, reading his friend's mind.

'I'm sure that's it,' John answered.

Yet despite a determined effort to push away disturbing thoughts, he still did not sleep well and was glad when Samuel rose at dawn in order to take a wherry back to London and open his goldsmith's shop at the Sign of the Crescent Moon in St Paul's Churchyard. Having seen his friend depart, John paid his bill and packed his bag, then borrowed one of the boats moored at Pelican Stairs and rowed across to Redriff in the early morning light, determined not to leave Wapping until he had found Kitty Perkins.

Certain that of all the people he had met it would be the mudlark who would know most about what was going on, the Apothecary headed upstream, staring at the bank as the spire of St Mary's Church and the outline of The Spread Eagle came into view. Sure enough, about two hundred yards from the hostelry, the upturned boat, an eccentric but merry looking little dwelling, came into his line of vision and he pulled inshore, splashing through the shallows to attach his craft to a wooden stump.

The tide was rising and Fred, taking advantage of the water creeping ever nearer to his home, was up and about his ablutions, which consisted of swimming naked through the swirling stream. He waved when he saw John, then shot into the hovel and came out again pulling on a pair of breeches.

'Caught me,' he said cheerfully.

'Good morning,' answered John. 'I thought I'd come and visit you early because, all being well, I hope to go back to London today.'

'Then step inside,' Fred continued, still beaming a smile. 'You won't never have seen nuffink like this.'

Bending low, the Apothecary stooped his way through the little door, then stood upright, his eyes widening at the sight of Fred's home. The wherry, long since taken out of service as it obviously had been, still consisted of good strong timbers well able to cope with the ravages of wind and storm. In fact there was something quite cosy about it, and the smell of the river and the spars combined was pleasing to the senses. By way of furniture there was a rusty old bedstead, clearly plucked from the jaws of the Thames, an old sea chest which served for a table, a chair with a piece of timber where once one of its legs had been, and, incongruously, an ornate mirror which hung, amongst other salvaged trophies, over the two points of the prow. Beside the bed, vast and rather frightening, was a ship's figurehead, this one depicting a bare breasted mermaid with staring eyes and curling yellow hair, a comb in one carved hand.

Seeing the direction of John's gaze, the mudlark said, 'That's the Sea Queen. She was beached after a storm. Reckon there'd been a wreck somewhere and she came in with the tide.'

'I think I'd get a fright if I woke in the night and saw her looming over me.'

'I like her,' said Fred, with spirit. 'She keeps me company, the Queen does.'

John stared round him. 'You've made yourself very comfortable here.'

'All of it come out of the river.'

'Including that chest?'

And the Apothecary looked down at the beautiful piece of wood which, in its day, had been artistically decorated with scenes of ships and even the owner's name, all painted on by hand.

'Yes, even that. But I'm forgetting me manners. Would you like a tot of rum?'

John shook his head. 'It's a little early, though thank you for asking.'

'You don't mind if I do? It's me breakfast time, see.'

And the boy produced from a basket, a great hunk of bread and cheese, a tin mug and a bottle of dark, powerful spirit.

'Please go on,' said John. His eye alighted once more on the sea chest. 'What do you keep in there? Your treasures?'

'Yes, everything that I find when I go scavenging.'

'May I look?' asked the Apothecary, and felt the thrill of premonition as he lifted the lid.

It was there, just as he had felt it would be, lying on top of everything else, clearly the latest acquisition, its ornate handle gleaming in the shaft of sunshine coming through the little door. John gasped, not so much in surprise but with delight at the beautiful craftsmanship of the implement which had killed Sir William Hartfield. Whoever had shaped the solid silver fox's head had been a master of his trade, while the dark glowing ebony, the wood from which the shaft of the great stick had been fashioned, was a tribute to the hands that had created it. In wonderment, John picked the cane up, silently offering a prayer of thanks, then he very carefully wrapped the head in his best linen handkerchief and tied the resulting package with a piece of string retrieved from an inner pocket.

'Where did you find this?' he asked the mudlark softly.

'It was washed up on the shore, just below here.'

'How long ago?'

'I can't remember exactly. About two weeks or so.'

'It wouldn't by any chance have been the morning after you saw the two drunkards on Church Steps?'

Fred stared at him suspiciously. 'Now you come to mention it, yes it was. Why?'

'Because I believe that this was the stick which killed the man I told you of. The one who was to have met Mr Randolph.'

'Oh my lawk!' said the mudlark.

John gave him an apologetic look. 'I'm going to have to take it away with me, I'm afraid.'

'But I scavenged it.'

'Fred,' the Apothecary said earnestly, 'I will try to return the stick to you if you really want it. But be assured that it is vital I get this straight to the Public Office in Bow Street.'

The mudlark's freckles glowed. 'But I like it, Mr Rawlings.'

'Who wouldn't? It is a beautiful thing. But it is also sinister and murderous and has been responsible for snuffing out a man's life.'

Fred nodded slowly. 'I suppose you're right. But I still want the stick back, mind.'

'Provided Mr Fielding agrees, you shall have it.' John looked at his watch, thinking that the much needed stroke of good fortune had come his way at last and now he could head for home. Then he remembered Kitty and his worry about her, and his jubilant expression vanished. 'Fred, do you know Miss Perkins, the oyster girl?' he asked.

'Yes, she comes to sell in The Spread Eagle sometimes.'

'Have you any idea where she lives?'

'In a lodging house in Star Street, just by King James's Stairs.'

'What number?'

Fred shook his head. 'That I'm not sure of.'

'Could you take me there?'

'I'm to be at work at half past seven.'

'That's in three quarters of an hour. Please, Fred. I think it could be important.'

They rowed back in the boat John had borrowed, the great stick lying safely on the bottom. But this time they did not moor at Pelican Stairs but went upriver to the next landing stage where the mudlark secured the boat, then jumped out.

'This is King James's. Come on, Mr Rawlings. The landlord will skin me alive if I'm late.'

The boy had such a sense of urgency about him that John found himself breaking into a run and was panting slightly when they stopped before a tall, seedy-looking house, badly in need of a coat of paint. There appeared to be no street door to the place and John found himself following Fred down a small passageway and into a kitchen. Beside a miserable fire sat a thin sour-faced woman in a grey dress and apron, while a haggard and wretched girl swept the floor.

'Morning, Mam,' Fred said, clearly having encountered the landlady before. 'This gentlemen come for Kitty.'

The woman of the house shot John a knowing look. 'Upstairs, first on the left,' she said.

'Is Miss Perkins home?' the Apothecary asked anxiously.

She mimicked his voice, 'Is Miss Perkins 'ome?' then roared with laughter. 'How would I know? I ain't seen 'er. Go up and try your luck.'

'Come on!' urged Fred.

'Do you want to go back?' John asked. 'I can manage now.'

'I'm sure you can,' the woman said with a leer.

He ignored her. 'I don't want to make you late.'

'I can stay another few minutes,' the mudlark answered, and led the way up a dark and dirty staircase.

'Poor Kitty. What a terrible place to have to live in,' the Apothecary said, staring round.

'It's cheap, Sir. Probably only a shilling a week.'

'Oh my God,' said John with feeling.

The landing was as dingy and foul as the stairs, and it was with some difficulty that John located the first door on the left, feeling his way along in total dimness. But eventually he identified Kitty's room and gave a tentative knock. There was no reply.

He turned to look at the mudlark, whose orange hair seemed to glow in the darkness. 'What shall I do?'

'Go in. She might be asleep.'

'Yes, she could be.'

'She won't mind you having to wake her, honest.'

Feeling like an intruder and not relishing his actions, John turned the doorknob and went in. Then he let out a breath of relief as he saw that Kitty *was* there, lying on a crude truckle bed, sleeping as Fred had predicted. Her back was turned to him and her dark hair was spread like black lace over the heap of shawls that served as a pillow.

'Kitty,' John called softly, 'wake up. I'm sorry to disturb you but I'm about to return to London and wanted to have a talk before I went.'

She did not stir and the Apothecary felt, rather than saw, the mudlark stiffen beside him, then cower in the doorway. Walking quietly, John approached the bed and put a hand on the oyster girl's shoulder. She turned beneath his touch, then fell back heavily so that she was staring up at the ceiling. Or would have done, had it not been for the fact that though her eyes were open, Kitty could no longer see. A trickle of dried blood ran from the corner of her mouth down to her chin, obscenely dark against the snowdrop whiteness of her skin. And round the oyster girl's neck, twisting like a thin black serpent, was the piece of knotted cord that had put an end to the life of Kitty Perkins.

Chapter Twenty

*T*he day that had started in the glow of early sunshine had by now turned into a nightmare. Only wishing that the Public Office had been near at hand but knowing that he would be failing in his duty if he delayed reporting his ghastly find, John had sent Fred running to fetch the constable. Then, left alone with Kitty's corpse, he had set about the grisly business of examining it. This was the first time in his experience that the Apothecary had been forced to study the body of someone who had been a friend, albeit of only short duration, and he found the experience grim and distressing. Yet look he must, for Mr Fielding would want to know everything there was to tell about the way the oyster girl had died.

Hastily and hating it, John sought for evidence of sexual molestation. But there was no ripped clothing or bruising of the privy parts, and his guess that Kitty had been killed in order to silence her, became a conviction. Oddly, there was no sign of a struggle of any kind, which led the Apothecary to conclude that the girl's attacker must have crept in while she was asleep and that poor Kitty would have woken to find the life already being choked out of her, too late to defend herself.

As soon as he had touched the body, John had discovered fully established rigor mortis, and from this had concluded that the oyster girl had met her death during the previous evening or, possibly, late afternoon. Had Kitty returned from fishing and taken a short rest before going to meet himself and Samuel? And during that sleep had either one of the five men involved in the fist fight in The Devil's Tavern or someone they had been able to warn, come creeping back to close her mouth for ever? Cursing the fact that he had not gone searching hours sooner, the Apothecary wept in the silence of the death room, a tear splahing down onto Kitty's cold cheek as he kissed her a final farewell.

Realising that he could now get caught in the spider's web of officialdom, John instantly informed the constable, who arrived puffing and harassed after an hour had elapsed, that he was working for John Fielding of Bow Street and was in the area investigating another death. He failed to mention, however, that he believed the two murders to be connected, fearing infinite complications and hours of delay might well result if he did.

'So how was it you come to be in this house, Sir?' the constable asked, showing a certain flair for the job, considering that he was a fishmonger reluctantly chosen by rote to fulfill the office for a year.

'I had arranged to meet Miss Perkins last night in The Devil's Tavern, where I have been staying with a friend. When she did not make an appearance I decided to come and look for her, but unfortunately too late to rescue her from her killer. By the way, I was in that friend's company throughout the evening and he can vouch for me completely.'

'And what makes you think she was murdered then and not this morning?' the constable asked.

'The body is cold as ice and completely stiff, suffering that condition known as rigor mortis. As rigor takes roughly twelve hours to wear on and lasts another twelve once it is established, I think it is safe to conclude that she was killed early last evening.'

The constable looked extremely surprised. 'Well, well! Are you a medical man, Sir?'

'In a manner of speaking. I'm an apothecary. Now, do you wish me to give you a statement about how I found her?' John asked wearily.

'I'm sure the Coroner will want to know. And you, boy, what's-your-name, you'd better make one as well.'

'I can't sign me signature,' said Fred, alarmed.

'Then you'll just have to put a cross, won't you. Now, I'd best get this poor creature taken to the mortuary before she starts to rot.'

The constable ushered them out but John turned in the doorway for one last look at the oyster girl, reflecting on her death in such squalid surroundings, and, indeed, her life in them as well.

'Fred,' he said impulsively, 'you must try and make something of yourself. Get away from here. Don't get caught in Kitty's trap.'

The mudlark stared at him blankly. 'But I'm happy as I am – and so was she. She weren't trapped.'

'But this terrible place. How could she stand it?'

'She only slept here,' Fred stated simply, as if he were explaining to a child. 'When she got up every morning she went straight to the river. Then she was all right again. We're water folk, see?'

John smiled harshly. 'Perhaps I do,' he said.

In the end, with the wretched business finally concluded, he had left Wapping in the late afternoon, by which time, the Apothecary had descended into a state of deep depression. Disregarding cost, he had ordered the wherryman to row him all the way to Hungerford Stairs, from which The Strand was but a moment's walk. From there, John took a hackney coach to Shug Lane, determined to have a few minutes alone and, even more importantly, to mix himself a potion to cure his mood of melancholia. Indeed, so dark were his thoughts, that the Apothecary had quite literally forgotten about Nicholas Dawkins and was momentarily surprised when he went to let himself into his shop, only to find the door unlocked.

'Who's there?' he called suspiciously, and felt every kind of a fool when Nicholas's pale face looked up at him from beyond the counter.

'Mr Rawlings!' the boy exclaimed. 'We were getting worried about you, Sir. You were away longer than you said.'

'I'm lucky to be here at all,' John answered, setting his bag and the great stick down on the floor. 'By God, things have become horribly ugly.'

'Come through to the back and sit down,' Nicholas answered anxiously. 'You look fit to drop. Here, I'll prepare a concoction to restore you.'

'Do you know how?' John asked, his whole manner melancholic.

'You showed me last time we were together, don't you remember?'

'I'm sorry, no. So much has happened.'

'Do you want to speak of it?'

'Not at the moment.'

Nicholas nodded but did not answer, busying himself with various bottles and jars and finally returning with a glass of extremely potable liquid which John, not caring whether he was being imprudent, gladly consumed. After he had drained every drop, the Apothecary asked what was in it.

'It is your recipe, Sir. Honey, sweet wine, and powder of dried feverfew, gathered and stored last year. Then I put in a special ingredient of my own.'

'And what was that?'

'Apparently my Russian great grandfather swore by corn poppy. So I chopped some and put it in.'

John smiled. 'Do you want me to fall asleep?'

'No, just to be more relaxed.'

'That's going to be difficult. I need to see Mr Fielding to give him this stick, then I have to talk to my father. And all I really want to do is go somewhere quiet and mourn for a girl who was being cruelly choked to death while I sat in a hostelry less than a mile away, enjoying myself and doing nothing to save her.'

'But how were you to know?'

'I think perhaps I should have guessed.'

'You're not a gypsy fortune teller, Sir. Meanwhile, may I make a practical suggestion?'

'Yes.'

'It's that you go to Bow Street, now, by hackney coach, and take the stick with you. Meanwhile, I will run to your home with your bag and ask Sir Gabriel to join you at the Public Office. Then all the right people can be together at the same time.'

John held out his glass. 'Mix another decoction and I'll go. I'm starting to feel a little better. It must be the corn poppy.'

'That's good news,' said Nicholas seriously, and started to bustle about his mixing once more.

An hour later, the Muscovite's plan had come to fruition. John sat in the Blind Beak's salon awaiting Mr Fielding's return from court and being cosseted by Elizabeth, who thought privately that she had never seen him look more grey. Meanwhile, the wheels of Sir Gabriel's coach could be heard on the cobbles below, followed shortly by his firm tread and Nicholas's limping gait ascending the stairs. And no sooner was John's father settled than Joe Jago hurried into the room to say that the Magistrate was on his way.

At that, Nicholas put his head round the door. 'Shall I serve punch, Mrs Fielding?'

Elizabeth fluttered. 'I don't like you acting as a servant, my child. Not now that you have found employment with Mr Rawlings.'

'But I couldn't just come and sit with you.'

'Why not?'

'Because until I'm apprenticed somewhere I'm still the boy you rescued from the streets.'

'A hint I believe,' said Sir Gabriel with an amused smile as the door closed behind the Muscovite. He turned to his son. 'My dear child, as soon as Mr Fielding comes you must tell your story and then let me take you home. You look fit to drop.'

'It has been a very extraordinary few days, I must admit.'

'Clearly a great deal has happened.'

They got no further. The door opened once more to admit the Blind Beak, his arm tucked through Joe Jago's.

'My good young friend,' he said, his manner direct. 'What has occurred that you are so distressed?'

'How did . . . ?'

'Joe said it is writ on your face for all the world to see. Now, unburden yourself.'

It was a command and John obeyed it, telling everything that had happened from the moment he and Samuel Swann had arrived at The Devil's Tavern till the terrible discovery that very morning, and its aftermath in the constable's house. When he had finished speaking, there was a moment of horrified silence, until John Fielding broke it.

'This killer has to be stopped before he or she strikes again, at you, Mr Rawlings.'

'But why should he do that?'

'The murderer may fear that he silenced Kitty Perkins too late. That she might have already revealed to you the name of the man she saw in the wrong place at the wrong time.'

'So the guilty party is definitely one of the five men involved in the fight?' asked Sir Gabriel.

The Blind Beak's wig swung as he shook his head. 'Not necessarily. I recall a conversation that you overhead at Kirby Hall, Mr Rawlings. If my memory serves me correctly, it was between a man and a woman whom you believed to be the twins. But just suppose it was two others, the killer and an accomplice.'

'But why could it not have been the twins?' said Joe Jago. 'Those two geminis play rum games.'

'They could quite easily be responsible for the crimes,' Fielding agreed. 'I am merely throwing into question the possibility of two people working together. A thing not unknown to us.'

John laughed harshly. 'Indeed not.' He handed the great stick to Joe Jago, pulling it out from under his chair. As he did so he turned to the Blind Beak. 'Sir, I think I may have discovered the murder weapon. The mudlark I told you of found it washed up on the morning after Sir William's murder. Its head is identical to the imprint that I saw on the dead man's forehead.'

'Have you examined it?'

'No, Sir. I was too preoccupied I fear.'

'Leave it here, then, and we'll let Joe take a look. If any trace of anything remains after the ravages of time and tide, he will find it.'

Jago, who had been carefully removing John's improvised protective covering, let out a whistle. 'It's a real beauty, Sir.'

'Expensive?'

'Very.'

'Does that rule out the two employees, Challon and Randolph?' asked Sir Gabriel.

'Not if the stick were a gift,' John answered. He steeled himself for one last effort to absorb information. 'Were the stories the family gave you at St James's Square checked, Sir?'

Mr Fielding rumbled a laugh. 'In the manner of a farce, yes they were. Listen to this. Lady Hodkin left her neighbour's house a good hour before she returned home, but we have got no further in discovering where the old wretch went in that time. The gypsy woman, whose clairvoyance Hesther sought, is no longer in residence, supposedly having sailed away with her husband. Maud's story that she was merely exercising is proving hard to dispute, though some seem to believe she has a lover. We sent a Runner to The Devil's Tavern, knowing that you would be busy with other matters, but nobody could recall seeing Luke there once he had delivered the blushing bride to her chamber. That same Runner crossed the river to Redriff and was able to confirm that both Valentine Randolph and the widowed Lydia were indeed prowling about the very spot where Sir William met his death, and at the correct time. And, further, that they spent the night together at The Angel. He also went to the Legal Quays and to Sir William's Wapping office, to try to discover the whereabouts of the captain of the ship that brought Hugh back from France, only to find that the man has returned to sea and therefore the account cannot be checked. Roger's man friend denies all knowledge of seeing him at the relevant time. And as to the twins, their versions of what they did on the night of the murder are as full of holes as a sieve. Incidentally, I *did* question Juliette merely to hear what she would come up with.'

'And?'

'The creature is a devious minx.'

John gave a deep sigh. 'So we are no further forward at all.'

'On the contrary. The killer has made a mistake, the death of the oyster girl proves that. Now all we have to do is discover what it is.'

'How?'

'By watching them all closely, Mr Rawlings. I intend to put Runner Rudge, whom you know of old, together with a carriage, at your disposal. That is, my dear friend, if you are willing to spare just a little more time from your shop.'

The Apothecary smiled wryly. 'Nicholas is excellent, there is no doubt of that, but he cannot prescribe for nor treat the sick.'

Joe Jago gave a small chuckle. 'If you will forgive my impudence, Mr Rawlings, I have approached one of your brotherhood who has recently given up his work due to advancing years. He has reason to be grateful to the Public Office for a favour we rendered him during the days of Mr Henry Fielding. Consequently, he has agreed to oversee your shop until you return.'

The Blind Beak interposed. 'He was contacted only as a precaution. I do not want you to feel you are under any obligation to continue with this search.'

'To give up now would be ridiculous. In fact I shall not rest until this vicious killer is brought to book.'

Sir Gabriel's voice cut across John's. 'My child, that is one of the most extraordinary remarks I have ever heard. Rest is the very thing you *must* do. If you do not get some sleep, urgently, you will make yourself ill and then the mystery will never be solved.'

'You're right of course,' his son answered, Sir Gabriel's very tone suddenly forcing him to realise just how sick the shock of Kitty's death had made him feel.

'Rudge will bring the carriage round tomorrow morning at ten o'clock,' said the Blind Beak. 'And Nicholas will open the shop as usual. I shall send word to Master Gerard – he is the grandson of the author of Gerard's Herbal incidentally – that his services will be required. Meanwhile, my young friend, I bid you good night and would like to say how grateful I am for all you have achieved.'

'But I feel as if I have done nothing.'

'Nonsense,' Mr Fielding contradicted roundly. 'I believe that you are on the point of the final solution.'

Chapter Twenty-One

*I*n order to help him sleep that night, John Rawlings took laudanum, a derivative of the white poppy, which did, indeed, render him unconscious as soon as his head touched the pillow. However, it also produced an extraordinary hallucination. During the small hours, the Apothecary thought that he woke and saw Kitty standing in his room, the pallor of death about her but other than that very much as she had looked in life. She said three incomprehensible words, 'The Belle Sauvage.' Then the vision vanished and he went back to sleep. When morning came, John knew, of course, that he had suffered a drug-induced delusion, yet the memory of it overshadowed him and he did not feel balanced and ready for the day until he had consumed several cups of coffee, that well-known cure for opiate overdoses, to say nothing of headaches and gout.

Greatly restored, John was ready punctually at ten when Beak Runner Benjamin Rudge, that bluff character with the ingenuous sense of humour, arrived, dressed in the guise of a coachman. With the nasty feeling that he was there to act as bodyguard as much as anything else, the Apothecary, recalling another occasion when Rudge had snored his way through a time of immense danger for John and, indeed, for Coralie Clive, hoped fervently that all their current missions together would be in the daytime.

'Good morning, Sir,' the Runner said cheerfully. 'I've brought the carriage up outside. Mr Fielding's orders are that I am to act as your driver and general factotum. So where are we bound for today?'

John, busying himself with putting on his hat and cloak, thought rapidly. 'Well, the Magistrate told me to keep watch on all of them so we may as well start with number thirty-two, St James's Square. Would it be possible for you to wait somewhere nearby?'

'Leave it to me, Sir.'

John stepped into the equipage, waved to Sir Gabriel, leaving the house for his morning perambulation, and they were off through the streets, this day freshened slightly by an early April shower. Leaning back against the upholstered interior, the Apothecary tried to formulate a plan. Questioning the Hartfields about their whereabouts on the evening of Kitty's murder was certainly one possibility. Yet something made him shy away from the idea. Better, John thought, to pretend that he knew nothing of it. After all, the Wapping constable was hardly likely to report the death of an oyster girl to the Public Office in the normal course of events. Therefore to plead ignorance was perfectly plausible. So, if he could somehow trick the killer into an error, an error that would at last reveal his or her identity, that would be by far the better scheme.

'I think I'll try following them individually,' he called up to Rudge, who sat on the coachman's box, looking the part superbly.

'What's that, Sir?'

John stuck his head out of the window. 'I believe we've got to start playing tricks with these people. Let's track them one by one.'

'A good idea.'

'So whichever comes out first, we'll trail. Then I'll affect that I was at the same place by the merest chance.'

But even as he decided what to do, John wished that there was some far more positive action he could take to apprehend the murderer, and had the dread feeling that all he was really doing was wasting valuable time.

The carriage drew up near the garden at the centre of St James's Square and Rudge loosened the reins as if he were allowing the horse to rest. John, meanwhile, kept discreet observation through the window. But their wait was to be of short duration. Within ten minutes the front door opened and Juliette appeared, dressed to go out. The Apothecary, narrowing his eyes, gave a small cry of triumph.

'We'll pursue this one, Mr Rudge. But take it slowly. I think she might be going to hire a chair.'

Sure enough, Juliette turned down towards Pall Mall and there hailed two chairmen to attend her. By dint of letting the horse plod along, the Public Office carriage kept the sedan within its sights, following it down Pall Mall, then The Strand, where its passenger alighted. Juliette, having paid the fare, promptly hurried down Salisbury Street, clearly heading for Salisbury Stairs and the river.

'You'll have to leave me here,' John called to Rudge.

'But Mr Fielding said I was to keep my eye on you.'

'I can't help that. I think she's going by water. Meet me at Nassau Street.'

'When?'

'Later today,' John said vaguely, and vanished in pursuit of his quarry.

Juliette was just stepping into a wherry as he caught up with her, but by dint of lurking in the shadows, unseen yet in earshot, the Apothecary overheard her say, 'Cuper's Gardens, if you please.'

Smiling to himself, John waited until the waterman had cast off, then stepped out of his hiding place to await the next hire boat that passed, delighted that Juliette was going to so public a place. For the Gardens she was about to visit were open to all. However they had enjoyed a somewhat checkered career in their time and it was still not considered *bon ton* for a young lady to be seen there alone with a gentleman, a fact which amused John considerably.

Originally started in 1691 by Boyder Cuper and situated on the south bank of the Thames in Lambeth, almost directly opposite Somerset House, Cuper's Gardens had been taken over in 1738 by Ephraim Evans, landlord of the famous Hercules Pillars. Evans had made many improvements including the erection of an orchestra stand, but unfortunately had died in 1740, when his spirited wife, known generally as The Widow, had taken over the running of the place. However, accusations had been made that the premises were often host to scenes of low dissipation and, in 1753, The Widow had not been granted a licence to open. Nothing daunted, she had continued to trade as a tea garden in conjunction with The Feathers, a waterside tavern connected to the grounds. Now, or so John had been led to believe, evening entertainments were to be held once more, though only for subscribers. But during the day the public at large were admitted, to roam the pleasant walks and woodlands or to sit in the arbours and drink bottled ale. None the less, Cuper's Gardens still maintained something of a seedy reputation and John felt highly intrigued by the choice of Juliette's rendezvous, for that, he felt certain, was what it was going to prove to be.

As he boarded his own wherry, the Apothecary could just see hers coming in to land at the ornamental jetty, complete with a little rotunda built beside it in which passengers could sit to watch the view or wait for their transport. However, safely moored,

Juliette ignored the pavilion, and the last glimpse John had of her was hurrying up the steps through the trees towards the entrance. Laying a small wager with himself about whom she was meeting, he followed at a leisurely pace.

Having paid his shilling entry fee, the Apothecary turned away from the main promenade, strolling the less well trodden walkways instead, and it wasn't long before his intuition was rewarded. Walking hand in hand, earnestly engaged in conversation and coming towards him, though they had not as yet seen who he was, were none other than Juliette and her companion.

'I was right!' said John out loud. He swept his hat from his head and gave a bow that would not have disgraced a court ballroom. 'Miss Hartfield, I do declare. And Lady Almeria, what a great pleasure. Why, I have not seen you since we were all at Marble Hall together.' He twitched his brows flirtatiously and smiled in debonair fashion. 'You're in fine looks, Miss Juliette, if I may say so. In fact I would go so far as to say that you grow a little lovelier each time I see you.' John's brows worked at double speed and he gave the slightest suspicion of a wink. 'I feel that it is high time we furthered our acquaintanceship. May I walk with you?'

Juliette flushed a deep angry red and when she spoke her voice was husky. 'Alas, it is not convenient today, Mr Rawlings. Lady Almeria and I have much to discuss.'

The Apothecary ran his eyes over Julian's sweetheart, taking in her determined mouth and tough little features.

'My lady, I throw myself on your mercy,' he said to her appealingly. 'How can I ever press my suit with Miss Hartfield? She is always in the midst of a merry throng and never has time for me. And I so long to be alone with her.'

Juliette was going redder by the second and John fought against a wild desire to laugh.

Lady Almeria seemed lost for words. 'I'm sorry . . .' she murmured.

'And so you should be,' the Apothecary answered, wagging a roguish finger. 'You ladies! Oh, how cruel are all your jests.'

'Are you drunk?' asked Juliette hoarsely.

'Yes,' John replied wildly. 'Intoxicated with your beauty and your charm. Oh Juliette, grant me the bliss of just one small kiss. Oh, fairest flower, be mine for an hour.'

'He's gone off his head.' Lady Almeria had found her tongue at last and was now glaring at the Apothecary furiously. She linked her arm through Juliette's. 'Come along, my dear, let's tarry no longer with this idiot. Why, I think he could be dangerous.'

John allowed his eyes to make full contact with the twin's. 'Oh yes, I could be very dangerous indeed,' he said softly, far from laughing.

Juliette's face contorted as she pulled a smile from somewhere. 'I'm sorry if I have upset you, Sir. I did not intend to do so but, alas, I am in no mood for frivolity today. Why don't you go and join my brother Roger? He announced his intention of visiting The Folly this afternoon in order to gamble. Perhaps his spirits might be more in tune with your own.'

The Apothecary bowed. The battle was his and he was now certain of everything that so far had only been conjecture. He could afford to be magnanimous.

'Then I'll bid you *adieu*, ladies, and hope that you enjoy the rest of your day,' he said politely, and, turning round, walked to the river without once looking back over his shoulder, very well aware that two pairs of anxious eyes were following his every move.

Close by Cuper's Bridge, the name given to the ornamental landing stage that led to the Gardens, was moored the most extraordinary vessel. It consisted of a large barge on which had been built a one-storeyed saloon, complete with a profusion of windows. The roof of this curious houseboat was formed by a deck platform surrounded by a balustrade, at the four angles of which stood a sizeable turret, another tower bearing a flag in the centre. Thus the whole whimsical structure gave the appearance of a floating castle and was known throughout London as The Folly. Created soon after the Restoration of Charles II, it was originally intended as a musical summer house for the entertainment of quality folk. But this delightful notion had been sadly dashed. Every whore, strumpet and draggle-tail in town had soon seen off the ladies of the *beau monde* and now it had become a centre for low class amorous intrigues and assignations, a rendezvous for illicit liaisons.

Yet, this decline in its fortunes had at least made the Folly available for poorer people, so that apprentice lads and their sweethears could afford to row there for an evening's amusement. Further, there was still some good gambling to be had at the Golden Gaming Table. While the long-sworded bullies who were the Folly's regular clientele, actually enjoyed being crowded together in the boxes and compartments of the saloon, smoking, swearing and drinking burnt brandy. So despite its rakish reputation and debauched atmosphere, The Folly did well enough for custom. And John, who had only been to the place once in his life, welcomed the excuse of spying on Roger which necessitated his going there.

Even though the notorious boat was only a few yards from Cuper's Bridge, there was no other way to travel than by water. Thus, John hired a wherry and was rowed towards it, an astonished grin crossing his features as he approached. For every doxy on the upper deck was scrutinising him, some leaning low over the parapet to call out, others dancing together yet watching him all the while, one lifting her skirt to give him a glimpse of a red garter. Shaking his head and calling out that he was in a hurry, John clambered up the gang plank and plunged within, wondering how long it would be before the more persistent of their number wandered down to find him.

Inside the saloon, all was total chaos. Booths were crammed with harlots and drunks, smoke from a hundred pipes choked the air, waiters sweated and fought to get round the tables, the smell of burnt brandy filled the nostrils, fighting for supremacy over all the other odious stinks. It was like a scene from hell and John was seriously wondering whether he really wanted to subject himself to it when he saw, not Roger, but Julian Hartfield, sitting at the Golden Gaming Table, white to the gills and obviously losing. So here was luck indeed, both the twins in one afternoon. Determined to add victory to triumph, the Apothecary, using elbows and feet, bucked his way through the mêlée.

'My dear Julian,' he said loudly, coming up unheard behind his quarry.

The twin jumped violently and peered over his shoulder. 'Oh, Mr Rawlings, it's you. The last person I would have expected to see. Whatever is a man of your profession doing in a hovel like this?'

'I might well ask the same of you.'

'Oh, I'm just whiling away a few hours with a little dice.'

'And I am continuing my studies.'

'Studies?' asked Julian, his voice squeaking. 'Into what?'

'Human nature and all its vagaries. Tell me, are you winning?'

'Not as yet. Perhaps you will change my luck.'

'Oh I wouldn't count on that,' John answered cheerfully. 'In fact,

I do believe that nowadays I am considered to be quite the bird of ill omen.'

A muscle twitched in Julian's beautiful face. 'Oh? Why is that?'

'I think it has something to do with the investigation into your father's death. I imagine that the killer thinks I am drawing ever nearer to him.'

'And are you?' Julian asked, throwing a dice.

'I am certainly close to unravelling several mysteries.' John took the seat next to Julian's, vacated by a rakehell who had just fallen onto the floor.

'Really?' said the twin, in a voice so deliberately casual that the Apothecary smiled to himself.

'Yes, really. Now, concentrate on your play. We cannot have you losing everything.'

'No.' Julian looked tense.

'But smile as you do so. Remember that a gentleman forfeits his money with ease and negligence, that is according to my friend the Masked Lady.'

Julian glanced up. 'Serafina de Vignolles? Do you know her?'

'Very well indeed. The only female in living memory who could take on the opposite sex at both cards and dice and beat them at what they believed to be their own game.'

'Why should women not be able to play as well as men?' Julian asked defensively.

'There is no reason,' John answered, his tone cheerful, 'except that, perhaps, they do not get as much practice. However, there are those unfortunates, presumably of both sexes, who simply have no talent for gambling and end up by blowing out their brains, in debt to the house for all they have staked.'

Julian shuddered. 'What an unpleasant thought.'

'Very. So be careful, my friend.'

'Are you saying that I might do such a thing? Never, I tell you.'

The Apothecary looked the twin straight in the eye. 'Just watch the path that you are treading, that is all. Often the most apparently innocent pastime can lead one into deep waters, believe me.'

Having delivered this dramatic warning and been rewarded by Julian's terrified stare, John stood up to go, but at that moment his gaze was caught by someone at the far end of the saloon. Having again abandoned mourning and resplendent in a dazzling coat, full mounted, fashioned in blossom-coloured velvet trimmed with gold lace, a gold waistcoat with purple spots beneath, breeches of delicate lilac hue completing the ensemble, Roger had just stamped his high-heeled way into the saloon and was staring about him to see if anyone he knew was aboard.

John waved, murmuring to Julian meanwhile, 'Why, there's your brother.'

The twin looked frantic, scrambling to his feet and forfeiting his turn. 'Oh great God, he mustn't see me. How can I get out?'

'There's a staircase over there which seems to lead to the deck. But why do you have to hurry away? He can't object to you indulging in play, surely?'

Julian did not answer, instead rushing madly for the stairs, on which he collided with two dollscommon coming down to see what custom they could drum up. John recognised one of them as the owner of the garters.

'Hello, my fine young buck,' she called.

The Apothecary hesitated, wanting to observe Roger unseen but equally having no wish to fall into the girl's clutches. In the end he decided that a tactical withdrawal was the only way. Waiting until Roger had stopped at a booth to chat to an acquaintance, he hurried past, his hat well down. Then, going to the top of the gangplank, John hailed a boatman from the many clustered around the houseboat.

'Where to, Sir?' asked the wherryman.

'Anywhere round here where we can watch the Folly but not be seen ourselves.'

The man nodded, unperturbed.

'I'm spying on a dog whom I believe to be dallying with my sweetheart,' John added by way of clarification. 'When he appears I want to pursue him to his destination and see what he's about. I'm sorry this is such an unusual request but there it is.'

The wherryman shrugged. 'Nothing unusual about it, you're the third this week, duke. Look, best I drop you at Cuper's so that you can sit in the pavilion in comfort. Then, as soon as the fellow shows up I'll come and get you.'

'But you don't know what he looks like.'

'I'm used to this,' the wherryman said briefly. 'Just describe him to me and he won't slip through my net.'

'As a matter of curiosity,' the Apothecary asked, intrigued, 'what happened to the other two fares?'

The wherryman laughed. 'Oh, the first one killed his rival as soon as they were put ashore at Tothill Fields. The second indulged in fisticuffs and gave his opponent as sound a thrashing as I've seen in many a day. I had my money on him and won handsomely off the other watermen who had come to watch. Sadly though, the man who was done away with was my passenger so I had no one to row home that night. But he was a gentleman and had paid me in advance.'

John was both amused and amazed. 'So following people is not uncommon?'

'An everyday occurrence, duke.'

Whether that was true or a piece of waterfolk's lore, the Apothecary could not be certain. But in the event he was glad to while away his time in the rotunda, consuming refreshments brought by waiters from the Gardens and conversing with other people waiting for transport, until, some hours later, his waterman appeared with much swishing of oars and winking of eyes. John immediately leapt to his feet and got aboard the boat, whispering, 'Where is he?'

'He's heading up river. Just in front of us. Take a look.'

John did so, wrapping his cloak round him and pulling down his hat, and feeling excitingly like a spy. Sure enough, Roger was in the wherry ahead, sitting perched high on the seat, the skirts of his coat spread neatly around him.

'So he's going back into town,' the Apothecary muttered to himself, and felt a quiver of disappointment that Roger was probably returning to St James's Square and that all his efforts had been wasted.

But having crossed to the north bank, the beau's wherry did not put in at Hungerford Stairs nor, indeed, at White Hall, the two obvious places for someone making for the area of St James's. Instead, Roger disembarked at Manchester Stairs, the landing place for those going in the direction of St James's Park.

An extraordinary idea took root in John's mind as his wherry slid smartly to a halt by the landing steps. And, having tipped the laconic waterman well and assured him that there wasn't going to be a fight worth watching, it grew even stronger as he mounted the Stairs in Roger's wake.

'It simply *can't* be,' John said to himself. But as he strode hastily along, never losing sight of the flamboyant figure hurrying ahead of him, he grew more and more convinced that the highly unlikely was about to prove to be the answer after all.

Chapter Twenty-Two

*T*he sun was just beginning to plunge behind the trees of St James's Park as John entered the noisesome confines of George Yard, certain that he knew where he was going but still hardly able to believe the proof his eyes were giving him. Ahead scurried Roger, using his beribboned cane to help him achieve greater pace. No rampant buck could rush to his mistress with greater despatch, John thought, marvelling at it all.

From the Stairs, John's unsuspecting quarry had cut down to Bridge Street, crossed King Street, and was now in the labyrinth of alleys that lay beyond the park's southernmost boundary. Keeping out of sight, the Apothecary had followed Roger all the way, growing more incredulous with every step. Yet by now there could be no doubt. The great beau was turning left through a mean twitten, a route which could only lead him to Queen Street.

'You duplicitous cull,' said John, and suppressed a hoot of laughter.

Roger entered Queens Square and having looked round, almost as if he were aware that he was being observed, went to Amelia's front door and let himself in with a key, an action that left the Apothecary gaping.

So this was an established liaison, he thought in amazement. Well, I'll give them an hour and then go back and see what they have to say for themselves. And this decision made, John retraced his steps and went to the Blue Boar's Head Inn, situated within the same maze of alleyways that he had just traversed.

As things turned out, the lovers had slightly longer on their own, the Apothecary having been drawn into a discussion about perfumes, a subject dear to his heart. The instigator of the conversation was a Frenchman, a handsome devil, in London to visit the great Charles Lillie, or so he said. Having heard that John was that rare thing, an apothecary who enjoyed experimentation into other related spheres, including the blending of fine scents, he begged leave to visit Shug Lane, and John gladly gave him his card. In this way, the Apothecary set off to interview the couple in rather a more tolerant frame of mind than he would have possessed normally.

As always, the sluttish maid answered the door. But even as she opened her mouth to speak, John forestalled her.

'I have come to see Miss Lambourn and Mr Hartfield and I will not be gainsayed by you or anyone else. Just tell them I am here and await them below.' And, so saying, he pushed past her and into the hall.

'You can't do that,' she screeched.

'I've done it,' answered John. He raised his voice. 'Mr Hartfield, this is John Rawlings. I have come to see you and Miss Lambourn on the business of Mr Fielding. Please be so good as to come downstairs.'

From the floor above came the sound of a startled shriek followed by the muffled tones of a male voice, this followed by a long silence, broken at last by the thud of steps on the staircase. John looked up and drew breath at the awesome sight of Roger, clad in a glistening scarlet turban and robe, making his way downward.

It was then, and only then, that the Apothecary had his first true sight of the other side of the great beau, a sight that he had glimpsed momentarily at Islington Spa, even though on that occasion Roger's heavy lids had suddenly concealed his eyes from John's inquisitive gaze. Now he saw that beneath the beautiful clothes and elegant wigs, the perfumed powder and the ornate jewellery, lurked something else. A sensual gluttony, an immense immorality, a grand licentiousness that was almost to be admired. Flamboyant and effeminate he might be, but for all that Roger seemed quite capable of making a woman fall in love with him. In the face of such deplorable depravity, John was silenced.

Roger took the initiative. 'So,' he said, with a careless shrug of a silk-clad shoulder, 'my secret is out, is it?'

The Apothecary recovered his composure. 'It has been out a while, in a sense. I have been aware for quite some time that Miss Lambourn had somebody else beside your father. Whilst Samuel Swann got an inkling of a hidden side to you at Sir William's funeral.'

'Did he now?' The beau poured himself a sherry and offered a glass to John. 'Then I must give him credit for his perception.'

'But though I agreed with him, I am frankly amazed that you

turned out to be Amelia's lover, Roger – you did ask me to call you that, if you remember.'

'Why? Because you thought me of another persuasion? How tiresome of you, John. Have you not heard of people who make their own rules when it comes to passion? I may be a frivolous, empty-headed profligate who squanders his life away at the gaming tables and other trivial pastimes, but let me assure you that my saving grace is a love of beauty.'

'I see.'

'No, you don't. Not at all. What I am trying to say to you is that I care not what form that beauty takes, in what body it is housed. Now do you understand me?'

'Of course I do,' John answered wryly. 'You are bi-sexual.'

'What a hideous word! And to admit such a thing would be to fall foul of the law. Let us leave it that I am a connoisseur of all that is fine regardless of its place of origin.'

The ruthless streak that the Apothecary usually suppressed, gained foothold. 'And does this elegance of judgement balk at murder in order to obtain its desires?'

Roger swallowed his sherry and poured himself another, the hand holding the decanter shaking very slightly. 'And what the devil do you mean by that?'

'I mean that your sexual mores are entirely your affair. I am not here to pass judgement on those. My concern is the investigation of a killing, the killing of *your father*, lest you had forgotten.'

Roger groaned and rolled his eyes, slumping back in his chair, the gorgeously turbaned head lolling slightly, giving it a strange puppet-like look. Then there was an eruption in the doorway as Amelia Lambourn flew in like a fury and rushed to her lover's side.

'There, now look what you've gone and done. He's come over faint! How could you, you heartless wretch?'

'No, no,' said Roger, reviving noisily and motioning her away. 'I'm perfectly all right. Don't make such a fuss.'

There was a silence during which Amelia, very pink in the cheeks but still displaying that fragile loveliness which set her apart from other young women of her background, gave Roger a fraught look. He returned it with a glance which John found inscrutable. Amelia, however, obviously read the signs for she let out a deep sigh and sank to the floor to sit at Roger's feet. He gently patted her head and the very movement spoke volumes. The beau could have been stroking anything, a pedigree hound, a handsome cat, a beautiful youth, or the woman with whom he had committed an act of enormous folly, it really was all one and the same to him. Yet again, John was consumed by a grudging respect for the blatant immorality of the man.

'You had better tell me everything,' he said. 'And I do mean *everything*.'

'We met five years ago,' said Roger, after consuming yet more sherry. 'I was thirty, Amelia ten years younger. I was involved with a group of bright young blades at the time – we called ourselves the Whisker-Splitters, as I remember it. In fact I was at Islington Spa with them that very night. Anyway, I saw Amelia and was so taken with her that I thought of her all next day. She became, for me, the butterfly that I had to have in my collection. To cut the tale short, I went back and captured her.'

'But surely Lady Hartfield was alive at that time?'

'Yes.'

'Well then, how did Sir William become involved?'

Roger actually laughed. 'I devised a plan to stop the poor old goat being so mournful. I thought that if he fell in love with Amelia he would cease to be so wretched and miserable. After all it wasn't easy for him, living with an invalid wife.'

'That has to be one of the most sinful statements I have ever heard.'

Roger laughed again. 'Oh don't be so pompous! It was not the credo of the Whisker-Splitters to be moralistic. Anyway, Amelia consented to the plan and I took my father to the Spa and introduced them. He fell in love with the girl at first sight and after a dignified courtship asked her to be his mistress.'

'Whilst remaining yours at the same time?'

'Certainly. A very erotic situation.'

'You are beyond redemption.'

'Yes,' said Roger, quite seriously. 'I truly believe that I am.'

'Everything was all right till Sir William asked me to marry him,' Amelia put in, her accent grating after her lover's cultured tones.

'So why, in God's name, did you say yes to him? Purely for material gain, I suppose?'

'Not quite,' answered Roger. 'To be honest with you I didn't have a mind for wedding myself. We Whisker-Splitters believed in roaming freely, taking our pleasures when and how we liked. Marriage did not enter into our thinking.'

'So?'

'So Amelia and I thought that we would give the old man a last few years of happiness with a young and beautiful bride.'

'With plenty of money for you both to squander and your own little arrangement unaffected.'

'Quite right.'

'Have you no shame?' John asked, torn once again between disgust and an awful sense of sneaking regard for such totally unprincipled behaviour.

'None at all,' Roger answered cheerfully. 'Do have another sherry.'

'One moment,' said the Apothecary, raising a staying hand. 'I have two more questions to ask you. The first is, have either of you ever heard a rumour that Sir William was being blackmailed?'

Amelia looked uncomfortable and stole another glance at Roger, who nodded. 'Yes, I have, and it was true. He told me so himself,' she said haltingly.

'But why. What was it all about?'

'Somebody was threatening to reveal the fact that he had a mistress to his fellow merchants. A terrible thing to him because he liked to appear respectable. You see, I think Sir William wanted to rise high in the world of commerce, perhaps become a man of some distinction. I don't really understand these things, but I do know that someone was making him pay to keep silent about me.'

'But he was just about to marry you so what was the point?'

'The blackmailer started to threaten while my mother was still alive,' Roger answered drily.

'I shall be reporting all this back to John Fielding, of course,' said John, trying to sound stern.

Roger instantly sprang to his feet and a large hand flapped. 'My dear, of course you will be. That is your duty, is it not?'

'Yes.'

'Well, it should certainly give the Beak something to think about. A respectable family man like him.'

John managed a smile. 'Tell me, what will the two of you do now?'

'In what regard?'

'Well, Amelia has been left penniless, while you have a share in a business, to say nothing of a considerable fortune. So who's going to keep the young lady now? Or is she going back to Islington Spa? What say the Whisker-Splitters to that little conundrum?'

Miss Lambourn turned an enquiring face to her lover. 'Yes, Roger. What *do* they say?'

'Er . . .' answered the great beau.

'Good night,' murmured John, and bowed his way out.

Chapter Twenty-Three

*H*is usual energy sapped by the day's events yet his mind teeming with all the extraordinary things he had learned, John had walked slowly home through the green of St James's Park, seeing none of its beauty, not even noticing the contentedly grazing cows who dwelled there, all of whom had looked up as he passed, mooed at him, then gone on eating. Almost in a trance, the Apothecary had made his way round the park's long pond and cut into Pall Mall, then turned off towards The Hay Market and Nassau Street. But there his reverie had been rudely interrupted. Benjamin Rudge, twitching with anxiety, was still awaiting him, not consoled at all by Sir Gabriel's assurances that it was highly unlikely his son had come to any harm.

'God's sweet life, Mr Rawlings. I'd almost given you up for dead,' he exclaimed as John walked into the library. 'I've been waiting for word since this afternoon.'

'I'm sorry, Mr Rudge, I really am, but there was no way I could communicate with you. One trail led to another and so it went on. But now I am all done, quite literally.' And he sank into a chair.

'Is there anything I should report to Mr Fielding?' asked the Runner, standing up, a slightly peevish expression on his face.

'Perhaps you could tell him that I will call on him tomorrow. There is so much to say that I think I should recount it personally.'

Rudge looked even more put out and Sir Gabriel said tactfully, 'What time will this be, John? Mr Rudge will obviously need to be there and it would be easier to tell him now.'

'Would eight o'clock be too early?' the Apothecary asked contritely.

'No, Sir, I am sure that will be in order,' Rudge said stiffly.

'Then I shall see you tomorrow and I do apologise again for your long and boring wait.' The Runner went out and John pulled a face at his father. 'Oh dear, he is not well pleased.'

'It can't be helped. Now, my dear child, tell me everything.'

What a pleasure it was, John thought, to sit in the familiar and well-loved confines of his favourite room and recount the story of the remarkable happenings of the last few hours to someone whose acute mind he considered equalled only by that of the Blind Beak. Indeed, even Sir Gabriel's sagacious nods were encouraging and the Apothecary warmed to his tale, finishing it with the words, 'Well, what do you think?'

'About the twins?'

'Yes.'

'That you are perfectly right.'

'But could their jinket have a more baleful purpose?'

'Indeed it could. I would watch them both very carefully.'

'And speaking of watching people, may I ask you another great favour, my very dear Father.'

'You want me to go to Kirby Hall again.'

'I do. Merely to observe the doings of the three weird women who inhabit it. I am sure you cannot find out their whereabouts at the time Kitty Perkins died, without arousing suspicion. However, any information would be useful.'

'I shall call on them the day after tomorrow in order to pay my respects.'

'Many thanks. Now, what do you make of Roger?'

'Much as I had thought, though I must confess I am surprised that he has turned out to be Amelia's lover.'

'He has collected her, so he says. He is an admirer of loveliness – in *all* its forms – and she proved irresistible.'

Sir Gabriel laughed robustly. 'What a blackguard.'

'Yes, but like the twins, could his longing for wealth and beauty have led him to kill?'

'More than likely,' said John's father matter-of-factly. 'Collectors – of anything – are known for their ruthlessness and eccentricity. Indeed, they are highly dangerous individuals, who would remove any obstacle in order to get their hands on the object of their desire.'

John nodded as the import of the words fully sank in, and with them the certainty that behind the mask of Roger's heavy-lidded eyes might well lurk a ruthless killer, prepared even to put down his own father in his search for perfection.

*   *   *

260

The Apothecary rose early the next morning and made a flying visit to Shug Lane to see that all was in order. For once he preceeded the redoubtable Nicholas, who came panting in some five minutes later with an extremely anxious expression on his face.

'Oh God's wounds, Mr Rawlings, I saw the door open and believed you had been robbed.'

'No, all's well. I just thought I ought to cast my eye over the place as I have a feeling I might be occupied elsewhere for the next several days.'

'Why, is the net closing round the villain?'

'I'd like to say yes,' John answered truthfully, 'but the fact remains that he or she still eludes me.' He changed the subject. 'Anyway, how is business? And what is Master Gerard like?'

'Old and pompous but full of interesting ideas and remedies. I've taken the liberty of writing some of them down.'

'Well done, I shall study those when I have a spare moment.'

'When,' said Nicholas, and smiled his thin-faced smile.

Walking very briskly, John reached Bow Street just as eight o'clock was striking and hurried in to find Mr Fielding awaiting him in his downstairs study. There was a fresh smell of lavender about the Magistrate this morning and John could see by a nick on his cheek that he had cut himself whilst shaving, a feat which he presumably accomplished by touch. Glad that he was looking smartly presentable even though he could not be seen, the Apothecary took a seat in the chair that the Blind Beak was indicating.

'I hear from Rudge that there is a great deal afoot,' said the Magistrate, not wasting time on pleasantries.

'Yes,' answered John, and started to describe all that had transpired.

The Blind Beak sat silently, the black eye cover turned towards the speaker, his hands motionless on the desk in front of him. Finally he nodded and said, 'You are proceeding apace, I believe.'

John shook his head. 'I don't feel as if I am. If anything, everything seems more confusing than it did at first.'

'Not at all. Continue as you are doing and very soon now you will find the link that connects the person concerned to the two murders.'

'I am glad you are so confident, Sir. I wish that I thought the same.'

The Magistrate's hands ran over the desk, feeling the various bits of paper that lay upon it. Eventually he identified one and handed it across the space between them.

'I received a letter last night from the constable in Wapping, an excellent fellow by the sound of it. He was checking that you were indeed working for the Public Office, a thorough move. Further he informed me that the funeral of Kitty Perkins takes place tomorrow. I thought you should attend.'

The Apothecary glanced at the piece of paper and saw that even though it was written in a somewhat ill-formed hand, it none the less asked all the right questions and contained every bit of relevant information regarding the laying to rest of one deceased oyster girl.

'As you say, Sir, a conscientious chap, this one.'

'It strikes me, my friend, that you would do well to go to Wapping straight away. Perhaps you might be able to have further words with Mr Randolph, or even Hugh. Take Rudge with you and see what the pair of you can discover.'

John smiled. 'You seem very keen on the Runner accompanying me everywhere. Is it your intention that he should act as my protector?'

'Yes,' said Mr Fielding bluntly, 'it is. You are too close to the murderer for comfort, as the saying goes. I want him there if anything untoward should happen.'

'A very kind thought.'

'Kind and practical,' answered the Blind Beak. He held out his hand. 'Now I must bid you adieu, Mr Rawlings. The court is sitting early today. Rudge is waiting in the Public Office, keen as a hound for an adventure.'

'Then I'll see how he fares on the waterway.'

'Yes. Good luck to you. Watch carefully at the burial. Oh, and by the way . . .'

'Yes, Sir?'

'Take the great stick with you and show it around. See if anyone can identify its owner.'

'Did Joe find anything on it?'

'No, it had all been washed away by the river. But do your best.'

'I will, Sir.' And with that assurance, John collected the stick and went off to find Benjamin Rudge, hoping that the Runner would be in a better mood than when he saw him last.

As it turned out a good night's sleep had done wonders for the man, and he greeted the Apothecary with enthusiasm.

'Good morning, Mr Rawlings. And where are we bound for today?'

'To Wapping, at Mr Fielding's suggestion. I am to attend the funeral of Kitty Perkins tomorrow, something I would have wanted to do anyway. However, I must go home first and collect my black clothes and an overnight bag.'

'I'll take you there in the carriage then I'll do the same.'

'Shall we meet at Hungerford Stairs in an hour?'

'Indeed we shall.'

'Oh, Rudge . . .'

'Yes, Sir?'

'Would it be possible to get a note round to Samuel Swann in St Paul's Churchyard? I rather think he might like to be at the burial.'

'If you can scribble it out, Mr Rawlings, I'll get one of the others to take it.'

'Good,' said John, and plunged into an hour of frantic activity.

It was almost a relief to take to the river again, even though the Apothecary had spent a great deal of time either on or near the water on the previous day. In fact so soothing was its influence that John found himself thinking yet again about a house near the Thames in years to come, a daydream that was becoming ever more important to him. Rudge, too, started to grin and relax, making John wonder just how effective he would be as a guard should trouble shortly break out. But all was calm as they climbed Pelican Stairs and headed into The Devil's Tavern, where the Apothecary booked two rooms for the night before taking a boat across to Redriff, or more specifically The Spread Eagle, in order to enquire the whereabouts of Valentine Randolph's lodging. On this occasion, John quite deliberately left Rudge behind, the Runner's task ostensibly to find out exactly where the late Sir William Hartfield's office was situated. In reality because another's presence might well inhibit Valentine should it come to an honest discussion.

The mudlark, who was washing up in preparation for the onslaught of custom due at any moment, greeted him with enthusiasm. 'How are you m'dear old duke? I see you've brought me stick back, you goodly fellow.'

John smiled but shook his head. 'I'm afraid you can't have it yet. I've got to show it around first. See if anyone knows who owns it.'

Fred looked crestfallen. 'Oh.'

'And I'd like to start with Mr Randolph. Have you any idea where he lodges?'

'Yes, he's with the Widow Greenhill, the end house in Elephant Lane. It's painted blue and white. Used to belong to Captain Greenhill who drowned at sea.'

'I should be able to find that easily enough.'

'I hope you can cos I ain't coming with yer. Remember what happened last time?'

'Only too clearly.'

'Anyway Mr Valentine won't be home yet. He generally rows across about six o'clock.'

'Then I'll come back.'

'Aren't you staying for a drink?'

'Not at the moment. I need to keep a clear head.'

Yet this wasn't quite true. In fact John wanted to go back to St Mary's and stroll about the churchyard, conjecturing what had happened on the night Sir William had gone to meet the blackmailer and instead had met his end by the grave of poor Elizabeth Wells, plucked from the cruel world at the age of fifteen. For, though they could never be quite certain, Joe Jago, after examining the scrapings of dried blood and the sad white hairs taken from the gravestone, had concluded with John that this had probably been the place where the dying man had fallen, never again to rise.

A glance at his watch told John that it was five o'clock and he turned his steps in the direction of The Spread Eagle, in order to watch Church Stairs for the return of Valentine Randolph. A balcony outside provided the ideal spot and it did not seem too long before a dot on the river grew larger and John recognised the long lean form and hawklike features of Sir William's office manager, dressed in sensible grey worsted, and rowing himself back home after a day at work. Keeping very still, the Apothecary watched Valentine moor his boat and make his way slowly up the stone steps. The man knew the river backwards, that much was obvious, and John thought back to the occasion when Kitty had called out that she had seen someone she recognised in a strange place, thus bringing about her own cruel death. That she knew exactly who Valentine was had been made clear on the night when John and Samuel had first met her. But surely all of the others must have been in Wapping at some time or another. Guilt did not necessarily rest on the shoulders of the local man. Glumly, John finished his drink, waited ten minutes, then followed Valentine Randolph to his lodging in the house of the Widow Greenhill.

He was shown into the downstairs parlour and a few moments later, the man he had come to see came through the door looking extremely puzzled.

'Oh, it's you,' he said.

'Yes. I do apologise for calling without prior warning. The fact is that Mr Fielding has asked me to speak to one or two people about the death of Kitty Perkins, the oyster girl. You knew her of course.'

'Yes, I did.'

'And you realise that somebody has killed her?'

'Yes. Redriff is a village, Mr Rawlings, and Wapping is too in its way. Everyone is talking about the girl's terrible end.'

'Did you also know there is a strong possibility her murder was connected to that of Sir William?'

Valentine Randolph looked astonished. 'No. That hadn't occurred to me.'

John decided that it was time to stop mincing words. 'Listen, Mr Randolph, let me warn you that you are in a very hazardous position. You were in Redriff on the night Sir William was murdered, and at the right time too. Further, you were with a possible accomplice. There is talk of blackmail flying about, money being extorted by someone who knew the dead man's private affairs. It seems to me that as far as your involvement is concerned, there are too many coincidences to be overlooked.'

Valentine gave him a bitter glance. 'And would he then have chosen me to be his bridegroom's witness? If I had been fleecing him all those years, would Sir William have asked me to stand up for him?'

'Quite true. But then, of course, Lydia Hartfield might have been the blackmailer and you could well have killed your employer to protect your mistress and her guilt.'

Valentine went white and his hand flew in the air as if he were going to land a blow. 'Don't call her that! How dare you do so! I am in love with that woman. I would give my life for her.'

'Be calm,' said John soothingly, wondering if he was going to have to defend himself, here in Widow Greenhill's parlour, full of pieces of delicate china and breakable little knicknacks. 'Think rationally. Admit that things do not look good for the pair of you.'

'I've already told you what happened that night.'

'But you've only told me half of it! The truth is that you met Lydia Hartfield wandering about, as were you. Then you took her to The Angel and there made love to her. That's what really happened, isn't it?'

Valentine sank onto the sofa, suddenly deflated. 'Yes.'

'So how did you know that she hadn't just killed a man when you came across her by the river? Or perhaps you *did* know. Mr Randolph, when I first met Miss Lambourn she told me that you had written to her, informing her of Sir William's death.'

'So?'

'There was a discrepancy in the timing of that letter. If what she said was true, you had written it *before* Luke Challon came to your office to tell you what had occurred. So how did you know that Sir William was dead? Was it because either you or Lydia, or both of you, had killed him?'

Valentine made a terrible retching sound. 'No! I swear it! The fact is that I never went to sleep that night at all, and left Lydia before dawn. I told you the truth about my movements, except that I lied about coming home. In reality, after I had checked at The Spread Eagle that Sir William had not spent the night there, I went straight to work, despite the earliness of the hour. As I rowed across to Wapping, a waterman came alongside, a man I knew well by sight. He told me of his grisly errand, to fetch a body from The Devil's Tavern and take it to the Coroner. When he described the corpse to me – he came from Redriff incidentally and would not have known Sir William – a terrible thought came to me. Then, when the bridegroom did not come to church, I guessed the ghastly truth, though I had no idea that the poor man had been murdered. I wrote to Amelia out of basic humanity, longing to remove from her the burden of having been jilted.'

'I see,' John answered quietly.

'Now I've told you everything.'

The Apothecary nodded, as if in agreement. 'Then I will take my leave. There is clearly nothing more to say.' He picked up the cane, still lying on the floor. 'By the way, is this yours?' he added casually.

The office manager shook his head.

'Then to whom does it belong? Have you ever seen it before?'

Valentine's lips tightened and his entire face became mask-like. 'No,' he said. 'I've never set eyes on it in my life.'

'Thank you,' answered John, and left the house, acutely aware that for reasons of his own, Valentine Randolph was once again lying through his teeth.

Obviously determined to enjoy himself, Runner Rudge had changed into a fancy waistcoat and black breeches by the time John returned to The Devil's Tavern that evening, to say nothing of having already consumed several pints of ale in preparation for a jolly time ahead.

'Ah, Mr Rawlings,' he said jovially, slapping the Apothecary on the back with a fist like a side of gammon. 'I'm glad to see you've returned safely. Otherwise it would have meant organising a search party.'

Not knowing whether to be irritated or amused, John kept his tone light. 'No need for that, Mr Rudge, I assure you. I wouldn't like to think that I can't go out without causing you worry.'

'You're my responsibility, Sir. That's how I look on you.'

'Well, give me certain freedoms, please do. Otherwise, like a naughty child, I might well run away.'

Rudge seemed to think this was terribly funny and clapped John on the back again.

'What would you like to drink, Sir?'

'A glass of good claret, please.'

'It shall be yours.'

So saying, the officer of the law pushed his way to the pewter bar, supported on its base of barrels, to stand shoulder to shoulder with the waterside lowlife who crowded the inn that evening. It was then, looking round for somewhere to go, that John spotted Luke Challon, sitting by himself as usual, looking on the verge of both tears and suicide. With a sudden surge of compassion, the Apothecary went over to join him.

'Luke, how are you? The last time I saw you you were fighting on this very floor.'

Sir William's secretary looked up and John saw that he had indeed been weeping. 'A bitter day that was, too,' he answered bleakly.

'You lost your employment through it?'

'Aye, it was a family decision that I should go.'

'Really?'

'Well, Roger is nominally now head of the Hartfields, but gives not a damn as long as he is left alone to pursue his perversions . . .'

Knowing Luke's adoration of Amelia, John gave an inward shudder.

'. . . but, anyway, he agreed. I have lost not only a job but also a home. I lived wherever Sir William did, you see.'

'What were your future plans, had this not happened?'

'I had hoped to stay on and work for the three brothers.'

'Have you no parents?'

'My father is a member of the impoverished minor nobility. I was his tenth child. He was only too delighted to see me make my way in the world and certainly couldn't afford to take me back now.'

'An ugly situation.'

'Fortunately, Sir William left me a small bequest which I shall receive in due course.'

'So what are you going to do meanwhile?'

'Valentine Randolph is hoping to find me another situation. He knows several merchant ship owners and is making enquiries amongst them. He is also trying to find me lodgings in Redriff. Meanwhile, I am living here, in the tavern.'

'Good gracious, I wouldn't have thought the place to have held happy memories for you.' John lowered his voice. 'Did you know that Kitty Perkins is dead?'

Luke looked uncomfortable. 'I never actually met her. Was she the girl who called something out while I was fighting?'

'Yes, that's the one. Did you hear what she said, incidentally?'

'No, not really. Something about somebody being somewhere?'

John smiled ruefully, aware that he was going to get nowhere with this particular line of questioning, then he remembered the stick that he still held in his hand. He held it out so that the handle was only an inch or so from Luke Challon's face.

'Tell me, have you ever seen this before?' he asked.

'I certainly have,' Luke answered promptly.

'Then whose is it?'

'Oh, surely you know. There's only one person who could own an ornate thing like that.'

'And who might it be?' said John, already guessing the answer.

'Why, the great beau himself. Roger Hartfield, of course,' Luke replied with a laugh, and drained his glass to the dregs.

Chapter Twenty-Four

*T*he skies wept on the day of Kitty Perkins's funeral. The Apothecary, waking early, looked out of the window of his attic bedroom to see that the Thames was swollen and grey, rushing at full spate, sheets of rain, so heavy that they appeared almost solid, adding to its volume. Cursing silently that he had not brought his umbrella with him, an invention from the Orient yet to become popular with the majority, John dressed in his black clothes, and went downstairs.

Yet for once the mighty breakfast served at The Devil's Tavern had not tempted him, too full of thoughts of the oyster girl's fresh young beauty being laid in the earth to corrupt and putrefy and then to seethe with worms. Instead, John had contented himself with a slice of toast and several cups of coffee while he waited for Benjamin Rudge, sleeping off the effects of a heavy night's quaffing, and read a note from Samuel sadly regretting that he could not attend the burial as business called him out of town. Restlessly, the Apothecary decided that he could wait no longer, and having scribbled a message for the Runner, he put on his hat and cloak and stepped outside.

It was a terrible morning for a walk, yet John had felt an overwhelming urge to get out of the confines of the tavern and breathe the river air. Almost without knowing it, he found his feet taking him down Wapping High Street, that area of contrasts where warehouses and offices stood side-by-side with taverns, brothels, and dens in which narcotic intoxication caused by smoking the derivative of the white poppy took place.

While John had been in Redriff on the previous day, Rudge had tracked down the whereabouts of Sir William's office, and now, despite the earliness of the hour, the Apothecary decided to call there, confident that Valentine Randolph would already be at work, and thinking to make some excuse in order that he might have a look round. Yet as he climbed the staircase beside a ship-chandler's, the window stocked with intriguing maritime gear, John heard voices and wondered whether he was going to be lucky enough to come across Hugh, and indeed fortune favoured him, for as he climbed higher the Apothecary identified the voice of Sir William's third son.

'. . . all seems to be in order. The ship can take fans, gloves, dresses, in fact everything desired by the ladies of Jamaica . . .,' Hugh was saying, then stopped as John knocked at the door. 'Who is it?' he called.

'John Rawlings, Sir.'

'Ah, how very nice of you to call,' Hugh answered, and opened the door, a broad smile lighting his tidy features. His face changed. 'Thank God you're here,' he whispered. 'I must speak to you. The matter's urgent.' His voice resumed its normal pitch. 'Do step inside.'

'Are you sure I'm not interrupting?' the Apothecary asked politely.

'Not at all, not at all. Valentine and I were just deciding on our latest shipment.' And he indicated a large ledger which lay open on a desk situated by a bay window, the office manager hovering over it.

John looked round the large pleasant room and saw to his surprise that in a chair by the coal fire, lit to ward off the chills of the day, Maud sat, sipping coffee from a delicate bone china cup. She gave the Apothecary a freezing smile, said, 'You're about bright and early,' then turned her attention back to the flames.

Hugh signalled with his eyes. 'I wonder if you'd be so good as to step into my sanctum, Mr Rawlings. There is a matter I would discuss with you privately.'

Maud's cup rattled violently in its saucer and Valentine cleared his throat.

'By all means,' said John, horribly aware of the sudden tension in the air.

'Then if you would come this way,' and Hugh opened a door leading off to the right and ushered John through.

He was in a room not much bigger than a cubbyhole, most of the space taken up by a desk and chair. Maps of the world and a great globe occupied what was left, and it was with difficulty that John squeezed his way through to the stool that Hugh was indicating.

'Oh damme,' groaned Sir William's son, even before the Apothecary was seated, 'I know she is being unfaithful to me. Her behaviour is going from bad to worse. Why she was missing a whole night recently and when I challenged her with it, demanded to know where she had been, she gave some feeble explanation about a dying aunt.'

'You're speaking of your wife?' John asked cautiously.

'Of course I am. Even in my hour of need she was not there.'

'I'm afraid that you are going too fast for me, Mr Hartfield. Pray tell the story from the start.'

'You were present when I was involved in that terrible incident with Challon?' John nodded. 'Well, afterwards, when I was bruised and bleeding, I came back to this office to recover and hired a messenger to fetch her from Kirby Hall to tend me, and would you believe that she was not at home?'

'Perhaps Mrs Hartfield had gone to the town house.'

Hugh's voice choked on what sounded suspiciously like a sob. 'No, because I returned there that night, when I had composed myself, and she had not been seen in St James's Square all week.'

A thought occurred to John and he had put it into words before he could stop himself. 'Were you acquainted with an oyster girl called Kitty Perkins, by any chance?'

Hugh stared at him. 'What a strange question. Yes, I think I know who you're talking about. A pretty little soul with bright blue eyes.'

'Yes, that's her. Well, she was murdered on the very night of your disagreement with Luke Challon. Mr Fielding believes the incident could be connected to your father's murder.'

Hugh went white. 'You don't think that my wife . . . Oh no, that could never be. She may be an adulteress but she could never . . .' He did not complete the sentence, was not able to in fact, for tears started to pour down his face and the wretched man became convulsed with sobs.

'Get a grip on yourself,' John whispered, acutely aware of Maud and Valentine in the next room.

'These awful suspicions,' Hugh gasped. 'How can I live with them?'

'They may well be unfounded.'

Hugh's reddened eyes suddenly narrowed. 'You know more than you are saying, I feel it.'

'Nonsense. The Public Office can find nothing against your wife.'

Recollecting the strange story of Maud's behaviour in the garden, John decided to keep it to himself.

'Nothing? Is that true?'

'Yes,' lied the Apothecary, and wondered whether Maud had indeed known Kitty Perkins.

Hugh wiped his face with a sensible linen handkerchief, took a nip of brandy from a hipflask, and pulled himself together. 'I apologise for that outburst, my friend. It was unforgiveable of me to burden you with my problems. Now. You obviously came here for a purpose. How may I help you?'

'I actually wanted to ask if you had ever seen this stick before.' And John produced the walking cane from the floor.

Hugh stared at it, then his face stiffened. 'It was my father's. I'd know it anywhere. Where did you get it?'

'It was found on the riverbank. It is believed to be the implement with which Sir William was killed.'

Hugh looked sick. 'Then take the hateful thing away. I can't bear to see it.'

John got up. 'I'm so sorry. I'll leave you in peace.'

Hugh rose from behind the desk. 'I apologise for my behaviour. I think that perhaps I need the sea air.'

'Are you planning another trip?'

'I thought I might take Maud to Jamaica. If there is another man in her life then that should put paid to his little schemes. You see, I still love her, Mr Rawlings. Perhaps on that romantic island I might woo her all over again.'

Thinking of the pair of them, the snapping-eyed shrew and the staid and stick-like Hugh, John's imagination took frenzied flight.

'I hope you have a pleasant voyage,' was all he could think of saying as he made his way to the door, supressing a scampish smile.

Scorning the vile morning and the drenching rain, Sir Gabriel Kent, aware that this was the day on which a poor girl who had befriended John was to be laid to rest, dressed in his best black clothes, for once not relieving this most dramatic of colours with white accessories. Then furtively taking an umbrella from a secret drawer, having declared to his son that he wouldn't be seen shot with such an effeminate and foreign contraption, Sir Gabriel placed a great tricorne upon his soaring wig and walked the few steps from his front door in Nassau Street to where his coach waited outside, completely blocking the narrow thoroughfare.

'Where to, Sir?' asked the coachman.

'To Kirby Hall. It is high time that I paid my regards to the ladies in residence.'

'Very good, Sir Gabriel.'

The coachman cracked his whip and the equipage set off at good speed, but nature and thirst being what they are a stop was necessitated at The George, where John's father caused a sensation as he stooped his way through the door of the low-beamed taproom.

'Allow me to prepare a private drinking place for you, Milord,' gasped the landlord, convinced that he was in the presence of a Duke, or at the very least a Marquis.

'No, pray calm yourself. I am only staying a few minutes. I am on my way to Kirby Hall.'

'Ah, Kirby Hall,' repeated Frederick Bull, looking knowing. 'I do hear that the old lady up there has been took bad, Milord.'

'Do you mean that Lady Hodkin is ill?' asked his visitor, adjusting a black lace cuff.

'So they say. Though she seemed right enough the last time I saw her.'

Sir Gabriel raised a brow. 'Oh? When was that?'

Frederick looked decidedly flustered. 'Well . . . er . . .'

'Don't worry, everything you say will be treated as confidential,' Sir Gabriel answered soothingly. 'I am an old friend of the family. Tell me, do our fears have any foundation? Does the lady have a weakness for drink?'

Mr Bull turned puce but said nothing.

'No blame will be attached to you, my good man,' Sir Gabriel forged on. 'You are in the business of selling a product. Who buys it is not your concern.'

'Then, to tell you the truth, Milord, Lady Haitch does have a leaning that way. Many a night she comes in here through the back door and goes into the Ram, one of our small private rooms, and there has her nightcap.'

'Lady Hodkin does this regularly?'

'No, only when she's been out visiting, Milord. Or so she tells us.'

'How very interesting.' Sir Gabriel passed Bull a coin. 'Pray, have some ale with me. I am most grateful to you. I will consider carefully all that you have said.'

'You won't mention my name?'

'Of course not.'

Sir Gabriel climbed back into his equipage, thinking that he had learned little new, yet wondering if Lady Hodkin's missing hour on the night when her son-in-law had been murdered might, in the light of what he had just been told, have a possible explanation. And he was still turning this over in his mind when a few minutes later the black coach with its team of snowdrop horses turned through the gates of Kirby Hall and set off down the drive.

A nervous looking servant answered the door and ushered Sir Gabriel into the small waiting room leading off the hall. To forestall any such terrible eventuality, the visitor assured the footman at once that he had absolutely no need of the private facilities and was perfectly comfortable and happy to wait until Miss Hesther could see him.

'Ah, there lies the trouble, Sir,' answered the man in an anguished tone.

'What do you mean?'

'Lady Hodkin is indisposed and Miss Hesther is somewhat preoccupied with nursing her.'

'Then pray tell them that I have called. Who knows but that a new face might cheer the invalid in her hour of sorrow.'

'Very good, Sir.'

The footman bowed and left the room, bearing Sir Gabriel's card on a silver tray. A few moments later he reappeared, looking decidedly relieved.

'Lady Hodkin says that you are to go up, Sir. She will receive you in her bedchamber.'

'How delightful,' answered the visitor, and inclined his head with its daunting wig in a gesture of acknowledgment.

They climbed the grand staircase, the footman leading the way, and solemnly proceeded down the landing, Sir Gabriel's features composed into the stern expression of one whose duty it is to visit a sick room. Yet the voice that answered the gentle knock seemed hale enough.

'Come in,' Lady Hodkin bellowed.

'Gladly,' Sir Gabriel replied, and strode through the doorway manfully, then froze for a moment, greeted by a sight that might well have frightened a lesser mortal.

Lady Hodkin sat propped on pillows in the middle of an ornate four-poster bed, complete with ostrich feathers above its canopy, hastily applying carmine to her lips. Beside her lay the pug, wheezing. On her other side, looking horribly lifelike, rested a wig, which Lady Hodkin hastily snatched up and slapped onto her balding pate, where it alighted slightly sideways. Sir Gabriel's eyes ran over the table by her bed, which groaned beneath an array of provisions: a bowl of comfits, another of marchpane, a decanter of brandy, some vintage port, several oranges, a selection of bonbons, and a large pink blancmanger, as yet in its virgin state and quivering slightly as if in anticipation of being gobbled down by the invalid.

'My dear Sir Gabriel,' Lady Hodkin gushed. 'What a pleasant surprise. Do please forgive my state of deshabillé. I've been quite cast down with my nerves of late. All this talk of murder ain't done me no good at all.'

'I'm quite sure,' her visitor murmured, spreading the skirts of his coat and taking a seat by the bed.

'Further, t'ain't right all this questioning and probing. That upstart Fielding should be horsewhipped in my view. Why, it's obvious that slattern of William's took a knife to him in order to get her hands on his money.'

'I thought she hadn't been left anything,' Sir Gabriel answered mildly. 'And wasn't he clubbed over the head?'

Lady Hodkin snorted. 'Be that as it may, she's responsible, mark my words.' She leaned forward, displaying teeth the colour of sulphur. 'Now, would you like a glass of French brandy, my dear Sir? Or some fine sherry from Spain? You will stay and chat a while, I trust. I can't tell you how pleasant it is to have some intelligent company at last. Hesther's so damnably dull, poor thing.'

Without waiting for her visitor's reply to this, the invalid picked up a handbell from beside the bed and rang it manically. 'Hesther!' she screamed. 'Come here at once.'

Sir Gabriel, who rarely allowed his temper to stray an inch, felt indignation on Miss Hodkin's behalf begin to rise in him. 'Really, there is no need for that,' he remonstrated.

'There's every need,' the beldame retorted. 'The wretched creature's taken my glass away, and besides I require another for my company. And what charming company it is, too.' She shot Sir Gabriel a roguish glance which made his blood run cold, then gave a peal on the bell that would have woken the dead. A moment later, Hesther appeared in answer to this summons, out of breath and looking totally exhausted.

'What is it now, Mother?' she asked wearily, then noticed Sir Gabriel, who had risen and was making an intricate bow. 'Oh, my dear Sir. I did not realise you were here. How very nice to see you again.' She curtsied.

'I want two glasses,' Lady Hodkin stated, with such a nasty edge to her voice that it occurred to Sir Gabriel she resented her own child. 'My visitor requires refreshment, as do I.'

'But your physician said . . .' Hesther protested.

'Damn my physician. Get me some glasses.'

Sir Gabriel fought to keep in control of an ice-cold fury that now threatened to possess him. 'You will be joining us of course, Miss Hesther?' he asked courteously.

The poor woman coloured up as he had so often seen her do before. 'Well, that would be very pleasant.'

'Pleasant for you but not for us,' snapped Lady Hodkin. 'You're dull company, my gal, not to mince words.'

'This is outrageous,' said Sir Gabriel, cracking. 'No mother should speak to her daughter as you do, Madam. Indeed, I'll go so far as to say you should apologise immediately.'

The harridan gaped in pure astonishment, making it perfectly clear that no one had ever spoken to her like that in her entire life. Then she got a grip on herself and her manner turned from one of waggish coquetry to that of glittering malice.

'Get out, Sir,' she hissed. 'How dare you insult me in my own house? And how dare you interfere in matters that are no concern of yours? I'll talk to my daughter exactly as I please. Be damned to you.'

There was a quivering silence during which Sir Gabriel drew himself together in order to make a dignified exit. Then Hesther spoke.

'No! Be damned to *you*, you horrid old woman. You long ago forfeited any right you might have to be paid the respect a mother should. So I'll bear no more of it. From this moment forward I am finished with you.'

'Bravo!' exclaimed Sir Gabriel, forgetting himself and clapping his hands.

'And further,' Hesther continued, ignoring him, 'I am leaving you to fend for yourself. I shall depart tonight for St James's Square and from there I shall make arrangements to find lodgings of my own.'

'Madam,' said Sir Gabriel, bowing deep, 'may I offer you the protection of a place in my home while you make your plans?'

'Ha ha!' shrieked Lady Hodkin triumphantly. 'A sinful liaison! I might have guessed. You have abused my hospitality, Sir. You have seduced my daughter whilst lodging beneath my very roof.'

'Alas, that pleasure was not mine,' Sir Gabriel answered smoothly. He offered Hesther his arm. 'Miss Hodkin, my carriage awaits outside. Pray do me the pleasure of accompanying me to town.'

She flashed him a smile more brilliant than he would have thought her capable of giving. 'Delighted to do so, Sir.' Hesther turned to Lady Hodkin. 'Goodbye, Mother. You can get a paid servant to fetch and carry from now on, and for all I care you can drink until you rot.'

'How could you leave a poor old defenceless woman on her own? Have you no heart?' whined her mother, suddenly changing her act to that of cringing supplicant.

'Absolutely none at all,' answered Hesther lightly, and putting her hand on Sir Gabriel's arm, swept from the room without a single glance backward.

They turned out in their dozens to honour the memory of Kitty Perkins, called to leave the world long before her time was due to do so. The people of Wapping, the river folk, the fishermen, the oyster women, the wherrymen, the mudlarks, packed into the church of St Paul's, Shadwell, until there was only room left to stand at the back. Then they formed into a long and solemn procession and accompanied her simple coffin to its final resting place, showing by their sheer weight of numbers how much they had loved and respected the good-hearted girl who had been born and brought up amongst them, and who had never done a day's harm to anyone in her life.

Walking amongst their number, John pondered the cruelty of death, withheld from those who suffered agonising illness, forced upon those too young and good to leave their loved ones behind. His thoughts became dark and bleak and he would have fallen into a mood of bitter introspection, had not an unexpected tap on his shoulder dragged his attention back to the present. Valentine Randolph was standing beside him, an anxious expression on his face.

'About the great stick,' he said without preface.

The Apothecary stared at the office manager blankly, his mind a million miles away.

'It's mine,' Valentine continued.

John snapped to attention. 'What's that you say?'

'The great stick. The one you showed me.'

'Yes?'

'It's mine.'

'Then why didn't you say so in the first place, you foolish man?'

'I thought it might incriminate me. It seemed you had enough suspicions of my whereabouts that night without adding anything further to them.'

'Oh for God's sake,' John answered angrily. 'We'll never get at the truth at this rate. Tell me from the beginning.'

'The stick used to belong to Sir William but I so admired it that he gave it to me. Then one day I left the thing in the office and never saw it again.'

'Are you saying it was stolen?'

'Yes,' said Valentine, a note of desperation in his voice.

'Very well. But if that is the case why did Luke identify it to me as Roger's?'

'Possibly because he doesn't like Roger and would gladly see him in trouble. Or maybe because the beau has one very similar, having admired his father's greatly and causing a copy to be made.'

'Are these the real facts?' asked John through gritted teeth.

'They are. I swear it.'

'Then the field is narrowed to someone who had access to Sir William's office because, sure as fate, that stick was used to kill him.'

Valentine turned pale. 'But they have all visited the office at some time or another, even Lady Hodkin.'

'I know,' said John morosely, wondering how much deeper the puzzle could get. With an effort of will he changed the subject. 'Which of the people here are Kitty's parents?'

Valentine made an effort to recover himself, swallowing hard before he said, 'She had none. She was an orphan.'

'Then who organised all this?'

'Her uncle, her only living relative. She used to sail on his fishing boat to get her oysters.'

'I think I'd like to have a word with him. Which one is he?'

'The dark, gypsy-looking man standing by the grave. He's known as Unkle, by the way. He spells it with a "k".'

'Can you introduce me?'

'I'll do so at the wake.'

'Which is to be held where?'

'In The Devil's Tavern.'

'Where it all began,' John answered harshly, and turned away to hide his tears as Kitty's small, pathetic coffin was lowered into the earth to vanish for ever from his sight.

It seemed that even death itself was subject to the rule of the mighty Thames. As the tide began to turn, so the riverfolk left the wake to proceed about their business; to row the people of London to their varied destinations, to go fishing, to head for the sea, to scavenge before the water level rose too high. And it was then, with the crowd thinning, that John Rawlings finally got his opportunity to shake the oyster girl's uncle by the hand and tell him how saddened he was by Kitty's death.

'I offer you my heartfelt condolances, Unkle.'

'I swear to God her killer must swing for this,' answered the gypsy. Then casting his eye over Benjamin Rudge, who had hovered discreetly in the background throughout the funeral, he added, 'The gossip is that that fellow is a Runner working for the Blind Beak, come here to search the villain out. Is it true, Sir?'

'Yes.'

'And what about you? Are you also present to bring a murderer to justice?'

'It is my avowed intent to do so.'

Valentine Randolph interceded. 'Unkle, this is Mr John Rawlings who does indeed work for the Public Office at Bow Street.'

'Then how can I help you find the man?'

John frowned. 'It's difficult really, because she probably said nothing. But I can't help wondering if Kitty mentioned anything to you about seeing someone in an unexpected place, somewhere that she wouldn't have anticipated that person to be.'

Unkle stared at him, his dark Romany eyes glowing. 'Yes, she did that right enough.'

John's heart leapt in his chest. 'Who was it? Did she say?'

'Alas, no. But I can tell you where it happened. In Gravesend.'

'Gravesend?'

'Yes. We had to hole up there one night because of a storm at sea that gave us a bit of a knocking about. Anyway, after we moored, Kitty went for a walk into the town, to visit The Belle Sauvage it was. Wanted to have a drink and sell some oysters. We'd been at Whitstable, you see.'

'The Belle Sauvage,' John repeated wonderingly, remembering his laudanum induced dream.

Unkle stared at him. 'Yes, that's right.'

'But you've no idea whom she saw there?'

'None. She come back laughing and muttering about "up to no good".'

'When was this?'

Unkle scratched his head. 'Can't really remember. About three or four weeks ago. Somewhen round then.'

'That fits with the killing of Sir William,' said John excitedly. 'Listen, will you take me there?'

'To Gravesend? I'm not bound in that direction.'

The Apothecary looked disappointed. 'But I thought you wanted to help me catch Kitty's murderer.'

'Do you think the person she saw is him or her, then?'

'Yes, I do.'

'In that case I'll change my plans. Can you be ready to sail in ten minutes?'

'I'm ready now.' John turned to look at the Runner. 'Mr Rudge, would you return to Bow Street and inform Mr Fielding of this development.'

'But he told me not to leave you.'

'I can't help that. It's most important that he knows what is happening.'

'Very well,' Rudge answered with resignation. 'But don't you get into no trouble, mind.'

'As if I would,' said John, his spirit of adventure soaring.

'Yes, as if you would,' the Runner repeated, and sighed.

As they went down to the sea, past the great shipyards of Deptford and Woolwich, the rain began to die away and a watery sun appeared, which grew stronger and stronger as the afternoon wore on. Then the river widened, as did John's eyes at the sight of so much vigorous waterlife. Sailing past Unkle's fishing boat were merchantmen, rigged with billowing clouds of canvas, bound for the Indies or other ports of exotic location. Whilst proceeding into London at a pace came their poor relations, fleets of colliers loaded with Newcastle coal for the fires of town. From the Kent coast, from Deal and from Sandwich, headed hoys loaded with local produce, while from Essex hurried smacks abrim with mackerel. On the port side, the common tilt boat went by, the ferry which took travellers from Gravesend to London at the charge of tenpence a head. As he saw it pass, loaded with sixty or so passengers, a thought struck John which refused to go away and instead grew like a seed in his mind.

The chalk-pits and marshes which lined the bank had given way to villages and shipyards, whilst midstream rode a queue of vessels, outgoing ships waiting for a final visit from Customs officials before they put to sea. Peering ahead, the Apothecary was at last able to glimpse their destination, a neat little town of fisherfolk's houses, perched prettily on the riverside.

'How long does it take from Gravesend to London in the ferry?' John asked Unkle, whose dark face was frowning with concentration as he navigated his way through the shipping lanes.

'Four hours with the tide in your favour. Why do you ask?'

'Curiosity, that's all. I don't really know this area, you see.'

Unkle gestured to a church spire, visible through the forest of masts. 'Then you won't know who's buried there.'

John shook his head. 'No. Tell me.'

'A Red Indian princess called Pocahontas. She died in Gravesend of fever on her way back to America, having married a Virginian settler, a John Rolfe, who brought her to this country. The inn Kitty visited is named after her.'

'The Belle Sauvage. Of course!'

'That's it over there.' And Unkle pointed to a hostelry not far from the water's edge.

John stared at it in the light of the dying sun, noticing the wide entrance to the courtyard behind it. 'Is the place a coaching inn by any chance?'

Unkle chuckled. 'Of course it is, Sir. That's where the stage and flying coaches from the Kent coast bring their passengers to catch the ferry to London.'

'Oh God's sweet life!' said John, and clutched his head.

'What is it?' asked Unkle, perturbed.

'It's the answer,' shouted the Apothecary, his voice ringing out in sheer exhiliration. 'Oh, my dear sweet man, it's the answer to the whole damnable mystery.'

Chapter Twenty-Five

*T*he Blind Beak sat in total silence, his puissant profile etched against the light coming in through the window, his extraordinary ability to remain utterly immobile never more clearly marked. Behind him, taking notes, was Joe Jago, his endearingly craggy face expressionless as he wrote down all that the Apothecary had to say. There was a stillness everywhere, the distant buzz of the household and the Public Office below it, strangely hushed, just as if the entire place was listening to the Apothecary's account of how Sir William Hartfield and Kitty Perkins met their death.

'And that, in my belief,' said John eventually, 'is how the first murder was done and why the oyster girl had to be disposed of.'

Mr Fielding remained still a moment longer before finally nodding his head. 'Yes, it all seems to fit. In any event, it is a strong enough argument to put to the test. Joe, can you get letters out calling all those involved together?'

'Certainly, Sir. But there's rum coves amongst 'em, some who won't be willing to oblige.'

'Threaten them with contempt, especially Lady Hodkin. In fact I think we should get Rudge to go to Bethnal Green and fetch her. By the way, where's Luke Challon living now that he has lost his situation?'

'I believe he's in lodgings in Redriff. But Valentine Randolph is bound to know. He was helping him find somewhere.'

'Good.' The Magistrate gave one of his melodious laughs. 'You'd best invite Samuel Swann to be present, too, or else he'll be mightily put out.'

'Indeed he will,' answered the Apothecary. 'He was out of town and missed Kitty's funeral, which made him very upset. But being there at the end of the story, so to speak, should restore his spirits.'

Joe made a note. 'Is there anyone else?' he asked.

'Don't forget Amelia Lambourn,' said the Blind Beak, and

laughed once more. 'I can't wait for you to describe the family's faces when they discover the truth about Sir William's betrothed and his eldest son.'

'Who turned out to be more Roger than Molly,' put in Jago, guffawing.

His laugh was so infectious that the other two simultaneously put their heads back and joined with him, so that for several minutes there was total chaos. Then Mr Fielding calmed down.

'Pray do ask your father to escort Miss Hesther Hodkin to the family gathering, my young friend. I would like him to be present. Incidentally, I find his habit of rescuing ladies in distress quite enchanting. I well remember how he once helped poor Mrs Harcross.'

John smiled. 'He did that very same thing for my mother and myself, many years ago.'

The Magistrate nodded. 'There is an innate kindness in Sir Gabriel Kent that his fellow men would do well to emulate.'

'Question, Sir,' said Joe. 'When do you want this gathering to take place? And where? And when?'

'Tomorrow at noon, and no later. We must not let the bird fly the nest. Call them to The Devil's Tavern, which I feel would be a fitting venue. Ask the landlord to reserve the cockfighting room. Let us complete the circle where it all began. Besides, I feel the need to quit Bow Street for a while and should much enjoy a journey by water.'

The clerk stood up. 'Then I'll get to it right away. I presume you'll want to sign the letters personally?'

'Indeed I will.'

Jago nodded and left the room.

'A great man, that one,' said the Magistrate as he heard the door close behind his assistant. 'My right hand. He has made himself indispensable to me, in fact I cannot contemplate a life without him.'

'A life without Joe,' John answered seriously, 'would be a colourless thing indeed.' And he sat in silence for a few moments, not even wanting to imagine such a thing.

'So,' said the Magistrate briskly, breaking the mood. 'What are you going to do with yourself until tomorrow, Mr Rawlings?'

'I am going home to write a letter and then I intend to call on the Comtesse de Vignolles. Tonight I am in the mood for a little gambling and sincerely hope that she will be pleased to accompany me.'

'Ah ha! Do I detect a plot to clip a pair or two of foolish young wings?'

'You most certainly do,' John replied, and once again both of them laughed, only this time more gently.

Having returned to Nassau Street and written his letter, John hailed a hackney coach and delivered the note personally to the Hartfields' house in St James's Square.

'You will make quite sure Mr Julian gets this as soon as he comes in,' he asked the footman, as he handed it through the door.

'Certainly, Sir.'

'And say that I look forward to seeing him at White's this evening and simply will not take no for an answer.'

The footman bowed. 'Very good, Sir. Will that be all, Sir?'

'Yes, for the present,' John said cheerfully, and returned to the hackney which had been waiting for him outside. 'To number twelve Hanover Square,' he instructed the driver, and felt the usual thrill of pleasure that the prospect of seeing Serafina always aroused in him.

Despite the fact that she was now in the seventh month of her pregnancy, this day the Comtesse radiated excitement as she stood at the top of the graceful staircase, waiting to greet him.

'My dear,' she called as John climbed upwards. 'I heard this morning that Sarah Delaney has given birth to a baby boy. Lord Delaney is said to be fit to burst with joy and is inviting the entire *beau monde* to celebrate as soon as the mother is fully recovered.'

'And does the baby resemble its father?' John asked, and winked an eye.

'According to my informant it is a fine child. Very dark and well made.'

'Enough said I think,' answered John, and arriving at the top, kissed her on the cheek.

'Now you are not to be naughty,' said Serafina, then laughed. 'Poor old fellow. I'm told he's as puffed with pride as a bull frog.'

'And Sarah? Is she well?'

'Sailed through her travail like a ship with the wind behind it.'

Serafina put her hand to her body. 'Let it be hoped that I can do the same.'

'Of course, you will,' said John. 'You have a robust attitude to life and that is half the battle, believe me.'

'Yes, Apothecary. Now, my dear, tell me about yourself. Have you solved your mystery yet? And have you seen anything of Coralie Clive?'

John smiled ruefully. 'Yes, to both. I believe the murderer is found, though that is yet to be proved. And the lady and I have met, only to part with no plans to meet again.'

Serafina smiled, her elegant face animated by her private thoughts. 'Give it time, my friend. As I told you once before, you and Coralie encountered one another too soon in your lives.'

The Apothecary sighed. 'Do you think we will ever become lovers?'

'Who knows? Fate has such strange twists and turns that one can never be certain of anything. But yet I do not believe that destiny has played its full game with the pair of you.'

John nodded. 'I hope you are right.'

'Now you are growing sad,' Serafina stated reprimandingly. 'Kindly raise your spirits and tell me why you have come to see me. There is a look about you that denotes mischief.'

The Apothecary brightened at the thought of the evening ahead. 'Well, there is a little game I want to play that only you can help me with.'

'Tell me of it,' ordered the Comtesse, and her twinkling smile deepened as John explained his plan. Then she sighed. 'You know how much I would adore to take part but, alas, I am so large I have withdrawn from public life.'

'Oh surely not.'

Serafina's smile ascended to her cheekbones. 'Almost but not quite. I shall put on a gown big as a tent and sally forth.'

'Will Louis accompany us?'

'Nothing would stop him once he hears what's afoot.'

'Then shall I call for you at nine o'clock?'

'No,' answered Serafina impetuously, 'go home and change then come to a late dinner. I intend to make this my last excursion until after the baby is born and I want to enjoy it to the full.'

'I think I can promise you an evening of fine play,' said John.

'Till seven o'clock,' answered the Comtesse, as they kissed and parted company.

White's gambling club in St James's had started its life as one of London's exclusive chocolate houses, the place in which the *beau monde* assembled to discuss the topics of the day. But it had not been long before its reputation as a meeting place for gamblers and spendthrifts had overtaken its other, more innocent, character. Eventually, the serving of coffee and chocolate had become of secondary importance, and White's had emerged as the place in which riches were lost or won, where suicides as a result of a night's gaming were a commonality, where great fortunes and estates changed hands at the turn of a card or the roll of a dice.

Yet White's had one eccentricity to which some diehards objected. In this all male preserve there was one solitary female who was allowed to enter and play. Serafina, Comtesse de Vignolles, who only a year previously had kept her identity concealed and had been known to fashionable society simply as the Masked Lady, had by her enormous flair and skill as a gamester, won herself a place at the tables at any time she wished. And this fine April evening with the place crowded by the noblest in the land and stakes running high, it was rumoured that her carriage had drawn up outside.

Just for the briefest moment, all play ceased, and every head turned towards the doorway. Then the Earl of Carlisle, an impetuous young blood, rose to his feet and applauded, leading the way to a standing ovation, as the lady herself, clad in a flowing scarlet robe and concealing her features with a domino of matching silk, entered on the arm of her handsome French husband, followed by an elegant but strange young man who was believed by many to be nothing more than a common apothecary.

Several of those present invited the Comtesse to honour them with her presence but she smilingly declined and made straight for the table at which sat a slight young man called Julian Hartfield, famous already for his ability to lose enormous sums with no hope of regaining his money.

'God help the fellow,' whispered Sir John Bland, the member for Luggershal, to his companion.

'This will probably finish him for good,' came the reply. Then everyone chuckled, some with sympathy, others with malice, as the

Masked Lady and her party took up the dice for a game of hazard and invited the poor unfortunate to join them.

'My dear Julian,' said John, as he picked up the dice box, 'it seems an age since I've seen you. When was it now? Oh yes, I remember. We were both at Cuper's Gardens.'

Julian flushed. 'No, I think not. We last saw one another aboard The Folly.'

'Of course, how foolish of me.' The Apothecary lowered his voice. 'You do realise who my companion is, don't you?'

Julian shook his head. 'No, I'm relatively new to White's.'

'Then you're in for an enormous pleasure. She is the famous Masked Lady whom you admire so much. The woman known the length and breadth of London as the finest and luckiest gamester of them all.' John rattled the dice and threw. 'You see, whenever she is present good fortune eludes me.' He handed the box to the twin. 'I sincerely hope that you fare better.'

Julian paled, threw, and lost.

'Let us raise the stakes,' said Serafina sweetly, pulling in the rouleaus of fifty guineas which had been wagered on the last throw. She looked at Julian. 'Sir, I am sure you will be willing.'

The twin gulped. 'Of course,' he answered, his voice feeble.

He was like a fly, caught in the net of a brilliant, glittering spider, terrified but unable to resist. In the end, everyone else at the table gladly dropped out of the game, leaving only Serafina and Julian to stare at one another over the dice box.

'One final throw,' she said. Then she laughed. 'I'm in a generous mood so let us play *deep*. My home in Hanover Square and all my jewels. What will you stake?'

Nobody moved and Julian's voice croaked into the silence, 'My house in St James's Square.'

'Is it yours to wager?'

'Yes,' Julian lied.

'Very well.'

The Comtesse threw the dice and a double six rolled out onto the cloth. There was a gasp of indrawn breath as Julian picked up the box, knowing that unless he drew equal all was lost. He shook, and a six and a four were revealed. The twin plunged his head into his hands and sobbed.

Serafina leaned across the table and said, very quietly, 'My dear Miss Hartfield, I have no intention of calling this wager in, but in return for my generosity I want you to honour two very simple requests. First, you must immediately stop masquerading as your brother and thereby causing no end of trouble; it is a dangerous game for any woman to play. And second, you must swear henceforth entirely to give up gaming for which, let me hasten to assure you, you have absolutely no talent whatsoever.'

Exactly one hour later, a sobbing saddened Juliette had been returned to her home and a note left at St James's Square for Julian to attend the Comte de Vignolles on a matter of the utmost urgency. Then, Serafina being utterly exhausted and having retired for the night, John and Louis sat up to wait for him, their manner not at all amused.

At just after midnight, there was a ring at the door, which they answered together.

'Damme, what's all this about?' the young reprobate demanded languidly, only to be seized by the collar and dragged into the hall by a furious John Rawlings.

'You ridiculous little man,' the Apothecary shouted, his eyes bright with anger. 'You deserve to be shot. By indulging in your stupid shabby masquerade, dressing up as your twin sister in order to have easy access to your lady love without the presence of a chaperone, you have placed Juliette in the greatest moral and physical danger. She wanders London dressed as a man, inviting all kinds of misfortune. Why, she could even be challenged to a duel. But her greatest peril is that she is totally addicted to gambling without the skill to go with it, and tonight came within a hair's breadth of losing everything.'

'I think,' said Louis, sounding very French, 'that a horsewhip is called for.'

'By all means,' the Apothecary answered him. He turned back to Julian. 'I intend to call on your sweetheart's father and tell him exactly how you managed to seduce his daughter in so despicable a fashion. No doubt, he will have his own methods of dealing with you.'

The twin looked so sick that John felt a momentary pang of sympathy for him. 'Oh no, please don't do that, I beg you,' he pleaded, his voice near to sobs. 'I promise I am going to do the right thing by her. We are running away to be married as soon as tomorrow's meeting with Mr Fielding is over.'

'Oh dear God spare us,' said the Apothecary, rolling his eyes, 'I do believe you have put her with child!'

'Yes I have,' confessed Julian, and burst into tears.

Remembering the knowing look on Lady Almeria Noel's tough little face, John felt his fury start to subside.

'That's all very honourable I'm sure,' he answered, slightly less harshly, 'but think of the cruel thing you did to Juliette by allowing her out and about dressed in your clothes.'

Julian wiped his eyes. 'I thought she would be all right, that her gambling was only a game, a pastime. I thought she would meet a worthy man who would protect her. Someone like yourself.'

Louis interceded. 'It is getting late and time that we concluded this conversation. Mr Hartfield, do I have your word of honour as a gentleman, that you will marry the woman who carries your child, and also that you will in future protect your sister not only from external dangers but those that she inflicts upon herself?'

'Yes, indeed,' said Julian in an earnest voice.

'Then that is all there is to be said.'

The twin looked from one to the other of them. 'I apologise . . .' he began.

'Save your words,' answered John abruptly. 'There'll be enough explaining for you to do when you get before Mr Fielding tomorrow.'

On Louis's insistence, the Apothecary took the de Vignolles's coach home, but rather than ask the equipage to turn into the narrow confines of Nassau Street, he alighted from it in Gerrard Street and went the rest of the way on foot, hardly noticing in his tired state that a dark shadow had detached itself from a doorway and was following him. In fact, if it had not been for a sudden cry from Louis's postillion, who had turned his head and seen the menacing state of affairs, the stick which crashed down within a few inches of his head might have hit its target and left John lying fatally injured. As it was, the servant jumped down from his place and gave chase while John recovered his wits.

'Did you get him?' the Apothecary asked, when the postillion eventually came running back.

'No, Sir. He lost me in the back streets. But I caught a glimpse of him and he didn't look like a footpadder or cutpurse to me. Too smart, if you take my meaning.'

'I take it very well,' John answered grimly. 'Tomorrow's meeting cannot come soon enough in view of this.'

'You keep a watch on yourself,' said the servant as he returned to the waiting carriage.

'From now on I shall travel fully armed,' the Apothecary assured him as he hurried into the safety of number two, Nassau Street.

Chapter Twenty-Six

*I*t was as windy as it had been on the day that John Rawlings first set foot in The Devil's Tavern. Great gusts of air blew through the streets of London, rattling the shop signs and blowing gutter detritus into the faces of passers by, while cloaks filled like sails and hats sped aloft irretrievably. On the waterway, passengers were having a hard time of it. The Thames was in a wild fury, waves whipping its surface and flying spume lashing the great ships and riverside houses alike. Travellers were arriving at their destinations green in the face and soaked to the skin, while the sale of restorative spirits in waterside inns rose dramatically.

The Apothecary had heard the tempest start up during the night and had thought how fitting it was that the sad affair was ending as it had begun. But even he, hardy sailor that he was, was not quite prepared for the anger of the river as he and Nicholas Dawkins, acting, or so John supposed, as some kind of bodyguard under the instruction of Sir Gabriel, attempted to board a wherry at Hungerford Stairs.

John's father, very wisely, had set forth with Miss Hodkin on the previous evening and had thus presumably enjoyed a calm and peaceful journey and a good night's sleep. How typical, John had thought fondly, wondering if he would ever become as wise and imperturbable as Sir Gabriel Kent. And now, attempting to get aboard the madly bobbing boat, he heartily wished he had followed the older man's example rather than spend time exposing the reckless prank played out by the Hartfield twins.

Nicholas, lame leg or no, gave a flying leap and managed to land in the wherry. He then held out his hand to John, who accepted it and clambered on board, wondering whether he was getting old. And at London Bridge, where the cataracts between the arches foamed and roared in the wind, the Apothecary conjectured the same thing as he went ashore and walked to the next landing stage, leaving the Muscovite to enjoy the perils of the waterfalls on his own.

The meeting at The Devil's Tavern had been called for midday and John had left plenty of time, considering the weather to be so atrocious that progress might be slow. And so, it appeared, had the Blind Beak. For as John and Nicholas alighted at Pelican Stairs, the Apothecary saw that not far behind them followed another wherry, this one bearing the Magistrate himself, sitting bolt upright, a broad piece of ribbon securing his hat onto his head, whilst Elizabeth Fielding, somewhat pale of complexion, dabbed at her upper lip and clutched the side of the boat for dear life. Scrambling ashore as best he could, John waited politely to help the couple up the steep wooden steps, by now periously wet and slippery as the waves of the Thames broke over them.

In the event, he was glad that he did. For it was no mean feat for a heavily built man who could not see, to heave himself up the saturated stairway, particularly as, for once, his redoubtable wife was clearly out of sorts. John and Nicholas were straining for all they were worth at Mr Fielding's arms, shouting orders at each other, when Joe Jago suddenly appeared as if from nowhere, called, 'One last gigg, Beak,' and the Magistrate sprung spryly ashore with only Joe's grasp to guide him. The Apothecary and his assistant looked at one another, shrugged, and went within.

Some of the company had already assembled. Valentine Randolph and Luke Challon were there, this last glaring at Hugh so violently that if looks could have killed, the head of the firm would have fallen dead at his wife's feet. Maud, meanwhile, ignored the situation and busied herself talking to Juliette, pale as ice beneath her burnished hair. Her twin, too, was totally subdued and sat staring moodily out of the window, observing the river which raced a mere few inches below. Slightly removed from all of them and sitting close to the fire was Hesther Hodkin, Sir Gabriel hovering politely close by.

'Tell me who is already here,' the Blind Beak ordered in a loud whisper, obviously meant to be overheard.

'Mr Hugh and Mrs Maud Hartfield, Miss Hesther, the geminis and the two employees, Mr Challon and Mr Randolph.'

'*Ex*-employee,' Hugh put in icily.

'There are more coming,' said Julian from the window, his voice flat and dreary sounding. 'Lydia is sharing a wherry with that friend of Mr Rawlings, and right behind them is Roger . . . God's teeth!' He broke off.

'What is it?'

'He's with Father's strumpet.'

Luke shot to the window. 'So he is . . . with Amelia, I mean.' He turned to Julian and they stared at one another blankly.

'Then we're only lacking Lady Hodkin to be complete.'

'I dread the thought of seeing her,' Hesther murmured.

'Courage,' answered Sir Gabriel and patted her shoulder, at which colour came into her cheeks.

'May I suggest, ladies and gentlemen, that we make our way to the cockfighting room? I shall start without Lady Hodkin if necessary,' Mr Fielding announced.

There was an unenthusiastic murmur of consent and slowly the party began to troop up the staircase, to be followed a few moments later by Lydia and Samuel Swann, she looking radiantly lovely, John thought, her damp clothes clinging to her and her hair wet from the spray. Last of all came Roger and Amelia, very pointedly ignoring one another and taking seats at the opposite ends of the room.

Oh dear, none of this is going to be easy, thought John, as his mind raced over the reputations that were about to be shattered.

The Magistrate, sitting in a sturdy oak carver set before the window, cleared his throat. 'Firstly, let me thank you for attending here today. I know it has not been a pleasant journey in this roaring gale for those who had to come any distance, or even for anyone who had to cross the river. However, I am aware that you all have a common interest in discovering why Sir William Hartfield was done so cruelly to death, and felt therefore that it was for the general good that the meeting proceeded despite the inclement conditions.' The Blind Beak turned his head as if he were looking round. 'I don't suppose that many of you realise that it was in this very room, once used for cockfighting, now as a place for bare knuckle contests, that Sir William's body was put for the night by the watermen who dragged it out of the Thames. And it was only by the merest chance that my friend Mr Rawlings, an apothecary, staying in the tavern that evening, happened upon Sir William's corpse and examined it, to find an indentation upon the dead man's skull distinctly bearing the mark of a fox's head. Had it not been for this, the murder of your father, employer, brother-in-law, might have gone undetected.'

'Why is that?' asked Hesther.

'Because as the body began to bloat, as those that have been in the water generally do, the mark would have vanished and with it the evidence of the blow that was struck.' The Magistrate paused, then said, 'Mr Rawlings, would you care to go on.'

John took up the story. 'I examined the mark of the fox's head by candlelight, as Mr Fielding has stated, but when, next morning, I returned to look at it again in the daylight, the body had gone, already taken to the Coroner as I was to discover later. However, the Magistrate soon became convinced that we had a case of murder on our hands and asked me to help him look for the victim's killer.

'As you already know, Sir William was to have been married to Miss Amelia Lambourn earlier that day, and most of you were in the church ready to make an unpleasant scene should this wedding have taken place. However, the poor man was already dead and therefore unable to keep his appointment, and the marriage party broke up in some confusion.'

Mr Fielding spoke again. 'Mr Rawlings's task was not an easy one for it was not long before he encountered a veritable maze of lies, deceit and half-truths. Everyone, or so it seemed, had something to hide.' His voice grew harsher. 'Let me start with the head of the family, Mr Roger Hartfield, a man of cutting fashion and a collector of all that is beautiful and rare. It may surprise those present to know that long before Sir William met her, Mr Roger had already *collected* Miss Lambourn, that they had been lovers for several years, and that it was Roger who introduced his mistress to his father in order to stop Sir William being so miserable.'

'God's wounds!' exclaimed Luke, who had gone very pale.

'Further, they planned to continue their adulterous relationship once Amelia was married.'

'I have never heard anything so disgusting in my life!' boomed a voice from the doorway, and every head turned to see that Lady Hodkin, complete with pug, had arrived. She glared about her menacingly. 'You're filthy fornicators, the whole damned lot of you. Heaven has punished me indeed by giving me such a detestable family.'

The Blind Beak ignored her entirely, merely saying, 'Would you now continue, Mr Rawlings,' to be echoed by Samuel adding, 'Damme, what a tale!'

John spoke again. 'I thought at first that Roger might have killed his father in a passion but it soon became obvious that this was not so. And the idea of Amelia murdering for gain was equally untenable. For the fact remains that Miss Lambourn has gained nothing. Under the terms of Sir William's new will, which he was to have signed on the night of his death, his wife was to have become his principal heiress. But Sir William never got to the lawyer's office because he was called away to meet someone. Someone who, according to Mrs Lydia Hartfield, had been blackmailing him for some while. Therefore, the decision the Public Office had to make was as to whether Sir William was killed in a fit of fury or in order to stop him signing the new will, a will which would, effectively, have taken both his fortune and his business out of family hands.'

'And which did you decide upon?' asked Julian curiously.

'Neither really, for we believe that the motive was a combination of the two.'

'Roger murdered him,' said Lady Hodkin forcefully, 'just so that he could have that dirty little doxie to himself.'

'Watch your language, Madam,' growled the beau. 'Mr Rawlings thinks differently.'

'He never said so.'

'Yes he did.'

'Quiet!' boomed the Blind Beak. 'Pay attention, all of you.' He took up the story. 'It was obvious to the Public Office that Sir William was murdered on the night before his wedding and it therefore became vital that we should discover where he went and whom he saw during those last fatal hours. Yet investigation showed that *every one of you* – and that includes yourself, Lady Hodkin – seemed to have something to hide during the relevant time. Mrs Lydia, for example, followed Sir William, ostensibly to confront his blackmailer, then disappeared for the rest of the night.'

'Murderess!' yelled the old woman.

'Oh be silent,' Lydia answered furiously. 'I spent that night in the arms of a good man and true, a man whom I love, so call me whore by all means, but a killer I am not.'

She turned towards Mr Fielding who, just as if he could see she was looking at him, said, 'Go on.'

'I had known for some time that my father-in-law was being blackmailed,' Lydia continued spiritedly. 'It started while Lady Hartfield was alive and my guess was that the threat was to reveal his illicit affair to the world. As the family already knew about it, but the business community did not, my suspicion alighted on Valentine Randolph. Oh forgive me, my darling.'

'My darling?' Roger repeated incredulously. 'Are you sleeping with Randolph then?'

'Of course I am,' she answered, her stunning mouth forming into a smile. 'I've told you, I love him. I would go to the ends of the earth with him.'

'Continue your discourse, Madam,' instructed the Magistrate severely.

'I followed Sir William to Redriff but there he vanished. In fact, I was lost, wandering about alone and rather frightened, when I suddenly came across Valentine, who took me to The Angel and there we spent the night together.'

'Didn't you regard it as suspicious that he was in the area?' Hugh asked.

'Not at all,' Lydia retorted angrily, 'he lives there, if you remember.'

Valentine interrupted. 'The fact is that I was looking for Sir William. He was to have met me in The Spread Eagle for a celebratory drink but did not arrive. Thinking he might have gone straight to The Angel, where he had booked to spend the night, I was making my way there to see if I could locate him.'

'I find that almost too much of a coincidence.'

'Would you also find it a coincidence that your grandmother went missing for an hour that very night?' John asked pointedly. 'That your brother Roger cannot satisfactorily account for himself? That Julian and Juliette were wandering round London disguised as one another? That Miss Hesther Hodkin's statement of where she was cannot be verified? That your own wife was seen stalking round the grounds of Kirby Hall just as if she were waiting to meet someone?'

Hugh looked abashed. 'I'm sorry. I didn't realise all that.'

'No, you wouldn't, would you?' said Luke nastily. 'So quick to put the blame on everyone else.'

'Gentlemen, please.' Mr Fielding's voice drowned all others. 'So, with so much deceit abounding, it was left to those trying to solve the puzzle to decide, firstly, who the blackmailer might possibly be, and, secondly, who would benefit most from Sir William's death, providing he did not sign his new will. There was another point too, the murder of the poor wretched oyster girl.'

'Surely that's not connected,' asked Amelia, speaking for the first time.

'Not only is it very closely connected,' answered John, 'it is the key factor in the entire mystery.'

'How so?' said Maud.

'During the brawl in The Devil's Tavern, the brawl between your husband and Luke Challon, the brawl in which Roger, Julian and Valentine were all attempting to intervene with varying degrees of success, Kitty Perkins, the victim, recognised one of the men and began to make a remark, a remark which she was never able to finish, but a remark to the effect that she had seen one of them in a place where she would never have expected him to be.'

'So?'

'So this evidence of hers, had she lived to give it, was obviously important enough to ensure that she must be silenced for ever.'

'Four key things then,' put in the Blind Beak. 'Who knew sufficient about Sir William's business and love affairs to be able to blackmail him? Who would lose all if the second will were to be signed? Who had sufficient access to Sir William's office to steal Mr Randolph's stick and use it as a murder weapon? Who was somewhere so strange that his very being there must name him murderer?'

Valentine Randolph spoke again. 'I suppose that I, as his office manager, knew most about his commercial ventures. And I was certainly aware that Sir William had a mistress. And the use of my stick makes things look very black for me, I realise that.'

Luke came in. 'I knew just as much. I was his confidential secretary. Further I had free range of the office at any time.'

Realising that everyone was staring at him, Roger said, 'Well, obviously, as I introduced them, I knew everything about his relationship with Amelia. But I didn't take the damned stick. I've got one of my own. Anyway, I understood little of Father's business dealings.'

'You understood enough to boost your funds by blackmail, you mollying dog,' screamed Lady Hodkin, silent for an unnervingly long time, but now clearly having gathered sufficient strength to come back in on the attack.

'I deny it,' shrieked the beau.

'Well, I may be the biggest fool in Christendom and thoughtlessly have put my sister at risk,' said Julian heatedly, 'but I would never stoop to extortion, particularly from my own father. As for the stick, I know nothing about it.'

'Never the less,' said the Blind Beak relentlessly, 'somebody did, and somebody killed, not one, but two people. Mr Rawlings.'

'Before the murder of Kitty a portrait was beginning to build in my mind, a portrait of someone both avaricious and ambitious, of someone capable of lashing out in a rage, of someone who above all loved power. Ideas began to come to me. Memories of a conversation I had overheard, in which a man told a woman that something had gone terribly wrong; of an eye witness declaring that a female had been acting strangely, only for that female to deny it; of a missing button by a gravestone, not fancy enough for most men to wear, only those who adopt a plain and God-fearing attitude to life.

'But, as Mr Fielding said, the real key lay with harmless little Kitty. She had seen someone somewhere out of place, so I determined to find out where that place might be. Her uncle told me that they had recently moored at Gravesend overnight, after a bad storm had shaken them up at sea. Kitty had gone ashore to have a drink and sell oysters, and had made for the inn, The Belle Sauvage. And it is to that particular inn that the coaches from the Kent coast come to drop their passengers to catch the ferry into London. So how easy it would be for anyone crossing the Channel to be put ashore at Dover, or anywhere adjacent, pick up a postchaise, then the common tilt boat, and be in London days before the ship on which he was sailing arrived at the Legal Quays.'

There was a terrible silence during which Benjamin Rudge loomed in the doorway leading to the staircase and Samuel Swann quietly rose to his feet.

Hugh burst out laughing. 'I take it that this fiction is directed at me?'

'Yes,' John answered seriously, 'it is. For only you answer all four of the criteria that the Public Office is seeking.'

'But I told you, I was at sea when my father was murdered.'

'No, you weren't. You were put off at the coast and you got to London in the manner I've just described. The only thing that went wrong was that Kitty Perkins, who knew you well by sight, saw you at The Belle Sauvage and wondered what you were doing there.'

'And Mrs Maud Hartfield is also implicated, being an accessory after the fact,' stated John Fielding. 'Do not deny it, Madam. You knew your husband was secretly returning from France in order to persuade Sir William, by force if necessary, not to sign his new will. However, you were not quite certain when. So you waited for him in the garden of Kirby Hall on the night he was about the filthy work of patricide. Then, when he *did* appear, you heard his confession that something had gone wrong and did nothing about it. You are as guilty as he is in the eyes of the law.'

'No, no,' Maud shrieked.

'Quiet,' Hugh snarled at her, and for the first time the Apothecary saw the wolf that lurked behind the crisply tanned features.

'Did you strike your father in order to stop him signing his new will or did you just lose your temper?' John asked. 'And did you deliberately steal the stick so that Valentine Randolph would be implicated, thus removing him from your path as well, or did you leave your own on the ship and simply take the first one that came to hand? Or don't you even know the answers yourself, you wretched man?'

'I deny the entire tale invented by this idiot,' Hugh answered.

'Deny away,' said the Blind Beak calmly. 'You're still going to swing at Tyburn.'

'What? On a thread of evidence that can never be proved? Don't be so ridiculous.'

'You've forgotten one thing,' said John, pulling something from his pocket.

'And what is that, pray?'

'The button from your coat, the button that you dropped by the gravestone where you murdered Sir William Hartfield. Even now Mr Fielding's Runners are searching your clothes press in St James's Square to find the garment from which it came.'

'And what if it is not there?'

'Then,' said John, taking an enormous gamble, 'I shall produce the potboy from The Spread Eagle who saw you taking Sir William's body down to the waterside, and ask him to identify you, face to face.'

The chance succeeded and Hugh let out a frantic cry, rushing not to the door leading to the staircase but to the balcony over the river.

'Stop him!' shouted John, but only Nicholas Dawkins had the wit to move quickly enough and dived immediately after Hugh into the river which, at full flood, ran only a few feet below them.

As if released from a trance, everybody surged to the parapet and stood looking downwards to where two heads bobbed in the wild water beneath. But though Nicholas had obviously learned to swim well he was no match for Hugh, who struck out downstream with a powerful stroke. And then, almost like a creature from some avenging myth, the mudlark appeared in his coracle, riding the surface of the waves like a gull.

'Which one?' he shouted to John through cupped hands.

'The man, not the boy,' the Apothecary called back.

Without further ado, Fred headed straight for the swimmer, swinging a vicious looking boathook and catching Hugh a crunching blow to the head with it.

'No more, you'll kill him,' John yelled.

Then he saw that revenge was indeed at work that day for the mighty river itself was taking charge of events. A freakish wave lifted Hugh's inert body high and crunched it into the hull of one of the tall ships dancing at anchor, splintering flesh and bone into pulp with the force of the blow. There was a terrible scream, though John was never sure afterwards from where it came, but at the sound of it most of the people on the balcony turned away their heads, so that only the Apothecary witnessed the moment when the mudlark hauled Nicholas out of the river and the two boys huddled together as Fred paddled furiously for the shore.

There was a sound behind him and John saw that Joe Jago had come to join him. The clerk's light blue eyes scanned the waterway. 'All over,' he called to the Magistrate, who had remained seated in his oaken chair throughout the uproar.

'Quite sure?'

'Yes, Sir.'

'"Full fathom five,"' quoted John Fielding.

'"Ding dong bell,"' finished Joe Jago, and shook his head in disbelief at the way in which fate deals out the cards.

Chapter Twenty-Seven

Dawn at Wapping, and the clear cold river reflecting the colours of the sky so vividly that it had transformed to a pink ribbon, as charming and delicate as any to be found on a pedlar's tray at a country fair. At first light the tide had swelled to full flood, so that now the mighty ships were hearing the call of the sea and were struggling to be set free from the moorings that held them captive. Up in the rigging, sailors were unfurling white clouds of canvas; the sightless eyes of figureheads surveyed the wild wide channel down which they must soon lead the way; and the air was full of the cry of gulls and the almost tangible sense of the great adventure that lay before them all.

Along the shore, at the bottom of the various Stairs, crowded small boats waiting to take passengers to the vessels which would carry them to their far distant destinations across the wide and dangerous oceans. And at the top of Pelican Stairs, standing with the friends who had come to bid them farewell, was a group of people brought together by the terrible events surrounding the deaths of Sir William Hartfield and Kitty Perkins.

Standing taller than them all was Samuel Swann, his arms flailing like the sails of a windmill as he swung them vigorously round himself to keep out the freshness of the breeze. Beside him, immaculate as ever despite the earliness of the hour, was Sir Gabriel Kent, his tricorne hat safely secured by a pearl-headed pin, his black velvet cloak swirling out like the sail of a funeral ship. Looking not quite as immaculate, in fact showing definite signs of needing a shave, his adopted son, John Rawlings, stood on the edge, the vivid blue of his eyes enhanced by the brilliant colours of the morning.

'So,' said Valentine Randolph, as the rowing boat from the ship *Sea Maiden* pulled up to the steps, 'we must finally say farewell.' He turned to Lydia, standing beside him, one lock of hair which had worked loose beneath her hat, flying out on the breeze. 'Are you ready, my dear?'

She smiled. 'Of course.'

Sir Gabriel drew Hesther Hodkin slightly to one side and put his hands on her shoulders. 'This is a very courageous thing you are doing,' he said gently.

She shook her head. 'No, it is a very sensible thing. I need to start my life all over again because, so far, I have had very little life to speak of. I shall be perfectly happy in Virginia with Valentine's kinfolk, the Randolphs and the Jeffersons. Who knows, I may even find myself a husband at long last.'

'Then he will be a very lucky man,' Sir Gabriel answered gallantly.

'And talking of lucky men, Lydia and I are to be married at sea,' Valentine informed anyone who wanted to listen.

'Congratulations,' said Nicholas Dawkins, yawning. He had already heard that particular piece of information a dozen times and was getting bored with it.

Luke Challon picked up the ladies' hand baggage, the rest of the luggage having already gone out to the ship. 'Best be getting along.' He shook hands with Valentine. 'Good luck, my friend. I hope your new life is everything that you hope it will be.'

Valentine cuddled Lydia close, an adoring expression on his face. 'With her beside me, how could it be anything else?'

John Rawlings kissed Hesther's hand. 'It has been a pleasure to meet you, Miss Hodkin. I wish you every success in the Colony.'

Sir Gabriel also bent over her fingers. 'You are a very fine woman,' he said.

'Thank you for everything, my dear,' she answered, and very briefly brushed his mouth with hers, before she climbed into the boat, from which she did not look back. Valentine helped Lydia into the swaying craft, then got aboard himself, and the pair of them waved continuously until they reached mid-stream.

'So,' said John, 'an ending and a beginning.'

'Not just for them,' answered Luke, making a grimace. 'Did you know that the great beau is emulating his eloping brother and is due to marry Miss Lambourn tomorrow? That is if he shows up.'

John's mobile eyebrows shot to his hairline. 'Good God! What *is* he trying to prove?'

'I suppose it doesn't occur to you,' said Sir Gabriel severely, 'that he might be genuinely fond of her?'

'No, it doesn't,' answered John cheerfully. 'He could never have exploited her the way he did if that was so. Besides, Roger is so madly in love with Roger that there's room for no one else in his heart at all.'

'Cynic!' replied his father, but Samuel guffawed.

Luke lowered his voice and spoke only to John. 'I shall be eternally grateful to you and Mr Fielding for not making my infatuation with the wretched woman public.'

'There was no need. So you have managed to come to terms with the fact that she's about to become Roger's wife?'

'I've had to,' Luke answered grimly, 'after all he and Julian are my employers now. They are continuing to run the company and have made me office manager.' He fingered his chin. 'Strange how it's all worked out.'

'With Hugh dead and Maud flown the coop, you mean?'

'Yes, I do. I wonder where she got to after that dramatic dash of hers.'

'Very probably Jamaica. She was damned lucky to escape as she did, though. If it hadn't been for the diversion caused by Hugh . . .'

'Well, he served her one good turn at least.'

'Probably more than he ever did in the rest of his lifetime, pretending she was unfaithful in order to throw dust into my eyes.'

'Any news of horrible Lady Hodkin?' asked Sir Gabriel, watching through his telescope as the *Sea Maiden*'s gangplank was raised and the capstan creaked into life and slowly began to haul up the anchor.

'I believe she's sending for some impoverished female who has been advertising in the newspapers for a position, to be her companion.'

'Heaven help the poor soul.'

'Look, they're moving!' called Nicholas.

John gazed at the pinched face, now filling out almost daily and developing a fine rosy complexion. 'Would you like to be on board?'

The Muscovite shook his head. 'No, indeed. Not now that you've made me your apprentice, Mr Rawlings, and Mr Fielding has paid for my indentures.'

'Then that's as well.'

The five of them fell silent. The square rigger was starting her stately journey down to the open sea. On board there was a flurry of waving white handkerchiefs and the notes of a fiddle playing a song of farewell was borne shorewards on the morning air. The sails began to swell with a lusty wind bound for the Americas and the powerful ship bobbed and dipped as the Thames led the vessel inexorably on towards the ocean, already casting its relentless spell upon her.

'They're on their way!' called Sir Gabriel, and the telescope passed from hand to hand as they watched the *Sea Maiden* grow smaller and smaller until she was finally hidden by the bend in the river and passed from their sight.

'They've gone,' said Samuel, a little sadly.

But John Rawlings shook his head. 'No. They are still there, just as are we. It is simply that now we can no longer see them.'

And so saying, he turned away from the river and set his face to the dawning day.

Historical Note

John Rawlings, Apothecary, was born circa 1731, though his actual parentage is somewhat shrouded in mystery. However, by 1754 he emerged from the shadows when on 22 August, 1754, he applied to be made Free of the Worshipful Society of Apothecaries. He did not succeed on that occasion and I thought it would be interesting to quote from the Worshipful Society's Court Book dated 13 March, 1755 (Ms 8200/7).

'Mr John Rawling, a Foreign Apothecary, attended the Court and desired to be admitted to his Freedom of the Company by Redemption on the terms mentioned in the Court of Assistants of 22nd August last but not withstanding the Order of this Court of Assistants of the 5th December last whereby the Fine for admitting Foreign Apothecaries was increased, he having attended at the Hall to take up his Freedom on the Private Court Day in August last but the Court was just broke up and he was prevented by business attending again before the 5th December last, which being taken into consideration. Ordered that on his paying a Fine of £7.10.0d. 40 to the Garden and Fees and passing an Examination he be made Free of the Company by Redemption. He paid the Fine.'

In this instance the word 'Foreign' means that he was apprenticed outside the City of London, and the word 'Fine' simply means a fee.

Here, then, is the authenticated record that John Rawlings was kept waiting at least seven months between ending his indentures and being made Free. On becoming a Yeoman of the Society, John gave his address as 2, Nassau Street, Soho, thereby linking himself irrefutably with H.D. Rawlings Ltd., Soda Water Manufacturers, who gave the same address over a hundred years later.

The Devil's Tavern still stands but these days is called The

Prospect of Whitby. Originally built in 1520 as a timber-framed country house, it opened as a tavern some time later and soon became the haunt of riverfolk and smugglers. In 1777 the landlord renamed The Devil's Tavern, calling it The Prospect of Whitby after the collier, The Prospect, which regularly moored off the tavern and became a local landmark. As well as The Devil's Tavern, both the other hostelries mentioned in this book remain. The Spread Eagle is now called The Mayflower, but has little sign of its historic past. The Angel, however, retains its original name and still boasts the balcony supposedly haunted by Judge Jeffreys. The Church of St Mary the Virgin, Rotherhithe, looking very much as it did in John Rawlings's time, also stands as a proud monument to the past.

DERYN LAKE

DEATH IN THE DARK WALK

A richly atmospheric and compelling Georgian mystery woven around the real characters John Fielding, the phenomenal sightless magistrate known as the 'Blind Beak', whose Runners formed London's early police force, and John Rawlings, the Apothecary reputed to have invented soda water.

Having just finished his indentures, Rawlings is celebrating in Vaux Hall Pleasure Gardens when he trips over the body of a young girl. Summoned to the magistrate's office as prime suspect, Rawlings not only clears his own name but impresses Fielding so much with his powers of recollection that he is asked to investigate the crime.

From gaming hell to fashionable house, Rawlings follows a trail of lustful liaisons and illicit intrigue which prove beyond a shadow of doubt that the girl has had quite a past . . . a past filled with threatening secrets.

HODDER AND STOUGHTON PAPERBACKS

DERYN LAKE

DEATH AT THE BEGGAR'S OPERA

John Rawlings, the apothecary with a talent for detective work, and John Fielding, the phenomenal blind magistrate whose Runners formed London's early police force, make a welcome return in this evocative Georgian mystery.

John Rawlings is among the beau monde enjoying a performance of 'The Beggar's Opera' in Drury Lane when the leading actor – the notorious philanderer Jasper Harcross – dramatically falls to his death on stage. As Rawlings and the Blind Beak hunt for vital clues, they discover a hotbed of rivalry both on and off the stage which produces numerous suspects and questions.

As the search takes on a new intensity, John Rawlings soon finds himself on an intriguing trail of obsession that leads to the dark heart of a cold-blooded murder.

HODDER AND STOUGHTON PAPERBACKS